Dermatology

Third Edition

Dermatology

Current Concepts and Practice
Third Edition

Edited by
Patrick Hall-Smith, MD, FRCP (Lond. & Ed.)
*Consultant Dermatologist, Royal Sussex County Hospital, Brighton
and Brighton General Hospital; Visiting Fellow, University of
Sussex*

R. J. Cairns, MB, BS, FRCP
*Consultant Dermatologist, Medway, Maidstone, Tunbridge Wells
and Gravesend Health Districts*

Butterworths
London Boston Sydney Wellington Durban Toronto

First Published 1981

© Butterworths & Co (Publishers) Ltd. 1981

British Library Cataloguing in Publication Data

Dermatology.—3rd ed.
1. Dermatology
I. Hall-Smith, Patrick   II. Cairns, R. J.
616.5   RC71   80–42218

ISBN 0–407–00208–1

Typeset by CCC in Great Britain by William Clowes (Beccles) Limited,
Beccles and London
Printed in Great Britain by
Butler & Tanner Ltd, Frome and London

Preface

Seven years have passed since the publication of the second edition of this textbook. In this period the growth of the specialty of dermatology has accelerated; there has been an increase in the number of specialist and research publications devoted to dermatology and to related subjects such as immunology, photobiology, biochemistry, genetics and various branches of pathology. For this reason the original authors have asked a number of colleagues to contribute chapters on those aspects of the specialty on which they are acknowledged experts. The aim of the editors, who themselves are contributors, is to produce a compact readable textbook and one which reflects current concept and practice in the specialty.

Dermatology is a visual discipline and so many colour plates have been included in the text, in addition to a number of black and white photographs and diagrams.

Two chapters, that on inherited cutaneous diseases and the one on photodermatoses, may be too detailed for the non-specialist. The editors decided however that the excellence and completeness of these contributions should permit their publication with only minor editorial abridgement and change in emphasis.

The book is above all aimed at providing the student and postgraduate with a basis in dermatology such as will be required for the final MB or MRCP examination and subsequent practice. It may in addition enhance interest in a subject which has an increasingly important place in general medicine.

Acknowledgements

Our profession, and none more so than those practising dermatology, is indebted to the pharmaceutical industry for their research programmes and their contribution to medical education. Without their cooperation and material help many congresses would never take place, symposia would remain unpublished and medical educational films would not be made. Among the leaders in these various activities are Messrs Glaxo Laboratories Limited, whose generosity has enabled us to publish over 160 colour plates. Without their liberal contribution this would not have been possible.

Mr S. T. Higgins, Clinical Photographer to the Brighton Health District, and his staff have been responsible for many photographs, though the various contributors have provided most of the illustrations for their sections.

Miss Joy Graham, Medical Artist at the Queen Victoria Hospital, East Grinstead, undertook the drawings in the chapter on plastic surgery.

Mr M. R. Geary, BVSc, FRCVS, Veterinary Adviser to Intervet Laboratories Limited, and Mr A. I. Wright, BVSc, MRCVS, of the Department of Veterinary Medicine, University of Bristol, have supplied many helpful facts contained in the chapter on parasitic infestations. This is information that is not easily accessible to the non-veterinary scientist.

Dermatologists, as do physicians in other branches of medicine, frequently require details of drugs and formulations from their hospital dispensary. We are indebted to Mr A. L. Goldstein, FPS, and to Mr P. A. Pannett, MPS, AKC, Brighton General Hospital, for their unstinted help in the chapter on the therapeutic guide and formulary.

The editors are especially grateful to Miss Maude Norman for her invaluable help in bringing order and balance to the text and without whose efforts the manuscript would never have got to press.

List of contributors

Martin M. Black, MD, FRCP,
Consultant Dermatologist, St. Thomas's Hospital, Senior Lecturer in Histopathology, Institute of Dermatology, London.

Desmond Burrows, MD, FRCP (Ed.),
Consultant Dermatologist, Royal Victoria Hospital, Belfast.

Nicholas M. Breach, MB, FRCS, FDS, RCS,
Consultant Plastic Surgeon, Queen Victoria Hospital, East Grinstead and East Sussex AHA (Brighton General Hospital).

R. J. Cairns, MB BS, FRCP,
Consultant Dermatologist, Medway, Maidstone, Tunbridge Wells and Gravesend Health Districts.

Rodney P. R. Dawber, MA, MB, FRCP,
Consultant Dermatologist and Clinical Lecturer, Oxford AHA (Teaching) and University of Oxford.

George Deutsch, MB, MRCP, FRCR,
Consultant Radiotherapist and Oncologist, East Sussex AHA (Royal Sussex County Hospital, Brighton).

Anthony du Vivier, MD, MRCP,
Consultant Dermatologist, King's College Hospital, London.

William F. Felton, MA, MB BChir,
Consultant in Genito-Urinary Medicine, Royal Sussex County Hospital, Brighton.

William Frain-Bell, MD, FRCP (Ed.),
Consultant Dermatologist, University of Dundee.

W. A. D. Griffiths, MA, MD, MRCP,
Consultant Dermatologist, St. John's Hospital for Diseases of the Skin, London.

Patrick Hall-Smith, MD, FRCP (Lond. & Ed.),
Consultant Dermatologist, Royal Sussex County Hospital, Brighton and Brighton General Hospital, Visiting Fellow, University of Sussex.

R. R. M. Harman, MB BS, FRCP,
Consultant Dermatologist, Bristol Royal Infirmary, Clinical Teacher, Bristol University.

Mark Hewitt, MB, FRCP,
Consultant Dermatologist, Cornwall and Isles of Scilly AHA (Royal Cornwall Hospital, Truro).

List of contributors

J. A. A. Hunter, BA, MD, FRCP (Ed.),
Consultant Dermatologist, Royal Infirmary Edinburgh, Grant Professor of Dermatology, University of Edinburgh.

Martin P. James, BSc, MB, MRCP,
Consultant Dermatologist, Royal Berkshire Hospital, Reading.

Ashley Levantine, MB, MRCP,
Consultant Dermatologist, Chichester and Worthing AHA (St. Richard's Hospital, Chichester, and Worthing Hospital).

Keith Liddell, MD, MRCP,
Consultant Dermatologist, East Sussex AHA (Eastbourne, Hastings and Bexhill Hospitals).

Donald M. MacDonald, MA, MB, MRCP,
Consultant Dermatologist and Director, Laboratory of Applied Dermatology, Guy's Hospital, London.

F. M. Pope, MD, MRCP (Lond., Ed., Glas.),
Consultant Dermatologist and Member of Scientific Staff, Medical Research Council, Clinical Research Centre, Northwick Park Hospital, Harrow.

T. J. Ryan, MA, DM, FRCP,
Consultant Dermatologist, Oxford AHA (Teaching) and Clinical Lecturer in Dermatology, Oxford University.

Denis E. Sharvill, FRCP,
Consultant Dermatologist, Canterbury & Thanet and South East Kent Health Districts.

Andrew P. Warin, MB, MRCP,
Consultant Dermatologist, Royal Devon & Exeter Hospital, Exeter, and formerly Consultant Dermatologist and Senior Lecturer, St. John's Hospital for Diseases of the Skin, London.

Contents

Contents

1 Anatomy, development and immunology of the skin

R. J. Cairns

The skin has evolved in land animals as a relatively impermeable surface layer to prevent the loss of essential watery substances into the surrounding gaseous environment, to form a protective layer from external hazards and to insulate against extremes of temperature. Thus the surface covering of land animals exhibits diverse degrees of complexity particularly adapted to suit the environmental surroundings. In man the skin forms a sheet-like single organ composed of a population of cells of diverse embryonic origin. The contiguous groups of cells at times betray their origin and their potentialities, although under normal conditions cells exist side by side in complete harmony as a complex mosaic.

Anatomy

A thin outer layer, the *epidermis*, is composed of *keratinocytes* (keratin producing cells) of ectodermal origin intermingled with melanin producing cells, the *melanocytes*, which arise from a specialized embryonic ectodermal tissue, the *neural crest*. The *dermis*, or stroma, that forms the main bulk of the skin is intimately bound with the overlying epidermis; fingerlike processes or dermal papillae project upwards into corresponding recesses in the epidermis. In contrast with the epidermis, the dermis is relatively acellular and predominantly fibrous, containing blood vessels; although of mesodermal origin it contains several structures derived from the embryonic ectoderm.

The skin, therefore, is a composite organ forming a bilaminar sheet covering the entire body surface. Knowledge of the mass migrations, fusions, foldings and minor rearrangements that occur to this complex cell population during fetal development helps our understanding of developmental errors (e.g. naevi, heterotopias) and gives some insight into the curious, apparently haphazard, reactions of groups of cells that occur in the diseased skin.

Epidermis

The basal layer of the epidermis forms a single row of columnar cells resting on a basement membrane (*see Figures 1.1* and *1.2*). Among

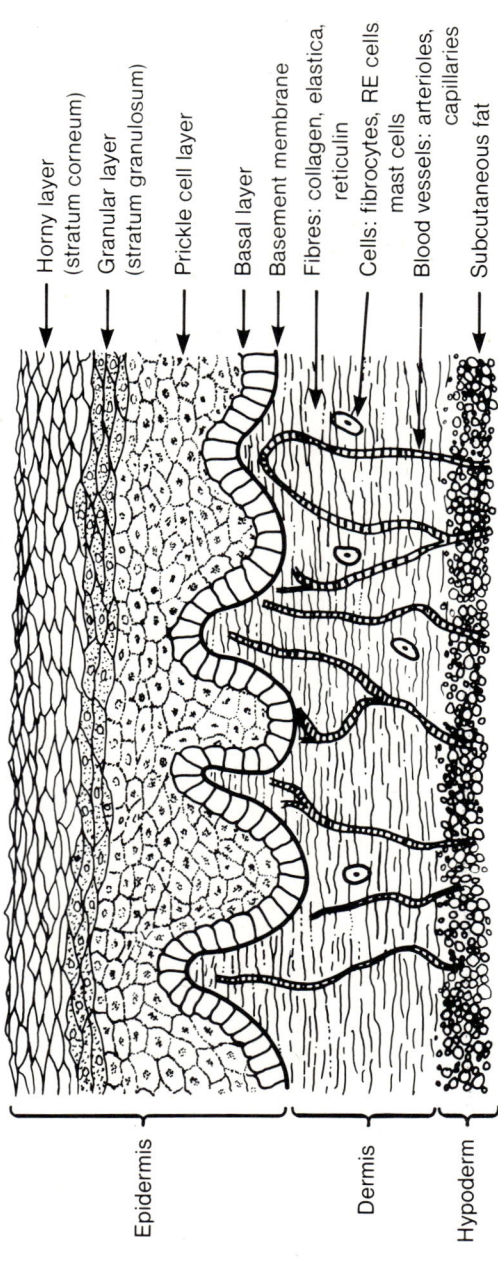

Figure 1.1 Anatomy of the skin

Horny layer
(stratum corneum)

Granular layer
(stratum granulosum)

Prickle cell layer

Basal layer

Basement membrane

Fibres: collagen, elastica,
reticulin

Cells: fibrocytes, RE cells
mast cells

Blood vessels: arterioles,
capillaries

Subcutaneous fat

Epidermis

Dermis

Hypoderm

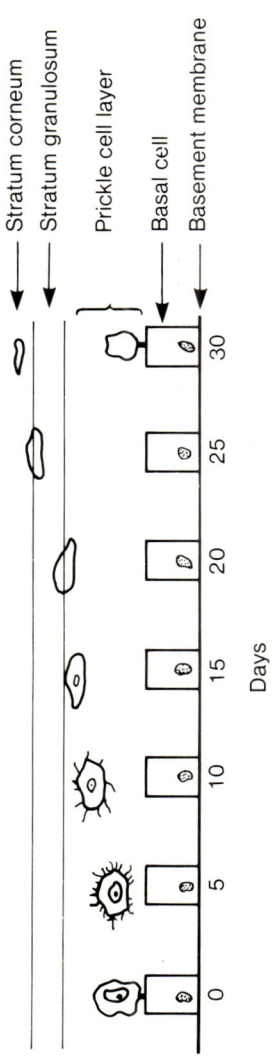

Figure 12 Epidermopoiesis

3

these cells are the pigmented melanocytes. The basal cells constitute a stem cell population that gives rise to a lineage of identical daughter cells, prickle cells, or keratinocytes, which slowly and inevitably pass towards the surface, mature, keratinize and are finally shed. Basal cells continue to divide throughout life and in this respect they resemble the ever active cells in the bone marrow and intestinal epithelium. Likewise melanocytes undergo continuous division throughout life, the daughter cells losing pigment before ultimately being shed from the surface. The process of maturation and keratinization of prickle cells (epidermopoiesis), normally takes about four weeks and as each cell passes towards the skin surface it first becomes granular before complete keratinization occurs. These sequential changes account for the different zones seen in the epidermis under the microscope. From the basement membrane outwards the following layers are recognizable: basal cell layer, wide prickle cell zone, narrow stratum granulosum and on the surface stratum corneum.

Specialized structures directly derived from the epidermis include hair, nails and cutaneous glands. These epidermal structures arise from proliferation of the undersurface of the epithelium as small bud-like downgrowths which subsequently differentiate. It follows that in the epidermis are several elements apart from the prickle cells; these include specialized cells ensheathing the sweat ducts and hair follicles, traversing the epidermis. (*Figure 1.3*). The so-called *poral* and *follicular epithelium* provide the tissue of origin of certain tumours.

Dermis

Fibres of two main types are seen in the dermis; both are fibrous protein. Collagen fibres which far outnumber elastic fibres are responsible for the main mass and resilience of the dermis. Collagen is disposed mainly parallel to the skin surface whereas elastic fibres form a subepidermal network and are only thinly distributed elsewhere in the dermis. The dermis and epidermis are nourished by blood vessels that pass upwards from the subcutaneous layer. In the dermis they form relatively small channels (arterioles) which pass towards the undersurface of the epidermis forming a rich capillary network in the dermal papillae. Other structures found in the dermis include veins, lymph vessels, sensory corpuscles, autonomic and sensory nerves. Hair follicles with their attendant hair muscles and cutaneous glands are also situated in this deeper layer of the skin. In this region cells are scanty although representatives of the reticuloendothelial system including histiocytes, fibrocytes and mast cells are found.

Cutaneous glands

Sebaceous glands are found adjoining and partly surrounding hair follicles. They form an appendage to the hair follicle and are composed

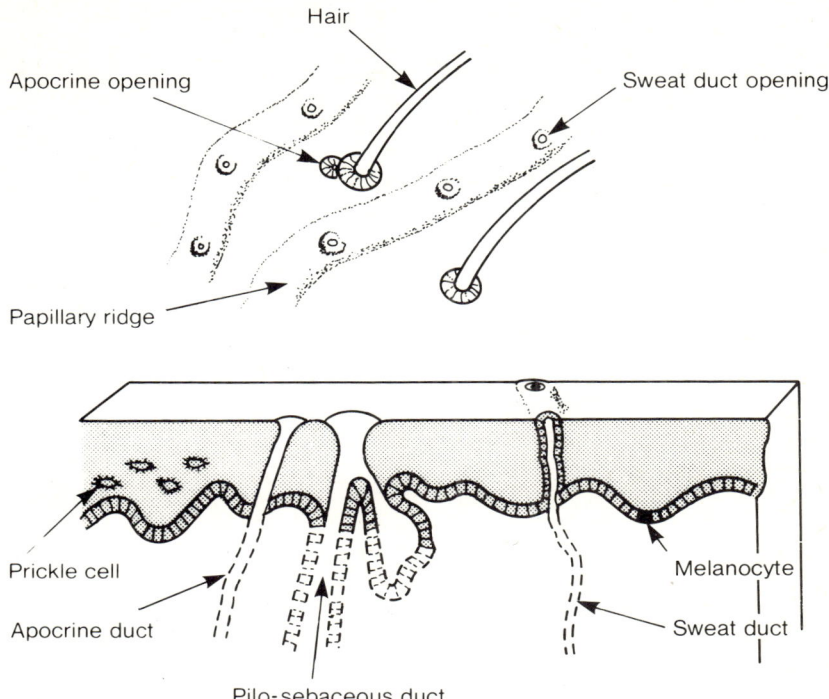

Hair

Apocrine opening

Sweat duct opening

Papillary ridge

Prickle cell

Apocrine duct

Melanocyte

Sweat duct

Pilo-sebaceous duct

Figure 1.3 *Composite structure of the epidermis*

of groups of lipid-containing cells. The glandular contents are discharged directly into the lumen of the follicle and the secretion, sebum—extends on to the hair shaft and spreads on to the skin surface. Apocrine glands are found in close association with hair follicles but are limited in distribution. They occur in the axillae, around the nipples and in the anogenital region. Activity only begins at puberty when the apocrine secretion is discharged on to the skin surface of the follicular lumen. Eccrine glands are widely distributed over the body surface and are particularly profuse on the forehead, axillae and palms and soles. They have a thermoregulatory function and are innervated by cholinergic fibres of the sympathetic nervous system.

Embryology and development (*Figure 1.4*)

The cells found in the adult skin have a dual embryological origin. The ectoderm forms the epidermis and the mesoderm the dermis. This fact is important in understanding genodermatoses, naevi and tumour formation. The somatic ectoderm in the embryo comprises the stratum germinativum. This gives rise over most of the body surface to the adult epidermis comprising the basal layer and overlying keratinizing cells with the ultimate formation of the

5

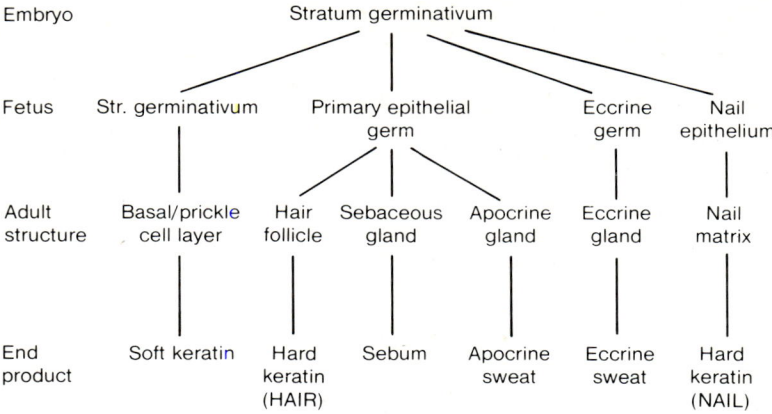

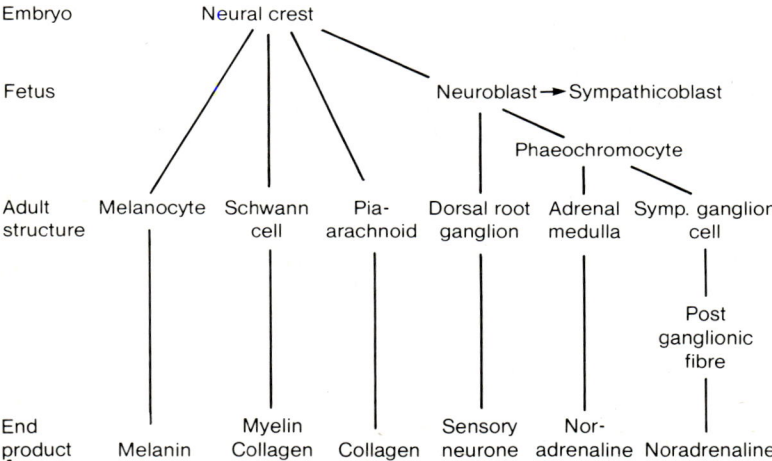

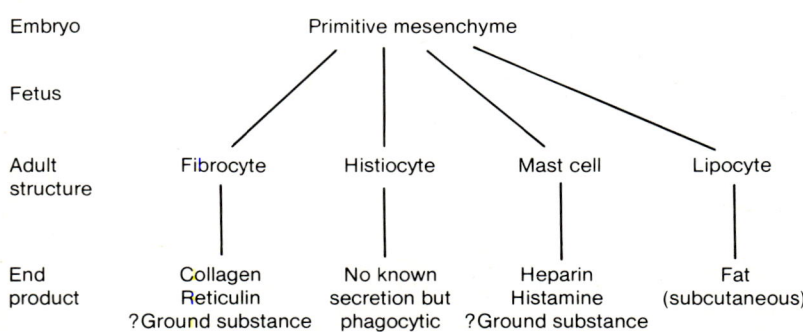

Figure 1.4 *Embryological development of skin components*

stratum corneum. During fetal life foci of epithelial overgrowth form as downward buds, the so-called primary epithelial germ. From this stem the hair follicle, sebaceous and apocrine glands. Other downgrowths ultimately differentiate into eccrine glands, whilst on the dorsal aspect of the terminal phalanges a specialized nail epithelium gives origin to the hard keratin of nails.

From the ectoderm there evolves in addition a single cellular system termed the neural crest which separates early in development from the somatic ectoderm and developing central nervous system. The neural crest gives origin to melanocytes found in the adult skin and the Schwann cells provide myelin that insulates the peripheral nerves. Neural crest tissue also gives rise to the dorsal root ganglia, sympathetic ganglia and the adrenal medulla.

The tissues of mesenchyme origin under the developing epidermis form fibrocytes, histiocytes, mast cells and fat storing cells known as lipocytes.

Immunology

The simple classification of Gell and Coombs divides into four groups the mechanisms causing immunological injury and disease.

Type I is the immediate or anaphylactic type of reaction based on IgE and antigen reacting on the surface of mast cells. Mast cell degranulation liberates histamine, serotonin and other inflammatory mediators, showing in the skin as a weal. Local or widespread urticaria is thus a feature of Type I reaction, with anaphylaxis, hay fever and allergic asthma representing non-cutaneous examples of this reaction.

Widespread urticaria is a feature of Type I sensitization to plant and plant products including many foods, drugs, chemicals and internal parasites. Contact urticaria appears from contact with animal and plant proteins. Prick tests with the appropriate antigen elicits an urticarial response within 10–15 minutes. Type I reactions are not complement-dependent.

Type II reactions are well illustrated by autoimmune drug-induced platelet damage. The antigen is fixed on the cell surface and the antigen–antibody reaction causes cytolysis. The target tissues for these reactions include the diverse mature and immature blood cells, and the basal epidermal cells in bullous pemphigoid. The desmosomes of the epidermal prickle cell are the target tissue in pemphigus vulgaris. There is some evidence that certain Type II reactions are mediated by 'killer' T lymphocytes. Type II reactions are complement-dependent.

Type III reactions are characterized by the formation of intra- or extravascular microprecipitates of antigen–antibody complexes. The so-called circulating immune complexes are the hallmark of the serum sickness type of the immune response. The antigen–antibody ratio largely determines the size, solubility and toxicity of the microprecipitates. Circulating immune complexes cause systemic disease and are particularly liable to become aggregated in the skin and renal glomeruli. Locally formed complexes result in localized disease—the Arthus phenomenon as occurs in erythema nodosum.

Neutrophil infiltration, acute small vessel vasculitis, microthrombi and infarction are common features of disease. Urticaria, papular purpura, haemorrhagic necrotic papules and nodules complete the common range of skin lesions. Extravascular deposition of immune complexes is accompanied by a sarcoidal or rheumatoid type of granulomatous reaction. Leucocytoclastic vasculitis, the vasculitis of systemic lupus erythematosus (SLE) and the exanthems of diverse bacterial diseases are based on Type III mechanism. Complement consumption is characteristic of this type of reaction.

Type IV is best illustrated by contact eczema and the Mantoux test. It is cell mediated immunity (CMI) which is the normal mechanism of protection against environmental allergens and micro-organisms, and for the rejection of grafts. It depends on the integrity of an immunological arc—the afferent limb comprising an effective antigen processing system by Langerhan cells and macrophages, and transport via the lymphatics of the processed antigen to regional lymph nodes. The central limb of the arc comprises the lymph node and in the paracortical zone T lymphocytes with specific surface immunoglobulins proliferate and emerge from the efferent nodal lymphatic to reach the blood stream. The blood stream represents the efferent limb of the arc and T lymphocytes 'home in' on their specific antigen in the epidermis (eczema) or dermis (intradermal test). Once the subject is sensitized the reaction develops 24–48 hours after re-exposure to the antigen—the so-called delayed response. It is reproduced by conventional patch test or by intradermal testing.

It should be noted that cell mediated immunity is a double-edged sword; it is both protective and tissue destructive. Depression of CMI may be produced by certain types of toxic drugs and corticosteroids. Similarly any 'lesion' of the immunological arc or interference with T lymphocyte maturation (pre-thymic, thymic or post-thymic) interferes with this protective immunological mechanism. Diminished or absent CMI predisposes to recalcitrant and persistent viral, bacterial and fungal disease, and depressed suppressor T cell function predisposes to an increased incidence of autoimmune disease and lymphoproliferative neoplasia. Granulomatous sensitivity as evidenced by the Mistuda and Kveim reactions and the delayed granulomatous response to beryllium and zirconium probably represents a variant of CMI.

Autoimmune disease

Many diseases are now recognized as representing an aberrant immune response against the host's own cells. Such disorders are dependent on part of the individual's tissue acting as an autoantigen. The changed tissue which fails to be recognized as 'self' may be a whole cell, e.g. pancreatic islet cell, part of a cell surface, e.g. a hemidesmosome in bullous pemphigoid, or a component of the cell nucleus, e.g. DNA in SLE. Sometimes an extracellular tissue such as cartilage, collagen or elastica is autoantigenic. The specific auto-antibodies are produced by B lymphocytes which circulate through-out the blood stream and bind on to their 'target tissue'. They are immunoglobulins produced in the same way as circulating antibodies concerned with humoral immunity. In certain autoallergic disorders T lymphocytes, as well as circulating immunoglobulins play a part in causing selective cellular or tissue damage with resulting inflammation.

The causes of autoimmune disease may lie centrally within the B cells which proliferate and produce abnormal immunoglobulins through lack of normal suppressor control from suppressor T cells. On the other hand, primary damage to the target tissue from chemicals, drugs, latent viruses or infectious agents may be the inciting event which causes an autoimmune reaction. Similarly, ultraviolet light (UVB) damage to epidermal cell DNA will in certain predisposed individuals provoke autoantibodies and SLE. A less common cause of widespread autoimmune disease is a defective complement system with failure to clear immune complexes from the circulation. We may recognize three groups of autoimmune disease relevant to the skin:

(1) Systemic:
    SLE, dermatomyositis, Sjögren's disease, scleroderma, polyarter-itis nodosa, polychondritis, Wegener's granuloma, mixed connec-tive tissue disease.
(2) Widespread cutaneous:
    Pemphigus vulgaris and pemphigus sub-groups, bullous pemphi-goid, herpes gestationes, Senear–Usher syndrome, erythroderma, autosensitization eczema.
(3) Localized cutaneous:
    Alopecia areata, Sutton's naevus, vitiligo.

A feature common to many systemic autoimmune disorders is the inflammatory process which is usually self-perpetuating and often represents a Type II reaction. Vasculitis based on immune-complex disease often accompanies the process; multisystem involvement is usual.

When autoimmune disease is confirmed attention should be directed towards elucidating precipitating factors, e.g. virus, etc. and predisposing factors, e.g. genetic, defective suppressor T cell function, complement defects, etc. Treatment is palliative and directed towards suppressing abnormal globulin production and damping down the local inflammatory process. Corticosteroids alone or combined with cytotoxic agents, e.g. azathioprine, cyclophospha-mide, are usually effective and sometimes life-saving.

The simple classification into four major groups by Gell and Coombs is useful, but many clinical disorders represent several different mechanisms occurring simultaneously or in sequence. The complexities of the problem are summarized below.

(1) Abnormalities of two or more types of reaction may coexist simultaneously:

Allergic granulomatous vasculitis: Type I and III;
Bullous pemphigoid: Type II and III;
Erythema induratum: Type II and IV;
Wegener's granulomatosis: Type III and IV;
Systemic lupus erythematosus: Type II, III and Type IV depression.

(2) One mechanism may inhibit or enhance another, or determine the localization of another:

Type I lesions may determine the site of Type III deposits;
defective Type IV enhances Type I, III and possibly Type II.

(3) Certain antigens cause sequential activation and inhibition of the diverse mechanisms over a period of years. This occurs with syphilis, leprosy and tuberculosis. Repeated antigen exposure, e.g. from repeated insect bites, first activates Type IV and then Type I immunity, the skin ultimately becoming tolerant or non-reactive.

(4) Localizing factors which modulate the final tissue damage and cellular response include the autonomic nervous system, the local microcirculation and polymorph and macrophage function at the site of the antigen–antibody reaction.

2 Examination and diagnostic procedures

Patrick Hall-Smith

'Listen! Listen to your patient:
He is giving you the diagnosis!' (Laennec)

The majority of medical students or practitioners tend to approach
a dermatological case with more diffidence and suspicion than they
would a patient with cardiovascular, chest or neurological symptoms.
This may in part reflect inadequate training in this specialty, but it
is also due to the mistaken belief that only absolute recognition of
the presenting skin picture allows of diagnosis.

History taking is essentially similar to that undertaken in any
general medical or surgical case. Common sense will indicate that if
a patient presents with a wart on the finger, time is not wasted on
superfluous note-taking. With an eruption of long duration detailed
questioning regarding the time of onset, past and family history and
response to past treatment may provide valuable information.
Assessment of the patient's personality, problems and possible
phobias, as well as the occupational and geographical history can
provide a vital clue to the diagnosis.

Drug sensitivities should be noted in red ink on the outer cover of
the notes.

Examination should be made under a good light; preferably
daylight or a daylight type electric bulb.

Modesty, laziness, or unmerited faith in the dermatologist's
diagnostic acumen make many patients unwilling to expose more
than a bare minimum of their involved skin surface. An untruthful
denial that there are areas affected other than a proffered forearm or
lower leg is not uncommon. The experienced dermatologist knows
that the general body pattern of an eruption is often more helpful in
diagnosis than the morphological minutiae of individual lesions.
This is frequently so in psoriasis, seborrhoeic dermatitis, pityriasis
rosea, herpes zoster, scabies, atopic dermatitis, dermatitis herpetiformis, contact dermatitis and light sensitivity eruptions. Close
inspection of individual lesions may be essential in cases of rodent
ulcer and other skin tumours, lichen planus, lupus erythematosus,
eczematous and lichenoid lesions and parasitic infestations.

Mention must be made of the importance of examining the patient's clothing. Features such as the degree of contamination with oils, cement, etc. enable assessment of the degree of occupational exposure. Likewise the presence of pediculi and 'flea spotting' on clothing can provide a useful diagnostic pointer. In cases of suspected clothing dermatitis, close examination of the garment may be rewarding.

A magnifying glass of good quality and magnification or a Berger's loupe should be a standard item of equipment.

Some basic equipment is shown in *Figure 2.1*.

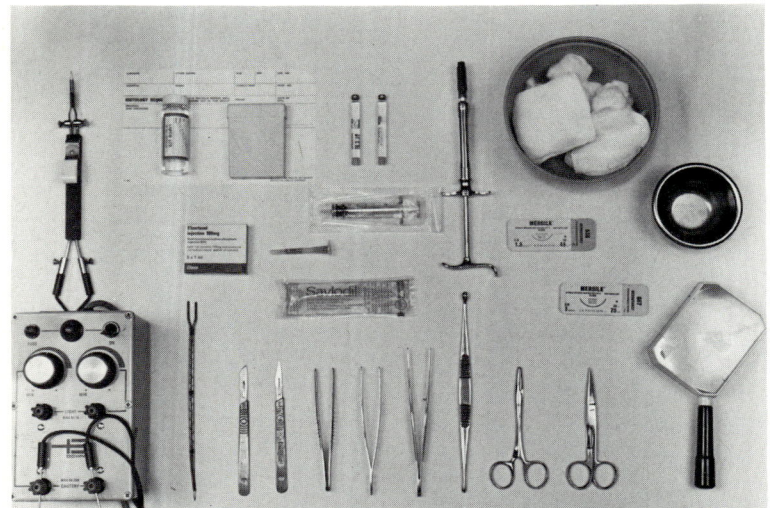

Figure 2.1 Dermatological trolley: note especially double ended curette, sharp pointed surgical scissors and Bard Parker scalpel, cautery points, cartridge loading syringe and Xylotox and cautery

Glossary of terms used in dermatology

Certain specialized terms are used to describe the gross morphology of a cutaneous eruption (dermatosis). Lesions encountered are subdivided into the primary and secondary type.

Primary lesions

Bulla: vesicle over 1 cm in diameter.
Cyst: an epithelium-lined cavity containing fluid or semi-solid material.
Macule: circumscribed non-elevated discoloration up to 1 cm in diameter; it may be erythematous, pigmented or depigmented.
Nodule: solid circumscribed dermal or hypodermal lesion often projecting above the skin surface and up to 1 cm in diameter.

Papule: small circumscribed superficial solid elevation up to 1 cm in diameter.
Patch: macule measuring over 1 cm in diameter.
Plaque: a disc-like lesion formed by the coalescence of papules or nodules, e.g. psoriatic plaque.
Pustule: pus filled vesicle.
Vesicle: papule containing fluid from 0.1–1 cm.
Weal: plaque-like oedematous elevation often surrounded by a zone of erythema.

Secondary lesions

Crust: mass of dried exudate—epithelial debris, blood, pus, serum.
Excoriation: superficial ulceration of traumatic origin—usually from scratching.
Fissure: linear breach of the skin bounded by abrupt sides.
Scales: collection of horny material ranging from small thin flakes to large sheets.
Scar (cicatrice): the connective tissue replacement following loss of dermal tissue.
Sinus: track leading to the surface.
Ulcer: irregularly shaped excavation of the skin.

Changes encountered in the skin

Alopecia: loss of hair.
Depigmentation: loss of melanin pigmentation.
Ecchymoses: extravasation of blood.
Erythema: redness resulting from vasodilatation, usually blanched by pressure.
Haemosiderosis: haemosiderin deposition with yellow-brown macules.
Hypopigmentation: diminution in melanin pigmentation.
Infiltration: palpable thickening or hardness.
Melanosis: darkening from increased melanocyte activity.
Oedema: thickening and pallor from extracellular fluid.
Purpura: extravasation of blood.
Telangiectasis: persistent vasodilatation, not blanched by pressure with a glass slide.

In clinical practice the technical vocabulary commonly employs word combinations that are self-explanatory; for instance, telangiectatic erythema, a maculopapular eruption, cicatricial alopecia, etc. would be appropriate for describing certain skin changes.

Microscopic changes in skin disease

Epidermis

Hyperkeratosis: hypertrophy of the horny layer (stratum corneum).

Parakeratosis: retention of nuclei in the horny layer from defective keratinization.

Dyskeratosis: disordered keratinization with groups of abnormal cells in the prickle cell layer.

Acanthosis: thickening of the prickle cell layer.

Atrophy: general thinning of the epidermis.

Oedema: intra- or extracellular collection of fluid. Intracellular oedema causes characteristic *balloon cells*, and extracellular oedema separation of prickle cells or *spongiosis*.

Dermis

Cellular infiltration: the aggregation of neutrophils, lymphocytes, mast cells, plasma cells and reticulohistiocytic cells.

Infiltration: the deposition of an abnormal substance in the dermis; this includes proteins, carbohydrates, fats and complex mixtures, e.g. mucopolysaccharides.

Regional location

Scalp

Acne,
alopecia areata,
boils,
epithelioma,
impetigo,
keratoses
(seborrhoeic,
senile and solar),
lichen planopilaris,
lupus erythematosus,
naevus verrucosus,
pediculosis,
psoriasis,
radioatrophy,
ringworm,
seborrhoeic
dermatitis,
tinea capitis,
verrucae.

Forehead, face and beard area

Acne,
alopecia areata,
boils,
chloasma,
contact dermatitis,
dermatophytosis,
drug eruptions,
eczema,
epithelioma,
herpes simplex,
herpes zoster,
hydroa
vacciniforme,
impetigo,
keratoses
(seborrhoeic,
senile and solar),
lentigines,
light sensitivity,
lupus
erythematosus,
lupus pernio
(sarcoid),
lupus vulgaris,
molluscum
contagiosum,
naevi,
perioral dermatitis,
psoriasis,
ringworm,
rosacea,
scleroderma,
sebaceous cysts,
seborrhoeic
dermatitis,
sycosis barbae,
syphilis,
verrucae,
vitiligo.

Eyebrows and eyelids

Alopecia areata,
blepharitis,
contact dermatitis,
dermatophytosis,
epithelioma,
hidradenitis
   eruptiva,
keratoses
   (seborrhoeic,
   senile and solar),
molluscum
   contagiosum,
meibomian cysts,
neurodermatitis,
pediculosis,
psoriasis,
seborrhoeic
   dermatitis,
styes,
sycosis vulgaris,
ulerythema
   oophryogenes,
xanthelasma.

Nose

Boils,
epithelioma,
herpes simplex,
keratoses
   (seborrhoeic),
lupus
   erythematosus,
lupus pernio
   (sarcoid),
naevi,
rhinophyma,
rosacea,
verrucae,
vestibulitis.

Lips

Angular cheilitis,
chancre,
contact dermatitis,
erythema
   multiforme,
epithelioma,
herpes simplex,
keratoses (solar),
lupus
   erythematosus,
mucous glands,
urticaria,
verrucae.

Ears

Chondrodermatitis
   nodularis helicis,
contact dermatitis,
epithelioma,
gouty tophi,
granuloma
   annulare,
impetigo,
keratoses
   (seborrhoeic,
   senile and solar),
lupus
   erythematosus,
lupus vulgaris,
psoriasis,
rheumatoid nodules,
seborrhoeic
   dermatitis.

Neck

Acne nuchae,
boils,
contact dermatitis,
dermatitis papillaris
   capilliti,
dermatophytosis,
epithelioma,
folliculitis,
keloid,
keratoses
   (seborrhoeic,
   senile and solar),
neurodermatitis,
papillomata,
syphilitic
   hypomelanosis,
tinea versicolor.

Axillae

Acrochordon (skin
   tags),
boils,
candidiasis,
contact dermatitis,
erythrasma,
Fox–Fordyce
   disease,
Hailey–Hailey
   disease,
hidradenitis,
hyperhidrosis,
intertrigo,
molluscum
   contagiosum,
pediculosis,
scabies,
seborrhoeic
   dermatitis.

Chest

Acne,
candidiasis,
contact dermatitis,
Darier's disease,
eczema,
epithelioma,
keloid,
keratoses
  (seborrhoeic,
  senile and solar),
lichen sclerosus et
  atrophicus,
melanoma,
Paget's disease,
pityriasis rosea,
psoriasis,
scabies,
scleroderma,
seborrhoeic
  dermatitis,
Senear–Usher
  pemphigus,
submammary
  intertrigo,
syphilis,
tinea versicolor,
urticaria.

Back

Acne,
Darier's disease,
dermatitis
  herpetiformis,
dermatophytosis,
eczema,
epithelioma,
keratoses
  (seborrhoeic,
  senile and solar),
lichen planus,
lichen sclerosus et
  atrophicus,
neurotic
  excoriations,
pityriasis rosea,
psoriasis,
scleroderma,
seborrhoeic
  dermatitis,
tinea versicolor,
urticaria,
verrucae.

Buttocks

Acne conglobata,
boils,
contact dermatitis,
dermatitis
  herpetiformis,
dermatophytosis,
eczema,
folliculitis,
herpes zoster,
lupus vulgaris,
scabies,
urticaria,
xanthomata.

Anal area

Candidiasis,
condyloma
  acuminata,
condyloma latum,
dermatophytosis,
haemorrhoids,
intertrigo,
lichen sclerosus et
  atrophicus,
Paget's disease,
pediculosis,
psoriasis,
seborrhoeic
  dermatitis,
threadworms,
vitiligo.

Abdomen

Contact dermatitis,
discoid eczema,
drug eruptions,
herpes zoster,
lichen planus,
pediculosis,
pityriasis rosea,
pityriasis versicolor,
psoriasis,
scabies,
seborrhoeic
  dermatitis,
urticaria.

Genitalia

Balanitis,
balanitis plasma
  cellularis (Zoon),
balanitis xerotica
  obliterans,
Behçet's disease,
candidiasis,
chancroid,
contact dermatitis,

epithelioma,
granuloma
    inguinale,
herpes simplex,
herpes zoster,
leukoplakia,

lichen planus,
lichen sclerosus et
    atrophicus,
lymphogranuloma
    venereum,
Paget's disease,

pediculosis,
psoriasis,
scabies,
sebaceous cysts,
urticaria,
verrucae.

Groins

Acrochordon (skin
    tags),
candidiasis,
contact dermatitis,
dermatophytosis,
erythrasma,

Hailey–Hailey
    disease,
intertrigo,
keratoses
    (seborrhoeic),
pityriasis rosea,

psoriasis,
seborrhoeic
    dermatitis,
verrucae.

Arms

Contact dermatitis,
dermatophytosis,
discoid eczema,
erythema nodosum,
keratosis pilaris,

keratoses
    (seborrhoeic,
    senile and solar),
leucoderma,
lichen planus,

oil folliculitis,
psoriasis,
urticaria,
verrucae,
xanthoma.

Wrists, hands and fingers

Actinic dermatitis,
atopic eczema,
candidiasis,
chilblains,
chronic fissured
    eczema,
contact dermatitis,
dermatophytosis,
erysipeloid,

erythema
    multiforme,
granuloma
    annulare,
hyperhidrosis,
keratoacanthoma,
mucous cysts,
palmar syphilide,
paronychia,

periungual
    fibromata
    (Koenen's
    tumours),
pompholyx,
psoriasis,
verrucae,
vitiligo,
xanthoma.

Knees and elbows

Atopic dermatitis,
Ehlers–Danlos
    syndrome,

epidermolysis
    bullosa,
psoriasis,

verrucae,
xanthoma.

Legs

Chilblains,
contact dermatitis,
eczema,
epithelioma,
erythema
    induratum,
erythema nodosum,
Kaposi's sarcoma,

keratoses
    (seborrhoeic,
    senile and solar),
lichen amyloidosis,
lichen planus,
necrobiosis
    lipoidica,
nodular vasculitis,

pretibial
    myxoedema,
prurigo nodularis,
psoriasis,
purpura,
urticaria,
varicose eczema,
varicose ulceration.

Feet

Actinic keratosis,
callosities,
chilblains,
contact dermatitis,
dermatophytosis,
eczema,

hyperhidrosis,
juvenile plantar
   dermatosis,
keratolysis
   punctata,

plantar syphilide,
pompholyx,
psoriasis,
verrucae.

Shape of lesions

The shape of individual lesions commonly provides a valuable clue to the diagnosis. Thus arcuate annular lesions occur in mycotic infections, granuloma annulare, tuberculoid leprosy, late secondary and tertiary syphilis, psoriasis and lichen planus.

Concentric rings are the characteristic lesions of erythema multiforme.

Bizarre ulceration with a serosanguinous exudate indicates dermatitis artefacta. Bizarre vesiculation occurs also from contact with certain plants and caterpillars.

Grouped urticarial lesions each with a central punctum suggest insect bites, whilst multiple patches of scarred alopecia with 'footsteps in the snow' pattern are seen with pseudopelade affecting the scalp.

Horseshoe shaped infiltrate patches are seen in mycosis fungoides and other skin reticuloses.

The appearance of skin lesions following trauma, particularly scratching, causes what is termed the 'Koebner phenomenon' and is seen in psoriasis and lichen planus.

A livid reticulate pattern is seen on the shins from exposure to heat. Similarly a reticulate pattern is seen on the limbs with polyarteritis nodosa and cutaneous vasculitis. Other circulatory causes include acrocyanosis and cryoglobulinaemia. A fine reticulate pattern is seen with poikiloderma of both exogenous and endogenous types.

Linear eruptions may be straight, curved or complex. Apart from the Koebner phenomenon linear eruptions are seen in dermatitis artefacta, striate dermatitis due to plants; linear urticaria is the hallmark of dermographism. Linear lesions from inoculation of virus are seen in some instances of viral warts, orf and the primary lesions of cat scratch fever. Linear scabs are likewise seen from scratching in impetigo. Linear warty vesicular and pigmented streaks characterize incontinentia pigmenti (Bloch–Sulzberger disease). Warts and sebaceous naevi commonly present as a linear lesion. Curved and complex lines are the feature of larva migrans; here the migrating larva leaves an urticarial track (*Plate 12.5*).

Oval erythematous discs with peripheral scales are the hallmark of pityriasis rosea. Many discs appear, particularly on the trunk, the long axes of the discs lying parallel to the skin creases.

An eruption of dermatome distribution is characteristic of zoster. However, herpes simplex and secondary carcinoma of the skin with perineural lymphatic permeation may also follow a zoster-like distribution.

Colour of the skin

Not only the location and pattern but the *colour* of the individual lesions forming an eruption and of the skin in general may be of diagnostic importance. Thus a bright red eruption commonly signifies a drug rash. Other bright red eruptions include the exanthem of scarlet fever and the facial flush seen in the carcinoid syndrome. A ruby red or tomato colour is characteristic of the tumour of mycosis fungoides and is typical in carbon monoxide poisoning; haemangiomata and pyogenic granuloma show a blood red tint. The generalized maculopapular eruption of secondary syphilis is characteristically dull red or ham-coloured.

Reddish brown to mahogany lesions are found with urticaria pigmentosa, haemosiderosis associated with venous stasis and the ecchymotic lesions sometimes seen in scurvy.

Fawn-coloured papules and nodules are seen with lupus vulgaris, sarcoidosis and acne agminata; the scales of tinea versicolor are sometimes fawn.

Yellow lesions on the skin are uncommon. The papules and nodules of xanthoma and the naevo-xanthoendothelioma are usually bright yellow. Yellow to red-brown lesions are seen in Darier's disease and Letterer–Siwe disease. Yellow discoloration is seen in jaundice, carotenaemia and from certain drugs such as mepacrine.

Green tumours are a distinct rarity and occur only with chloroma, a rare reticulosis.

Blue lesions include tattoo marks, blue naevi and the blue cellular naevus. Cyanosis has many pulmonary and cardiac causes.

A brown-grey pigmentation is seen with haemochromatosis.

Red-violet or plum-coloured lesions are uncommon. However, fixed drug eruptions and lichen planus are characteristically violaceous, while the nodules and plaques of sarcoidosis may be violaceous rather than fawn. Distinctly violet erythema around the eyelids character-izes a dermatomyositis, and the striae seen in pregnancy and Cushing's syndrome have a purple coloration.

Melanosis is characteristic of a variety of disorders, both systemic and cutaneous. Particular mention should be made of Addison's disease, haemochromatosis, pituitary disorders, hepatic cirrhosis and visceral malignancy. Café au lait macules are seen in neurofibro-mata and Albright's disease, while chronic photomelanosis is seen in porphyria, pellagra and intoxication with certain metals.

Brown to black macules include lentigo and junctional naevi. Slate-grey to black macules or nodules usually signify malignant melanoma. Gunmetal grey purpura are characteristic of meningococcaemia.

Depigmentation of the skin may be partial or total and hypopigmentation sometimes follows an inflammatory process. Off-white hypopigmentation is seen with tinea versicolor, pityriasis simplex and in leprosy. Snow white areas are characteristic of vitiligo and albinism. Morphoea shows white waxy infiltrated patches. Areas of milky white depigmentation in young children are characteristic of epiloia.

Not only the colours but the sequence of colour changes and the presence of different colours in multiple lesions may be of diagnostic importance. Thus the colour sequence of red-purple to green and yellow is commonly seen in erythema nodosum and the nodules of secondary carcinoma; the tumours of mycosis fungoides show a wide range of colours from lesion to lesion.

Ulcers

Ulceration of the skin commonly poses difficult diagnostic problems. Here again both the shape and colour of the lesion may provide helpful diagnostic clues. The major characteristics are summarized below:

Arciform with islands of normal epithelium within the ulcerated area: arteriosclerotic or syphilitic.

Shallow with an erythematous surround: diabetic.

Arciform with dusky cyanotic halo: rheumatoid.

Circular with normal surrounding skin: neurotrophic.

Shallow ulcer with white atrophy surrounding: cryoglobulinaemia.

Shallow ulcer with surrounding scleroderma: morphoea, systemic sclerosis, Werner's syndrome.

Ulcer with surrounding livedo racemosa: polyarteritis nodosa.

Necrotic nodule: Bazin's disease.

Ulcer with surrounding cyanosis and pustules: pyoderma gangrenosum.

Bizarre shaped ulcer: dermatitis artefacta.

Ulcer surrounded by haemosiderosis: stasis ulcer, polycythaemia.

Ulcer surrounded by brown-grey and black pigment: malignant melanoma.

Ulcer surrounded by pustules, erosions and green pus: pseudomonas pyocyaneus infection.

Ulcer with raised edge: possible squamous epithelioma.

Ulcer with membrane: tropical ulcer, diphtheritic ulcer.

Ulcer with 'wash leather' base: gumma.

Ulcer with yellow exudate: sickle cell anaemia.

Two of the commonest findings associated with ulceration, particularly leg ulceration, are eczema surrounding the lesion caused by contact sensitivity to topical medication and a glazed atrophy or deep ulceration from the over-use of powerful topical steroids.

Diagnostic procedures

Biopsy

Skin biopsy for diagnosis is a simple procedure. It provides a definitive diagnosis in a wide variety of diseases. The lesion selected should be fully developed and representative of the eruption. In the case of a large lesion the biopsy can be taken from the edge and should include some normal skin.

Lignocaine 1%, with adrenaline, is used as a local anaesthetic; ideally the anaesthetic should be infiltrated into skin around the lesion and not into it. The incision should be elliptical and about three times as long as it is wide. A Bard-Parker No. 10 or 15 blade is recommended. Mersutures No. FSE-324 are useful for suturing the wound. A 2–5 mm biopsy punch is a rapid alternative method of obtaining biopsy material. When a punch is used bleeding can be controlled by a single suture or the galvanocautery. The specimen, however obtained, is placed in a solution of 10% formal saline.

Patch testing (*see* Chapter 5)

This is a method for determining which of a number of suspect substances might be responsible for a contact (allergic type) dermatitis. The possible offending substances include plants, industrial chemicals, drugs, articles of everyday use, clothing and cosmetics; literally 'anything under the sun, including the sun'.

The patch test consists of the application to normal skin of a non-irritant concentration of the suspect substance. The upper back is the preferred site. The allergen can be applied to a 1-cm square of lint, which in turn is covered by a square of polythene, kept in place by strapping. Most hospital skin departments, however, use a set of allergens proposed by the International Contact Dermatitis Research Group, which can be obtained from Trolab AC, A.N. Hansens alle 6B, 2900 Hellerup, Denmark. A roll of aluminium foil-backed patch test squares can be obtained from Astra Hewlitt Ltd, King George Avenue, Watford, Herts. These are kept in place by zinc oxide strapping or, for patients known to be allergic to the plaster, Micropore or Dermicel.

A new method of applying suspect allergens is by means of the Finn Chamber (Associated Hospital Supplies, P.O. Box 4, Pershore, Worcestershire). These are shallow metal chambers. Ten metal chambers on Scanpor (non-woven microporous adhesive tape) are practical for testing with a large number of substances, e.g. with routine tests (*see Figures 2.2* and *2.3*). Used singly with small pieces of Scanpor tape they are suitable for a small test series and for separate tests. The substances, incorporated into petrolatum, are applied directly into the chamber, filling slightly more than half its volume (*Figure 2.4*). For solutions a filter paper disc is first placed in the chamber and then saturated with the solution, but without surplus. When removing the tests after 24–72 hours' exposure, a ring-shaped depression around the test area indicates the success of the tests (*Figure 2.5*).

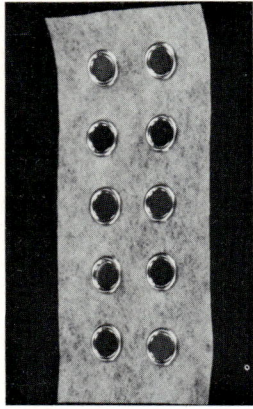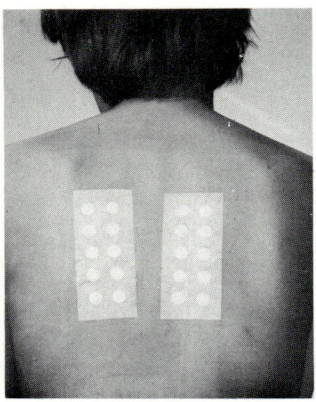

Figures 2.2 and 2.3 *Patch testing with a number of substances (routine tests) using the Finn Chamber method*

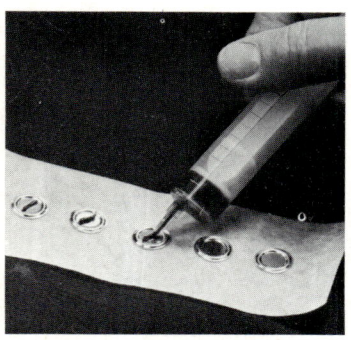

Figure 2.4 *Patch testing—applying individual allergens to Finn chambers mounted on Scanpor tape for a small number of separate tests*

Examination for fungus

The lesion should be cleansed of ointment with spirit. The overlying scales or superficial layers of the epidermis are scraped away with a Bard-Parker No. 10 blade, paying particular attention to the advancing edge of the lesion. The scales are then placed on a microscope slide, covered with a coverslip and one or two drops of 10% potassium hydroxide are allowed to seep beneath the coverslip. The slide is gently heated over a bunsen burner and, on cooling, the specimen is examined under a microscope using low power magnification. A scraping can easily be put into an envelope and sent through the post to a mycology laboratory for examination and culture.

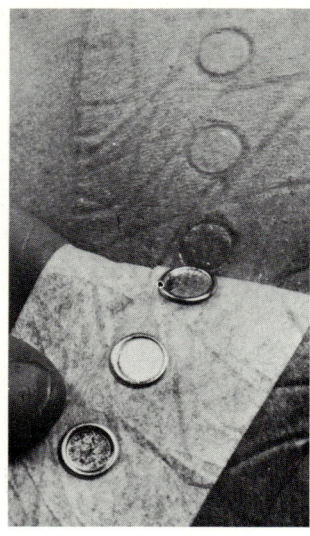

Figure 2.5 *Showing ring shaped depressions on removal of chambers, indicating positive tests*

Ringworm of the scalp is seen in prepubertal children and can be examined by means of a Wood's Light. This is an ultraviolet lamp with a nickel–cobalt filter. Examination of infected scalps in a dark room will reveal fluorescence of the patches of hair infected with human (*M. audouinii*) or domestic animal (*M. canis*) small spore fungus. Microscopic and cultural examination should also be undertaken. Skin affected with erythrasma gives a pale pink fluorescence and tinea versicolor a pale yellow coloration.

3 Histopathology of the skin

D. M. MacDonald

Introduction

A knowledge of skin histopathology, however rudimentary, is an important factor in understanding skin disease; more advanced knowledge is an invaluable aid in diagnosis.

Clinical examination of the skin allows only a view of the surface morphology but with experience gives valuable clues to the underlying pathological process. Increased surface scaling, for instance, suggests involvement of the epidermis; erythema may imply increased vascular flow; a brown colour may be associated with an excess of melanin or haemosiderin in the tissues, and a diffuse smooth lump suggests that the pathological process is occurring in the dermal or subcutaneous tissue. The third dimension of the skin may be directly visualized in histological sections of biopsy material. However, it is important to realize that histology shows the tissue in a single vertical plane at one particular moment in time. The techniques of skin biopsy have already been briefly described (Chapter 2).

The normal histology of the skin shows specialized features appropriate to its function. Basically, it comprises an outer epidermal layer with its specialized appendages of hair, sweat and sebaceous glands and an inner dermal layer composed of ground substance containing a supporting scaffolding of collagen and elastic tissue. The dermis also contains a network of nerves and vessels and a variety of other cells including reticuloendothelial cells and mast cells. Before embarking on a study of skin histopathology, a knowledge of the normal skin anatomy is essential.

The principles involved in the histopathological examination of skin tissue differ little from those associated with the pathology of other organ systems. Nevertheless, disease processes affecting the skin occur on a background of a unique anatomical structure and give rise to characteristic changes whose diagnostic value ranges from the non-specific to the pathognomonic. In common with other tissues, the skin reacts pathologically in a limited number of ways, each of which is characteristically identifiable in tissue sections, and which will be described below. The presence of one or more of these features in combination contributes towards the histological diagnosis. This, in turn must be considered in relation to the clinical data. It is of paramount importance to provide the histologist with an adequate piece of tissue and full clinical information.

Terminology of pathological processes in the skin

Hyperkeratosis

The stratum corneum consists of a normally anuclear superficial layer of the epidermis. It varies in thickness in various sites of the body, being thick and compact on the palms and soles and thin and loose on the face. Hyperkeratosis implies increased thickness of the stratum corneum over that which is appropriate for the site. It is a prominent feature of lichenified chronic eczema, or any condition where friction to the skin occurs, but it is also common in lichen planus (*Figure 3.1*) and a number of genetically determined conditions, particularly the ichthyoses. As a single feature its diagnostic value is poor, but in association with other pathological changes it may provide corollary evidence for a particular diagnosis.

Hyperkeratosis may occasionally be confined to, or be more prominent in, follicular openings. This is seen frequently in discoid lupus erythematosus and lichen planopilaris.

Hyperkeratosis may be associated with skin tumours, either as a primary event where there is hyperplasia of epidermis giving rise to the excess keratin as in squamous cell epithelioma, keratoacanthoma or virus warts, or as a secondary friction-induced event as sometimes occurs over histiocytomas and other benign tumours.

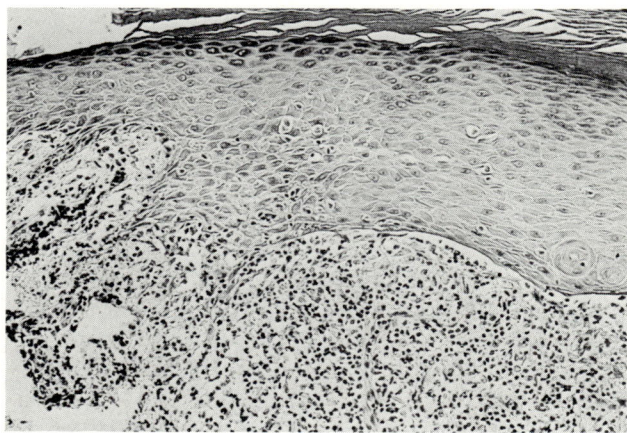

Figure 3.1 *Lichen planus: there is hyperkeratosis, hypergranulosis, acanthosis, liquefaction degeneration and incipient subepidermal bulla formation. An upper dermal infiltrate of lymphocytes and some histiocytes is present*

The term epidermolytic hyperkeratosis is applied to a specialized form of hyperkeratosis which is encountered in bullous ichthyosiform erythroderma and some cases of ichthyosis hystrix, epidermal naevi and congenital keratoderma. Hyperkeratosis is found in association with intracellular oedema of the granular layer of the epidermis which may be sufficiently severe to cause disruption of the superficial epidermis and bulla formation.

Parakeratosis

The stratum corneum is normally devoid of nuclei except on mucous membranes. Retention of nuclei or their remnants in the stratum corneum is termed parakeratosis. The nuclei take the form of small, elongated, darkly staining structures. It occurs in many inflammatory skin diseases which affect the epidermis. It may be seen in eczema, but is virtually always seen in psoriasis and certain other dermatoses including pityriasis lichenoides chronica and the active phase of secondary syphilis. Parakeratosis denotes an abnormality of cellular metabolism, particularly an increased rate of cell replication.

The morphological pattern of parakeratosis may be helpful in diagnosis. Actinic keratoses show an alternation of columns of parakeratosis and hyperkeratosis, the former arising from dysplastic epidermis and the latter from the more normal epithelium of hair follicles. In the porokeratoses the parakeratosis occurs at the margin of the lesion and histologically resembles the plume of a feather, the so-called cornoid lamella. In Darier's disease (*Figure 3.2*) the parakeratosis is also characteristically focal and the parakeratotic nuclei are larger and plumper.

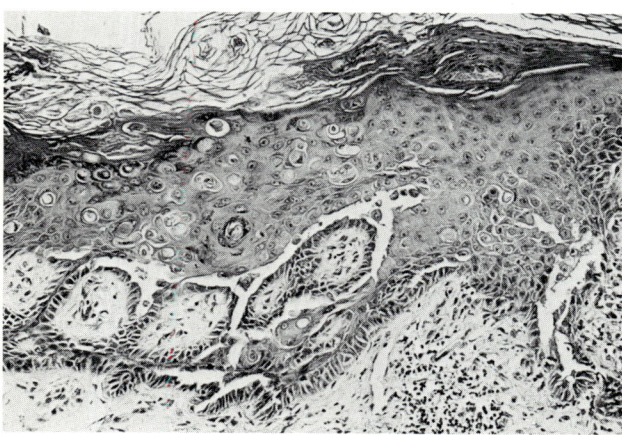

Figure 3.2 *Darier's disease: an area of parakeratosis is present. Numerous dyskeratotic cells are scattered within the epidermis and a few rounded acantholytic cells are present within the epidermal cleft*

Physiological parakeratosis occurs in mucosal sites. Cells of the stratum corneum appear ballooned and possess rounded nuclei. It is important to realize that this change is not pathological on mucosae.

Parakeratosis is accompanied by loss of the granular layer at the same site. It is not uncommon for hyperkeratosis and parakeratosis to be associated.

Hypergranulosis

The granular layer (stratum granulosum) of the epidermis lies immediately below the stratum corneum and appears as one or two layers of flattened cells which stain deeply basophilic owing to the presence of keratohyalin granules. Increase in thickness of this layer is termed hypergranulosis. It is found in situations where the epidermis as a whole is thickened (*see below*) and therefore occurs in circumstances where the skin is subjected to frequent rubbing or scratching as in lichenification. It is also a prominent feature in lichen planus. Hypergranulosis is frequently associated with hyperkeratosis.

Acanthosis

Thickening of the prickle cell layer (Malpighian layer; stratum spinosum) is termed acanthosis. Various patterns of acanthosis may be recognized. A common type seen particularly in chronic eczema comprises thickening of the epidermis with overall preservation of the rete ridge pattern. If rubbing and scratching has been prominent there may be apparent fusion of rete ridges. This appearance may be seen as a reactive change over benign tumours. Reactive hyperplasia with massive acanthosis may sometimes be seen in association with chronic inflammatory skin lesions and certain benign neoplasms—a situation referred to as pseudo-epitheliomatous hyperplasia.

Another type of acanthosis is typically seen in psoriasis—hence frequently termed psoriasiform acanthosis. There is gross elongation of the rete ridges with concomitant increase in length of the dermal papillae. The suprapillary epidermis is reduced to one or two cell layers. In this type parakeratosis is frequently present and the granular layer consequently absent.

Tumour-like acanthosis may be found in benign hyperplasias or neoplasias of epidermis such as in epidermal naevi or seborrhoeic warts. Viral invasion of keratinocytes may also induce tumour-like acanthosis as in virus warts and molluscum contagiosum.

The term acanthosis is not usually applied to frankly malignant epidermal proliferation.

Acantholysis

Acantholysis is a pathological process affecting the epidermis, in which keratinocytes become separated from each other as a result of loss of or damage to the connecting desmosomes. The so-called acantholytic cells take on a characteristic rounded appearance which is readily recognized in sections or even smears of tissue. The loss of cohesion between the keratinocytes results in an intra-epidermal blister.

These histological changes are exemplified by the pemphigus group of disorders in which an antibody is directed against intercellular components. In pemphigus vulgaris (*Figure 3.3*) the split usually occurs just above the basal layer while in pemphigus foliaceus the blister is usually situated at a higher level in the granular layer.

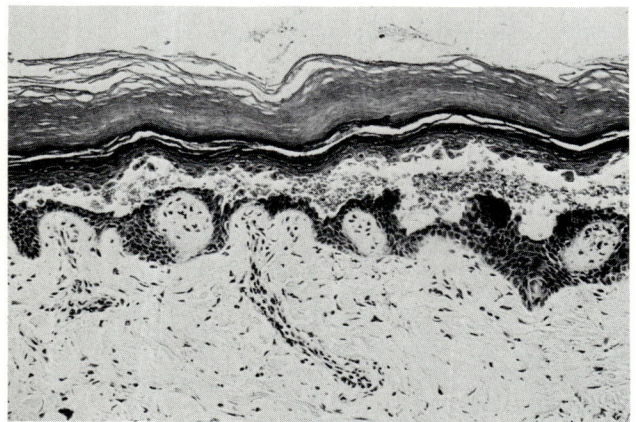

Figure 3.3 *Pemphigus: an intraepidermal bulla with acantholysis. Hyperkeratosis is an incidental feature*

Acantholysis also occurs in the dominantly inherited genodermatoses, Darier's disease and benign familial pemphigus.

The abnormal malignant keratinocytes of actinic keratosis and squamous cell epithelioma occasionally produce abnormal desmosomes with consequent 'malignant' acantholysis.

Dyskeratosis

Dyskeratosis refers to abnormal or premature keratinization of individual epidermal cells. This occurs in several genodermatoses including Darier's disease and benign familial pemphigus. Keratinization of cells is seen as increased cytoplasmic eosinophilia, and pyknosis of the keratinocyte nucleus. The cells often appear larger than their neighbours. In the completely dyskeratotic cell the nucleus is likely to disappear totally.

The phenomenon is seen prominently in epidermis which has been sunburnt.

Not surprisingly dyskeratosis is frequently found in malignant epidermis, for instance in actinic keratoses, Bowen's disease and squamous cell epithelioma. Large bizarre dyskeratotic cells with abnormal mitoses and other features of cytological malignancy may be evident.

Spongiosis

Spongiosis implies intercellular oedema of the epidermal cell layers with consequent widening of the intercellular spaces. When this occurs the desmosomes of the keratinocytes become readily visible as intercellular prickles. With more severe intercellular oedema the desmosomes become ruptured with separation of keratinocytes from each other giving rise to a spongiotic vesicle. This change is seen particularly in eczema (*Figure 3.4*), tending to be minimal or even absent in chronic eczema but much more prominent in acute disease.

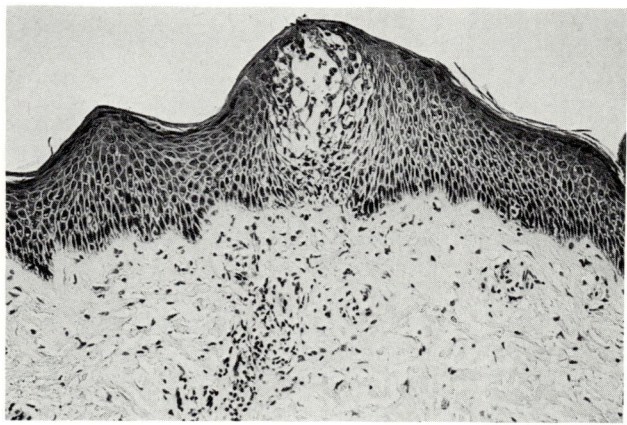

Figure 3.4   *Eczema: marked spongiosis leading to frank vesicle formation is present in the epidermis*

Ballooning (reticular) degeneration

Ballooning or reticular degeneration refers to a specific change affecting the epidermis in which both cell cytoplasm and nucleus become grossly distended and eventually rupture giving rise to vesicles or bullae. This appearance is seen in several viral infections of the skin including herpes simplex and herpes zoster. These changes may be mimicked by degenerative epidermal changes caused by other factors such as may be seen in thermal burns and erythema multiforme.

Liquefaction degeneration

Liquefaction degeneration is the term applied to a specific degenerative change occurring in the basal cells of the epidermis. There is loss of the orderly palisading arrangement of the basal layer. Individual cells may swell, become pale or show vacuolar change or may appear teased out and attenuated. Eventually the cells disintegrate and disappear. These changes occur in two important dermatoses, namely lupus erythematosus and lichen planus. Similar but milder changes may be found in lichen sclerosus et atrophicus, poikiloderma atrophicans vasculare and certain degenerative inherited conditions such as poikiloderma congenitale.

In association with liquefaction degeneration of the basal layer, the melanocytes which are situated in this layer are frequently damaged with consequent loss of pigment, known as pigmentary incontinence. This may be reflected clinically by hypopigmentation or alternatively hyperpigmentation may ensue as a result of granules of melanin being phagocytosed by macrophages which lie in the superficial dermis.

Papillomatosis

The lower surface of the epidermis shows a characteristic regular undulating configuration when viewed in vertical skin sections. Accentuation of this pattern with elongation and apparent bifurcation of the epidermal rete pegs is found when the papillary processes of the dermis are enlarged. This papillary hypertrophy and consequent changes in epidermal architecture is termed papillomatosis. This is seen in psoriasis and also in the focal lesions of Darier's disease. The premalignant epidermis of actinic keratoses and also benign and malignant epidermal tumours may also show this feature. Papillomatosis is a very non-specific histological change which may appear as a reactive process consequent on other pathological changes.

Colloid bodies

Small, more or less round amorphous eosinophilic bodies are found in the superficial dermis near the epidermal basement membrane in several skin diseases. These have been named colloid bodies or alternatively cytoid bodies or Civatte bodies. They are of approximately similar size to keratinocytes and are thought to arise as a result of degenerative changes in basal or suprabasal epidermal cells which drop into the adjacent dermis. Colloid bodies are most prominently seen in lichen planus and lupus erythematosus. In the latter prominent thickening of the basement membrane is frequently evident.

Microabscesses

Several types of microabscesses may be encountered in histological sections of skin either in epidermis or dermis. They comprise small collections of polymorphonuclear or mononuclear cells whose precise type and position may provide diagnostic information. So-called microabscesses of Monro comprise small collections of neutrophils in various stages of degeneration situated in the upper epidermal and corneal layers of psoriatic skin. Pautrier microabscesses are seen in mycosis fungoides and are composed of abnormal mononuclear cells (now known to be malignant T lymphocytes) occurring as focal collections within the epidermis. In dermatitis herpetiformis papillary microabscesses of neutrophils and frequently some eosinophils are confined to the tips of the dermal papillae at the sites of blister formation. Obviously, small neutrophil or eosinophilic abscesses may be found in dermis or epidermis as a result of bacterial or parasitic infection.

Occasionally foreign material or damaged skin tissue may be extruded through the epidermis to the exterior, a process termed transepidermal elimination. In biopsy specimens, such material on its way through the epidermis superficially may resemble an intraepidermal abscess. The phenomenon may be seen in a 'stitch abscess' or may occur spontaneously in such conditions as perforating collagenosis or elastosis perforans serpiginosa.

Bullae

Blisters over 1 cm in size are termed bullae. In histological interpretation the precise level in the skin where the bulla forms is of paramount importance. This, coupled with observation of the associated features can usually provide a diagnosis. In the pemphigus group of disorders, the bulla is always intraepidermal and is associated with acantholysis. Intraepidermal blistering is also found in bullous impetigo and staphylococcal scalded skin syndrome where the level of splitting is very superficial; other histological features such as collections of neutrophils or bacteria and absence of prominent acantholysis may be helpful in differentiation.

Bullae may also be seen intraepidermally in acute eczema as a result of coalescence of vesicles. Spongiosis is always present in the epidermis adjacent to the bulla.

Subepidermal bulla formation occurs in a much wider variety of diseases so that the associated pathological features become extremely important. In pemphigoid (*Figure 3.5*) there is usually clear cut separation of a relatively large area of epidermis from the underlying dermis with an associated dermal infiltrate of eosinophils. Cicatricial (mucous membrane) pemphigoid may be very similar but additionally frequently shows features of scarring in the upper dermis. The subepidermal blister of dermatitis herpetiformis (*Figure 3.6*) may occasionally be difficult to differentiate from early lesions of pemphigoid, but the separation usually covers only the area of a papillary tip and is associated with the neutrophil papillary tip microabscesses previously mentioned.

Epidermolysis bullosa, a group of inherited blistering disorders,

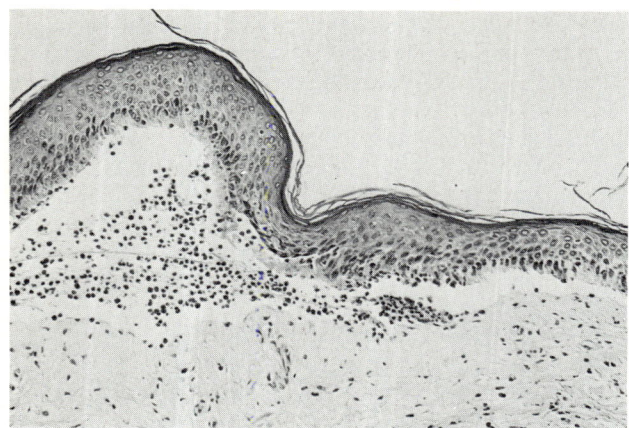

Figure 3.5 *Pemphigoid: a large subepidermal bulla is associated with an infiltrate of eosinophil leucocytes*

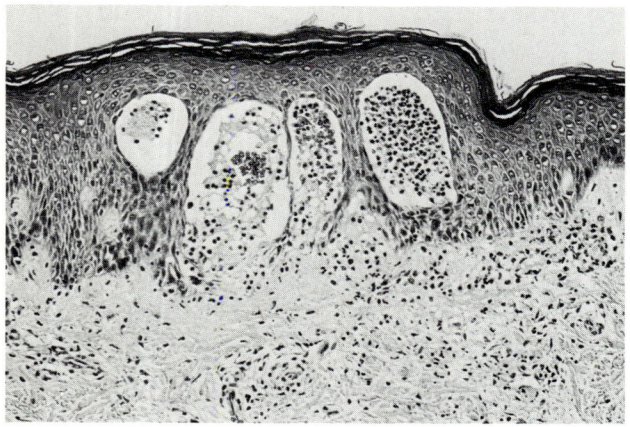

Figure 3.6 *Dermatitis herpetiformis: subepidermal bullae are forming at the sites of papillary tip microabscesses comprising predominantly neutrophil leucocytes*

show subepidermal bulla formation with an absence of inflammatory infiltrate. Dermal scarring may or may not be present depending on the precise anatomical location of the genetic disturbance. The porphyrias also result in subepidermal bullae frequently with scarring and relative paucity of inflammatory infiltrate. However, the dermal vessels are seen to be surrounded by amorphous eosinophilic material which stains positively with periodic acid–Schiff reagent. Subepidermal bullae may also arise as a result of epidermal necrosis as in erythema multiforme or certain viral diseases. The characteristic degenerative changes in the epidermis will be evident.

The process of observation and interpretation of the features of the histopathology of the bullous disorders exemplifies the principles involved in differential diagnosis in dermatopathology.

'Metabolic infiltration' of the skin

In addition to infiltration of the skin by inflammatory or other cells, which will be discussed below, the dermis is sometimes the site of infiltration by metabolic products.

Lipid may accumulate as a result of inflammation or because of excess circulating levels. The lipid is engulfed by phagocytic cells giving the appearance of foamy macrophages in the dermis. Mucin may also occur in the dermis and is not phagocytosed actively. It may be found in many inflammatory or neoplastic processes but occurs specifically as a major pathological feature in pretibial myxoedema and rare conditions such as lichen myxoedematosus and scleroedema. Accumulation of glycosaminoglycans occurs in the skin fibroblasts and other cells in the mucopolysaccharidoses giving rise to the respective cutaneous features. In primary systemic or myeloma-associated amyloidosis, amyloid deposits may occur in the dermis and in blood vessel walls causing the waxy plaques and purpuric lesions seen clinically. In primary localized cutaneous amyloidosis, small deposits of amyloid are found in the dermal papillae in the absence of any systemic disease. The porphyrias are characterized histologically by the deposition of an amorphous material around the blood vessels of sun exposed skin. A very similar deposition around vessels is seen in the rare congenital disease lipoid proteinosis.

Histological examination of the skin is important in the diagnosis of all these metabolic disorders. Special histochemical staining techniques allow differentiation of these various 'metabolic infiltrates' but occasionally more sophisticated experimental methods including electron microscopy may help in elucidating the specific diagnosis.

Cytology and cellular infiltrates

In discussing the basic pathological processes which affect cutaneous tissue, specific cell types such as eosinophil leucocytes and lymphocytes have been mentioned and reference has been made to absence or presence of inflammatory infiltrates.

As in other tissues the presence of cells not normally resident in the skin implies inflammatory or neoplastic (benign or malignant) infiltration. The dermis is more commonly and more prominently affected than the epidermis.

Neoplasia may involve any type of cell which may be derived from skin components or metastatic from some distant site. In inflammatory processes one may encounter a wide variety of cells including neutrophil and eosinophil polymorphonuclear leucocytes, lymphocytes, plasma cells, histiocytes, epithelioid cells and giant cells. Mast cells and fibroblasts are also frequently found in association with both inflammatory and neoplastic infiltrates.

The study of individual cell types consequently assumes great importance and it is necessary to return to normal histology to learn cellular morphology.

Granulomatous infiltration of the skin

Granuloma formation in the skin implies a chronic inflammatory process in which the cellular infiltrate comprises histiocytes, epithelioid cells and frequently giant cells arranged in more or less localized masses in the dermis. Lymphocytes and plasma cells are often present in variable numbers.

The differentiation of the conditions giving rise to granuloma formation depends on the composition and architecture of the granuloma, its distribution and specific associated features. Special staining techniques or microscopic methods may be helpful in diagnosis. In sarcoidosis, for example, the granulomas occur in a 'pure' form with neat rounded masses of epithelioid cells and histiocytes with very few mononuclear cells of other type. Granulomas of such pure cytology may be referred to as 'sarcoidal' in type. The infiltration affects the dermis while the epidermis and most superficial papillary dermis are only exceptionally involved. Despite this characteristic histology, sarcoidosis may be difficult to differentiate from other granulomatous conditions, particularly tuberculoid leprosy.

In the latter the granulomatous masses are also well circumscribed and frequently contain few lymphocytes. However the infiltrate occurs particularly in association with nerve bundles in the dermis giving the clue to the diagnosis. The presence of acid-fast leprosy bacilli though frequently difficult to detect, should always be sought by Ziehl–Neelsen or Fite–Farraco staining.

Lupus vulgaris is another granulomatous skin condition which must be considered in the differential diagnosis. Unlike tuberculous lesions in other tissues caseation only rarely occurs. The superficial dermis is usually prominently involved with secondary damage to the epidermis. The granulomas tend to be significantly less discrete than in sarcoidosis or leprosy and there is a more mixed population of infiltrating cells including, of course, epithelioid cells and histiocytes with numerous giant cells but also an irregular infiltrate of lymphocytes. This type of histology may be considered as 'tuberculoid'. Again, staining for the presence of acid fast organisms is important.

The deep mycoses give rise to granulomatous infiltrates of mixed inflammatory type which may extend deeply to the subcutaneous tissue but also frequently affect the epidermis sometimes causing pseudoepitheliomatous hyperplasia and verrucous change. The granulomatous infiltrate is usually extremely irregular and mixed with an abundance of lymphocytes and histiocytes. Small neutrophil abscesses may be present in the vicinity of fungal organisms. The periodic acid–Schiff stain and other specific stains for fungi may be valuable in the detection of organisms. A somewhat similar histology of irregular mixed granulomatous infiltrate is seen in foreign body reactions in the skin. Doubly refractile material associated with the foreign body may be visualized by polarization microscopy.

Associated features may be helpful in the interpretation of cutaneous granulomatous histology. The presence of vessel wall damage may be associated with a granulomatous infiltrate in tertiary syphilis or in Wegener's granulomatosis. Histiocytes, and perhaps giant cells, focused around an area of collagen damage or necrobiosis is suggestive of one of the palisading granulomata, such as granuloma annulare, necrobiosis lipoidica or rheumatoid nodule.

The differential diagnosis of granulomatous infiltration of the skin is much wider than is implied by the examples briefly described above. In general terms the diseases of the skin giving rise to granulomata can be classified according to the type of granulomatous infiltrate as illustrated in *Table 3.1*. This account however is designed not to be exhaustive but to illustrate the principles involved in the evaluation of cellular infiltrates.

Table 3.1

Sarcoidal	*Tuberculoid*	*Histiocytic*
Sarcoidosis	Lupus vulgaris	Leishmaniasis
Tuberculoid/borderline tuberculoid leprosy	Tuberculoid leprosy	Lepromatous leprosy
Berylliosis	Gummatous syphilis	Wegener's granulomatosis
Wegener's granulomatosis		

Palisading	*Mixed inflammatory*
Granuloma annulare	Deep mycoses
Necrobiosis lipoidica	Sea urchin spines
Gummatous syphilis	Foreign body
Rheumatoid arthritis	Ruptured cysts, etc.
Gout	
Cat scratch fever	

Vasculitis

Inflammatory vascular disease of the skin has been confused by a wide range of terminology based on variations of the clinical features.

Vasculitis is not itself a finite diagnosis but merely a manifestation of a basic pathological process.

Many tissues are liable to be affected by vasculitis, but the particular morphology of the cutaneous vasculature makes the skin (particularly of the lower limbs) a common site of clinical and pathological expression of vessel damage.

Three basic processes are most likely to give rise to vessel wall damage with inflammation. These are firstly deposition of immune complexes within the vessel wall, secondly defective fibrinolysis of microthrombus on the luminal surface or between endothelial cells of the vessel wall and thirdly direct secondary involvement of vessel wall by an acute or chronic inflammatory process, e.g. an abscess or trauma.

Deposition of immune complexes between vascular endothelial cells is the most important cause of vasculitis. The result of this deposition is activation of the complement pathway with resultant liberation of histamine, chemotaxis of polymorphs, activation of clotting and fibrin deposition. Subsequently limitation of the process is brought about by phagocytic histiocytes and suppressor T cells which limit the local production of antibody. The severity and therefore the speed of development and morphological form of clinical lesions depends on various factors including the size of the antigen load and the size of the immune complexes. Skin biopsy is likely to be undertaken when clinical lesions are evident and will show the histological changes at a single moment in time. Consequently, the histology will reflect just one stage of the dynamic process outlined above. The early stages of vasculitis tend to be seen in acute lesions, the vessels involved often being capillaries in the upper and mid-dermis. The later stages of vasculitis are found in chronic lesions usually affecting somewhat larger vessels in the deep dermis and subcutaneous tissue.

Acute vasculitis is exemplified by Henoch–Schönlein purpura. The small vessels of the papillary and upper reticular dermis show various degrees of damage, ranging from endothelial swelling, sometimes with luminal occlusion, to complete disintegration of the vessel wall with replacement by fibrinoid material. Neutrophils are present in considerable number permeating the vessel wall and lying in the surrounding dermis. The polymorph nuclei are frequently fragmented, a process termed leucocytoclasis, giving rise to so-called nuclear dust. There is also considerable extravasation of erythrocytes, causing the lesion to be clinically purpuric, and dermal oedema. Pathologically, this process is best called leucocytoclastic vasculitis. Histologically, a similar process is seen in polyarteritis nodosa except that the vessels involved comprise small to medium sized arteries. There is fibrinoid necrosis of the arterial wall with an associated infiltrate of neutrophils, eosinophils, lymphocytes and histiocytes. The arterial nature of the vessels can be demonstrated by identifying the internal elastic lamina with special elastin stains.

Nodular vasculitis on the legs is representative of chronic types of vasculitis. The histological picture is variable. Frequently, there is vessel damage in the deep dermis and subcutaneous fat evidenced by endothelial swelling and a surrounding infiltrate of lymphocytes and histiocytes. In the earliest lesions there is an acute inflammatory infiltrate comprising neutrophil leucocytes with fat necrosis consequent on vessel damage. The fat necrosis subsequently gives rise frequently to a granulomatous infiltrate consisting of histiocytes, epithelioid cells, giant cells and lymphocytes. Thus, a variety of histological appearances may be found in nodular vasculitis and the evidence of vasculitic damage is frequently difficult to demonstrate conclusively. It must be remembered that a blood vessel, if affected by an area of fat necrosis, is liable to be damaged resulting in a secondary vasculitis. The presence of a damaged vessel does not therefore necessarily implicate that vessel in the pathogenesis of the lesion.

4 Genetics, HLA type and disease

F. M. Pope

More than a quarter of the 5000 catalogued human inherited diseases affect the skin. Sometimes the abnormality is entirely cutaneous but mostly the skin is only one organ affected in a generalized process. Hereditary influence upon disease was recognized and observed for centuries before its essential orderliness followed from Mendel's description of transmitted inheritance. He showed that hereditary factors are transmitted through generations in an ordered pattern. The term 'gene' was invented in 1908 to denote a specific hereditary unit. We now know that structural genes specify particular protein chains and more than 100 000 (10^5) are possessed by each one of us. Garrod first suggested that chemical abnormalities can be produced by hereditary factors (genes) which control enzyme production. Faults or mutations in such enzymes allow the accumulation of intermediary compounds, or in certain cases a complete deficiency of other compounds, depending upon whether the metabolic pathway is blocked or diverted. This is the concept of the inborn error of metabolism which can affect protein, carbohydrate lipid, nucleic acid or any other bodily constituent. The fundamental mechanism is genetic. The next great step was the recognition that genes are chemical entities rather than vague philosophical control mechanisms. In 1940 deoxyribonucleic acid (DNA) was shown to transfer the specific qualities of one bacterial strain to another quite distinct one. Watson and Crick, in 1952, revolutionized the chemical understanding of inheritance in showing that DNA consists of two intertwined helical strands of nucleic acid polymers, each the exact complement of the other. They recognized that adenine always paired with thymine on the opposite chain and guanine always with cytosine. From this observation stems all the present day DNA and RNA biochemistry including the revolutionary technology of genetic engineering. Genes are particular segments of the total (very long) DNA content of a cell and can direct the synthesis of particular cell products. (The gene for ichthyosis, for example, results in the production of abnormally flaky skin.) Since DNA is a polymer of purine and pyrimidine chains (linked with phosphate) and particular bases in one chain always pair with complementary bases of the other, it follows that each chain is the chemical complement of the other. The information in the nuclear DNA (chromosomes) is transferred to the cytoplasm where another similar molecule (RNA directs the final synthesis of particular cell products. RNA is very similar to DNA except that thymine is replaced by uracil (but still pairs with adenine). An exact (equivalent) RNA copy of DNA (gene) is then made. This particular RNA (called messenger or mRNA) then carries the information from the gene to the cytoplasm. Here it is transformed into the various cell products. The conversion of information contained within DNA into its mRNA equivalent is called 'transcription' and the change of mRNA into final cell product 'translation'. The change from mRNA to product involves the participation of two further forms of RNA; transfer RNA (tRNA) and ribosomal RNA (rRNA). Transfer RNA is a remarkable molecule which has the ability to bind the equivalent amino acid which corresponds to a particular base triplet within the mRNA. (Each of the 21 common amino acids is coded by a sequence of three bases within the DNA and its mRNA equivalent.) The mRNA sequence is recognized at one end of the molecule and the amino acid binds to the other. The tRNA then allows the assembly of amino acids corresponding to the sequence of bases contained in the mRNA. The actual assembly of amino acids takes place when a third variety of RNA, rRNA draws through the mRNA chain, each tRNA then transporting the appropriate amino acid to the growing protein chain. Particular nucleic acid triplets (codons) within the mRNA tell the chain synthesis to start and other instruct it to stop. The initiating sequence is always AUG (adenine, uracil and guanine). All sorts of mistakes are possible in the translation process and are called mutations. Sometimes a single base is altered—the codon thus being altered and a different amino acid inserted during translation (missense mutation). At other times the terminator codon is inserted too early (nonsense mutation) or a single amino acid is added or removed. Chain termination mutations occur when the full stop codon mutates. Translation then proceeds to the next full stop. (Haemoglobin Constant Spring is an example in which the normal 141 amino acid haemoglobin chain is increased to 172 residues.)

Types of genes

There are two varieties of genes; those which produce various biochemical products such as haemoglobin, collagen or keratin, and those which control their rate of production and destruction. The former are called structural genes and the latter regulatory genes. In general, structural gene abnormalities are autosomal dominant and regulatory genes are autosomal recessive.

Chromosomes

DNA is packed within a supportive protein framework of histone proteins to form chromosomes. Chromosomes are evenly distributed between dividing cells. In somatic cells the number of chromosomes is precisely reproduced so that each daughter cell contains the same number as the parent. In germ cells on the other hand, the distribution of chromosomes is half that of the parent cell. Various faults can occur in the process of sexual (meiotic) and somatic (mitotic) division, and duplication (doubling) fusion (sticking together), deletion (omission), conversion (faulty assembly) and translocation (the sticking of one chromosome part to another) can produce dramatic clinical abnormalities. Mongolism is perhaps the best known clinical example, in which faulty transfer of chromosome 21 results in a gamete with two such chromosomes. Either there can be an extra 21 alone or there is a translocation of a 21 chromosome to a 15 chromosome. In either case the result is mongolism. The important difference is that the 15/21 translocation can affect young mothers who repeatedly pass on the mutation, whereas the 21 duplication is an isolated event in older mothers.

One half of the 46 human chromosomes are maternally derived, the other half paternally derived. Genes occur in pairs (one for each chromosome half). Any particular gene has a number of alternatives or alleles and generally large populations have the largest number. Any individual has a maximum of two alleles for any one gene. Those expressed when both are identical are called homozygous (recessive). Those expressed in preference to their coalleles are heterozygous or dominant. An intermediate or codominant gene is expressed when heterozygous but is even more obvious when homozygous; sickle cell anaemia is an excellent example. Allelic variation is the whole basis of genetic variation within populations. Mutations at any given allele may then alter nothing, greatly benefit or greatly disadvantage particular individuals. The result is Darwinian evolution (survival of the fittest depending upon circumstances).

Classification of genetic disease

Genetic diseases are conveniently separated into single gene, polygenic and chromosomal defects. These differ only in degree and form a spectrum of causation ranging from a single point mutation (affecting one DNA base) to chromosome deletions (affecting thousands of genes). Surprisingly, the deletion of whole chromosomes can sometimes be advantageous as has apparently occurred in man who, with 46 chromosomes, has evolved from his anthropoid ancestors who had 48.

Single gene disorders

Genes are sequences of DNA bases situated upon one of 44 autosomes or either of the two sex chromosomes. Eukaryotes (plant and animal) have maternal and paternal chromosomes arranged in pairs (each chromosome is partially maternal and partially paternal). Genes occur in particular positions (loci) along the chromosomes, each locus having several alternatives or alleles, within the general population. Single gene disorders result from specific changes in gene composition (mutations). Thus, sickle cell haemoglobin which follows the replacement of glutamine by valine at position 6 in the haemoglobin β chain produces a protein with radically altered properties which sickles in conditions of oxygen depletion. When both alleles mutate then the patient gets sickle cell anaemia (homozygous, severe disease). A single gene mutation (heterozygous) produces the less severe sickle cell trait. Mutated genes produce three possible genetic patterns: autosomal dominant, recessive and codominant. Dominant defects are those expressed to the full in heterozygotes, recessive defects are only expressed when both alleles are mutated in the homozygous state. Codominants are expressed as heterozygotes but are even more obvious as homozygotes. Each type of inheritance can occur in either the sex chromosomes (sex linked inheritance) or on any of the other chromosomes (autosomal inheritance). Disease patterns within families result from the type of inheritance and have characteristic family patterns. Confusion arises either when single new dominant mutations occur, or when excessive interbreeding allows apparent autosomal dominant patterns in autosomal recessively inherited abnormalities. The particular family characteristics for the various patterns are shown below.

Autosomal dominant (*Figure 4.1*)

The following typical features may be observed:

(1) Several generations are affected.
(2) Males and females are affected equally often.
(3) Transmission is not influenced by sex.
(4) On average 50 per cent of affected individuals have affected children.
(5) Unaffected individuals do not transmit the trait.

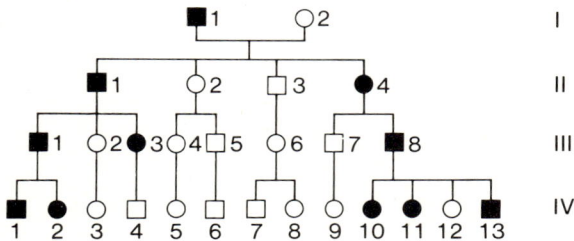

Figure 4.1   Typical autosomal dominant pedigree showing transmission through several generations, unbiased by the sex of patients

41

Autosomal recessive (*Figure 4.2*)

Both maternal and paternal genes are mutated (homozygosity).

(1) Usually, single generations are affected.
(2) Parents are unaffected carriers.
(3) Siblings of affected individuals have a 25 per cent chance of being affected themselves.
(4) Children of affected individuals are unaffected carriers of the trait (unless the affected homozygote marries a carrier heterozygote).
(5) Consanguinity (family connections) within small communities allows several affected generations. Conversely, for rate recessive disorders the parents of affected individuals are more often consanguinous than chance allows.

Autosomal recessive

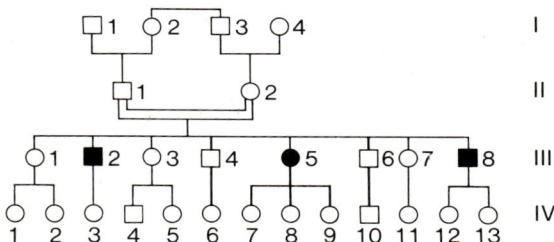

Figure 4.2 *Typical autosomal recessive pedigree showing consanguinity of generation II with homozygous affected individuals in generation III. Both the parents in generation II are heterozygous unaffected carriers as are two of the four grandparents. I_2 and I_3 are brother and sister and presumably the initial gene carriers*

Sex-linked recessive inheritance (*Figure 4.3*)

Sex-linked recessive

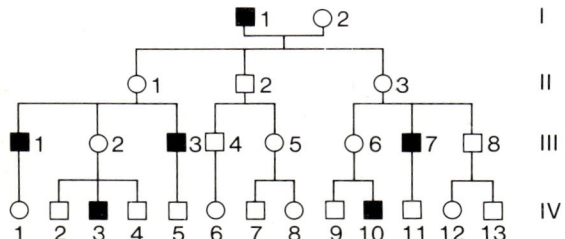

Figure 4.3 *Sex-linked recessive pedigree showing transmission of the gene through female carriers of affected fathers*

The mutation is carried in the X chromosome and so:

(1) Several generations may be affected.
(2) Female carriers do not express the disease.
(3) Females transmit the trait to half their sons and half their daughters are carriers.
(4) Sons do not transmit the trait to sons, but half their daughters are carriers.

Sex-linked dominant inheritance (*Figure 4.4*)

This is an unusually rare inherited pattern.

(1) Several generations are affected.
(2) Affected women transmit the trait to half their sons and daughters.
(3) Affected men have affected daughters and unaffected sons.

Sex-linked dominant

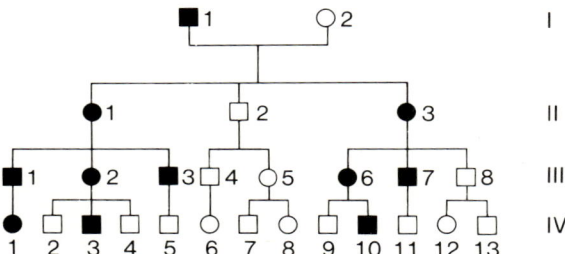

Figure 4.4   Sex-linked dominant pedigree showing father to daughter, daughter to son, but no father to son transmission of the gene

Y linked inheritance

With the exception of hairy ears, none are known. Affected men would transmit the trait to all their sons and none of their daughters.

Polygenic inheritance

Here the transmitted disorder results from the interaction of several genes. Certainly some single gene disorders are also modified by other autosomal genes and autosomal dominant diseases are somewhat variable. Thus, the alternative partner allele may influence phenotypical expression, and so may some other non-allelic genes. Polygenic inheritance on the other hand results from the interaction of many genes. Such abnormalities cluster within families but the inheritance is atypical and does not follow any of the simple dominant or recessive patterns described earlier. High blood pressure, height, intelligence, rheumatoid arthritis and psoriasis are perhaps inherited this way.

Gene interaction with environment

Diseases have a spectrum of causation ranging from the purely genetic to the completely environmental. Classic autosomal diseases such as neurofibromatosis are almost entirely genetic, whereas infectious diseases such as pneumonia are almost entirely environmental. Cancer is an excellent example in which predisposing factors to harmful environmental agents are modified by genetic inheritance. Dark skinned races have a lower frequency of skin cancer compared with fair skinned who have a relatively low frequency in Britain but high frequencies in Australia, South Africa and the southern USA. On the other hand, patients with xeroderma pigmentosum, ataxia telangiectasia and Bloom's syndrome have an exceptional predisposition to light induced skin cancers. The relationship between genetic disposition and susceptibility to disease is clearly complex and tangled. No doubt many genetic relationships await discovery, but an excellent and illustrative recent example is the connection between HLA type and disease susceptibility.

HLA type and disease

The HLA system in man defines a series of leucocyte antigens which are exceptionally heterogeneous. Four loci with multiple alleles at each site have been detected at the so-called A, B, C and D sites. Analogies with the mouse suggest a close relationship between the HLA system and the so-called immune response (Ir) genes. The H_2 loci in mouse are reliable predictors of transplantation rejection frequency. Closely matched mice are much more likely to tolerate grafts than badly matched animals. Such a complex and variable system, however, did not evolve as a hindrance to transplant surgeons and has important implications in the relationship between infection and disease. The system is essential both for the efficient functioning of lymphocytes when presented with antigen and T cell receptor diversity and interaction. So diverse is the system that according to Bodmer, 300 million separate individuals could have different combinations of the known HLA loci alleles without once repeating themselves. Only 10 per cent of those would have differences detected by current techniques. An enormous untapped pool of disease associations remain. He thinks that HLA polymorphisms have preferentially evolved because particular HLA types have conferred selective advantages in resistance to common epidemic human diseases such as smallpox, TB, cholera, malaria and leprosy. Possible means by which HLA types give protection include molecular mimicry between HLA types and certain pathogens. Then the possession of an HLA type resembling a pathogen predisposes that individual to infection with it, and conversely the possession of other types protects against this. Darwinian evolution could favour either the efficiency of T cell response or other immune responses. No doubt such selective pressures have allowed the flourishing of certain HLA types which by chance are susceptible to other less lethal but more chronic diseases which do not affect genetic fitness (the efficiency of producing offspring). Such individuals have sufficient time to breed before or even when the disease affects them (in contrast to premature death by epidemic disease). Recently, many diseases have been shown to be HLA associated. Notable examples are Hodgkins disease with B5, BW 35 and B18, ankylosing spondylitis and Reiter's syndrome with B27, acute lymphoblastic leukaemia with A2 and B12, nasopharyngeal cancers with BW 46 and oesophageal cancer with B40. Juvenile onset insulin dependent diabetes is associated with A1, B8 and B18, A2, B15 and B40. Latterly these have been shown to be in linkage disequilibrium with DW 3 and DW 4 immune response antigens. Some forms of psoriasis are closely associated with DW 6 and have secondary associations with B13, BW 16 and 17. Psoriasis is unusual because, unlike most of the other HLA associations that we have mentioned and according to Bodmer it cannot be explained satisfactorily on the basis of an altered immune response. Instead, we must assume that the HLA genes are close to those which control cell turnover and replication. Other dermatological diseases connected with HLA haplotypes include dermatitis herpetiformis and B8, discoid lupus erythematosus B7, 8; systemic lupus erythematosus B8, BW 15, A2; pemphigus B13; and atopic eczema A1 and B8. This complex interaction between the immune response and various diseases illustrates the interaction of inherited and environmental factors in disease.

5 Dermatitis–eczema and associated conditions

Desmond Burrows

The dermatitis–eczema group comprises about 25 per cent of all skin diseases seen at hospital skin clinics and includes both contact dermatitis and constitutional dermatitis of various patterns, namely, discoid, atopic, seborrhoeic, pompholyx of the palms and soles, varicose and generalized exfoliative dermatitis.

Dermatitis or eczema—terms which are used interchangeably—is an inflammatory condition of the skin produced by a variety of external and endogenous factors of which the characteristic feature is oedema (spongiosis) of the epidermis.

Histopathology *(Figure 3.4*, p. 29*)*

The findings depend on the stage of the condition. The first change is focal oedema of the epidermis (spongiosis) with dilatation of dermal vessels and an increase in mononuclear cells. Oedema in the epidermis may increase rapidly to produce visible vesicles which may rupture. As the eczema becomes more chronic the prickle layer increases in size (acanthosis), the horny layer thickens (hyperkeratosis) and nuclear debris may remain (parakeratosis).

Classification

Exogenous:
    Primary irritant
    Allergic

Endogenous:
    Atopic
    Discoid
    Pompholyx
    Seborrhoeic
    Varicose

Exogenous eczema *(see Table 5.1)*
Primary irritant *(Plates 5.1–5.4, 5.6–5.8)*

Noxious substances show a wide range of irritant properties when in contact with the skin. Some require minimal contact with the skin

Table 5.1 Exogenous eczema

	'Weak' irritant dermatitis (cumulative insult dermatitis)	*Irritant dermatitis*	*Allergic dermatitis*
Pathological mechanism	Multiple sub-threshold exposures	Infrequent exposure to a noxious concentration of offending chemical	Repeated exposure to allergen
Physicochemical— multiple factors:	(a) abrasion (b) degreasing (c) desiccation or maceration (d) microtrauma	Factors such as degreasing are rarely important	Immunological— initial contact with sensitizing substance must be followed by eliciting exposure
Preceding signs	Dryness, soreness, fissuring, precede eruption	No preceding drying or fissuring	No preceding eruption
Onset	Slow, over days, months or years	Sudden, occurring within half an hour to five days of exposure	Sudden, appearing within 48 hours in previously sensitized subjects
Physical signs	Hyperkeratosis, fissuring, erythema, vesicles	Erythema, vesiculation, exudation and rarely necrosis	Erythema, vesiculation, oedema and exudation. Patches well marginated
Commonest sites	Hands, e.g. detergents, shampoos, oils, etc.	Hands—acids, caustic soda, cement, epoxy resin	Hands and face, e.g. hair dye, nickel, rubber, medicaments
Patch tests	Negative	Positive—of irritant type. Patch test in controls also positive therefore not of value and not recommended	Positive Controls negative

to produce an irritant eczematous reaction, e.g. strong acids and alkalis, solvents or white spirit. Others with only minimal irritant properties, e.g. detergents—require more prolonged contact with the skin. Reaction is also determined by the site of contact. When the hands are exposed to a noxious irritant, the palms and palmar aspects of the fingers, protected by a thicker horny layer, will require more prolonged contact than more vulnerable parts. The signs of reaction will probably first appear on the finger webs, spreading to the backs and sides of the hands and front of the wrists, with involvement of the palms and finger pads following only after prolonged exposure.

Oils sometimes produce a pattern which resembles discoid eczema.

Rarely secondary spread to distant sites not in contact with the irritant can occur and this can cause diagnostic problems unless a careful history is taken to determine the initial site of the eruption.

Allergic

Allergic contact eczema is mediated by delayed (Type 4) hypersensitivity. Allergens vary in their sensitizing potential from negligible, e.g. hydrocortisone to high, e.g. dinitrochlorbenzene (DNCB). Failure of an individual to become sensitized to DNCB is a reliable indication of a failure of Type 4 sensitivity. To sensitize, the substance must be able to penetrate the skin and form a compound with a skin protein. The Langerhan cell probably processes and passes on the antigen-protein complex to the T lymphocyte. The frequency with which an individual substance causes allergic dermatitis depends on both the sensitizing potential and the opportunity of contact with the skin. Some examples of the commoner sensitizers are listed below.

Nickel

Nickel is the commonest cause of contact dermatitis; 10 per cent of women are affected. Diagnosis is usually easily made by a distribution under metal articles, jewellery or clothing, but some cases of hand eczema are caused by allergy to nickel where there is no other history to suggest nickel sensitivity. The majority of cases can easily be dealt with by eliminating nickel from jewellery or clothing but when it presents with dermatitis of the hand it can be very intractable. This may be due to hidden sources of contact with metal or exacerbations by oral ingestion (in food or from saucepans).

Hip replacement with a metal prosthesis raises the question of whether previous nickel sensitivity is important prognostically. All the evidence suggests that preceding metal sensitivity is not a contraindication. Neither does this type of prosthesis commonly initiate sensitization.

Chromium

While not such a common cause of dermatitis as nickel, chromium is important because it produces a very chronic dermatitis. Common sources are cement, chrome plating and tanning.

Cobalt

This metal is nearly always found in association with nickel and concomitant sensitivity is therefore common.

Metal induced dermatoses are an exception to the general rule of distribution of contact dermatitis occurring on the backs and sides of the fingers and finger webs. In nickel dermatitis on the hands for instance, the distribution is often palmar. Chromium dermatitis can produce a discoid eczema pattern.

Rubber

Natural latex does not sensitize but antioxidants and vulcanizing agents which are added to rubber do. Irritated skin is particularly prone to sensitization by rubber gloves.

Medicaments

These will particularly sensitize when applied frequently and to broken skin. Most cases are seen in the lower legs following treatment of varicose eczema and ulcers, and on the perianal area where proprietary medicaments and anaesthetic creams are applied. Preservatives such as parabens and formaldehyde as well as the medicament itself can sensitize.

Plastics and glues

Plastics and glues, when completely polymerized do not sensitize and so epoxy resins are only likely to cause trouble prior to mixing with the hardener. Acrylates have become a more common cause of dermatitis with their more frequent use in industry, e.g. printing.

Plants

In the USA poison ivy is a very common cause of contact dermatitis but in the UK, apart from *Primula obconica*, plants seldom cause trouble.

Patch testing (*see* Chapter 2)

Sensitization to a substance is demonstrated by placing a suitably dilute sample under occlusion for 48 hours and then examining for redness or redness and swelling. Severe reaction may produce vesiculation, providing strong evidence that the patient is sensitive to the substance. Correct dilution of the test substance is important because if tested in too high a concentration under occlusion many substances can cause a reaction which does not indicate allergy, and the reverse can be also true; very often substances need to be tested in higher concentration than may be present in the offending contactant. Therefore, patch testing should only be carried out by those with experience in interpretation of results and knowledge of types of substance which are useful for patch testing and dilutions in which they should be applied. As a result of much research the International Contact Dermatitis Research Group have drawn up the following list of chemicals which are common sensitizers and the dilution in which these should be tested. These are available commercially from Trolab AC, A. N. Hansens alle 6B, 2900 Hellerup, Denmark. Potential contact sources are shown in brackets.

potassium dichromate 0.5% (cement, anti-rust agents, plating, dyes, bleaches, photographic chemicals, laboratory chemicals)
cobalt chloride 1% (dyes, cement, clay, anti-corrosion agents, animal feeds)
nickel sulphate 5% (cheap jewellery, metals, plating)

formaldehyde (in water) 2% (preservatives—cosmetics, shampoos, adhesives, leather tanning, photography, laboratory fixative, anti-fungus, disinfectant, anti-perspirant—powders, solutions, inner soles)

p-phenylenediamine 1% (anti-oxidants, photographic chemicals, cosmetic dyes)

balsam of Peru 25% (perfumes, medicaments)

neomycin sulphate 20% (ointments)

parabens (methyl-, ethyl-, propyl-, butyl-, benzyl-, 3% each) 15% (preservatives in medicaments or cosmetics, food preservatives)

chinoform 5% (medicaments)

colophony 20% (adhesives in strapping, polishes, printing ink, violin rosin, filling material, soap, rubber and plastics)

wood tars (pine, beech, juniper, birch, 3% each) 12% (woods, medicaments)

wool alcohols 30% (lanolin, cosmetics, medicaments)

epoxy resin 1% (adhesives, flooring, anti-rust paint)

mercapto-mix (mixture of four chemicals, 0.5% each) 2% (rubber accelerator, oils)

thiuram-mix (mixture of four chemicals, 0.25% each) 1% (biocides—fruit, nuts, mushrooms, rose sprays—rubber accelerator)

PPD-mix (mixture of three chemicals; 0.10%, 0.25%, 0.25%) 0.60% (anti-oxidant, rubber, oils)

naphthyl-mix (mixture of two chemicals, 0.50 each) 1% (rubber)

carbo-mix (mixture of three chemicals, 1% each) 3% (rubber accelerator)

ethylene diamine dihydrochloride 1% (medicaments)

fragrance-mix (mixture of eight chemicals, 2% each) 16% (perfumes)

Diagnosis

The rash is eczematous and diagnosis is made by evaluation of the following:

(1) Distribution—In some cases the diagnosis is easy, for instance, when it occurs under ear-rings or bracelet, under a shoe or sandal or in the exact area where a rubber glove is worn. On the hand distribution is usually finger webs, backs and sides of fingers and wrist. Nickel and chromium can produce a palmar pattern. Secondary spread from sites of contact is particularly common in allergic dermatitis.

(2) History—Frequently a painstaking history is necessary to elucidate the cause, particularly where the distribution is not diagnostic, for instance on the hands. The patient is often his own best detective when he is given guidance. The history of improvement at week-ends or holidays may indicate a work related cause.

(3) Patch testing may elicit the cause of allergic dermatitis but is of no value in 75 per cent of cases where the cause is an irritant. Nevertheless, all hand eczemas should be patch tested to the international battery.

Treatment

Either removal of the cause from the patient's environment or the patient from the cause is usually sufficient. If the cause is encountered at work, a period off or a change of job may be needed. It is difficult to avoid some agents, such as nickel or chromium and so these cases can become chronic. The dimethylglyoxine test can be used to detect nickel in the environment. Local steroid ointments may suppress the eruption. In severe cases, a short course of systemic steroid may be necessary.

Endogenous eczema

Discoid eczema *(Plate 5.9)*

Discrete, coin-shaped erythematous plaques studded with vesicles occurring particularly on the extensor aspects of the extremities and especially the dorsa of the hands are characteristic. The thighs and legs may be affected and occasionally patches appear on the trunk and face. Oozing may result in crusting. The condition usually runs a course of one to two years before becoming quiescent. Atopic and discoid eczema have many features in common and may be variants of the same disease.

Differential diagnosis

(1) Contact dermatitis sometimes resembles discoid eczema particularly in chrome and oil dermatitis. However, it tends to occur at the areas of maximum contact; the legs may be spared. A careful history of the periodicity of the rash may indicate some outside factor.
(2) Fungal infections often involve exposed sites and show central healing with peripheral extension. Widespread distribution is unusual. Microscopy reveals mycelia.
(3) Spread from an acute contact dermatitis or varicose eczema often produces a discoid pattern but the prime cause can be recognized when the whole of the patient's skin is examined.

Atopic dermatitis *(Plates 5.10 and 5.11)*

(Synonyms: Besnier's prurigo, asthma–eczema complex, flexural eczema, infantile eczema.)

Aetiology

About 30 per cent of patients with this condition have a family history of either asthma, hay fever or atopic dermatitis. The atopic individual has a genetic tendency to produce reaginic antibodies, IgE and to develop hypersensitivity reactions of the urticarial type.

51

There are two theories of aetiology:

(1) Immunological—The atopic individual has a tendency to produce IgE reaginic antibodies. There is also both clinical and laboratory evidence of T cell dysfunction.
(2) Autonomic imbalance—Partial β-adrenergic blockade has been suggested by abnormal response to catecholamines of cultured atopic skin, abnormal vascular reaction and altered sweat gland responses to various pharmacological agents.

Clinical features

Atopic dermatitis is one of the commoner types and occurs particularly in infancy and childhood, though it can persist or appear in adult life for the first time. Infantile atopic eczema first appears about the second or third month with an erythematous or scaly eruption generally on the cheeks, though other areas, especially the wrists, outer aspects of legs, arms or the neck may be involved (*Figure 5.1*). The lesions usually clear in a few months though may relapse at times of stress, for instance during teething. In other children the

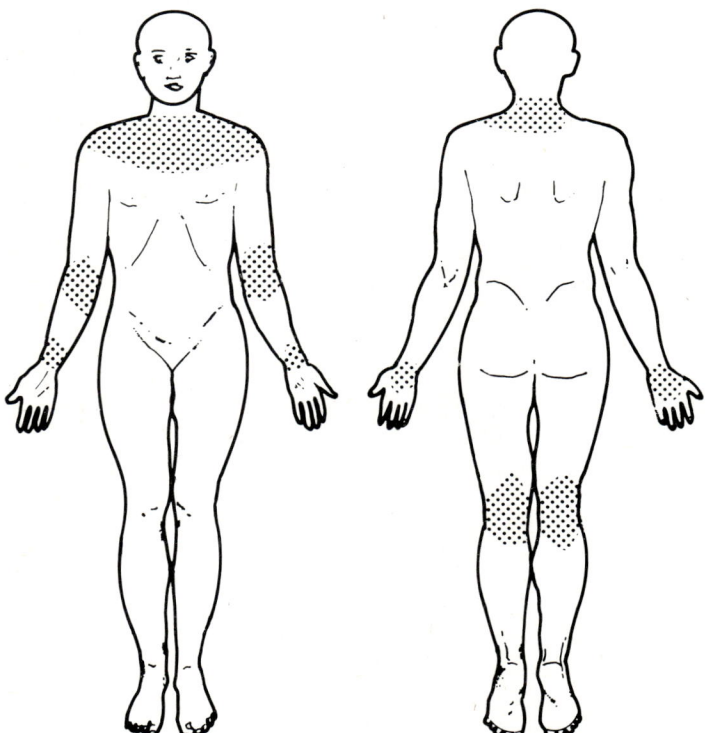

Figure 5.1 *Atopic dermatitis: characteristically affecting the limb flexures—acute, subacute and lichenified eczematous patches*

disease persists without remission, but the majority will clear before adulthood. A few unfortunate individuals will have eczema for the rest of their lives. Many atopics have associated ichthyosis or dryness of the skin.

In children and adults the involvement of the antecubital and popliteal fossae is characteristic and diagnostic. Other typical sites are the eyelids, front and sides of the neck, the forehead, chest and sometimes the knees and elbows. This dermatitis may affect a single area or a few isolated sites, or it may become generalized. The predominant symptom is itching which may at times be intense. Most of the eruption is a result of scratching, which causes lichenification, haemorrhagic crusting and secondary infection.

Pompholyx *(Plate 5.12)*

Aetiology

Some cases are due to nickel or chromium; fungal infections of the feet can also produce a pompholyx-like rash but in most cases the cause is obscure.

Clinical features

The eruption is characteristically vesicular, often producing larger blisters than other forms of eczema and usually occurring in the centre of the palm or sole of the foot, spreading to the rest of the palm and the palmar aspects of the fingers. It runs a recurrent course over some months or years, at times almost settling, then flaring up again with blisters. It may become chronic with a thickened scaly rash in the centre of the palms or soles.

Seborrhoeic dermatitis *(Figure 5.2* and *Plate 5.13)*

Aetiology

Seborrhoea denotes an increase of sebum production by sebaceous glands. It is doubtful whether 'seborrhoeic' dermatitis has anything whatever to do with sebaceous glands or over or under production of sebum. The name arose from the distribution; it occurs in those areas where sebaceous glands are largest and most numerous. The cause is unknown but there is sometimes a family history.

Clinical features

Relatively localized stigmata of seborrhoeic dermatitis are usually present. Rarely does it occur in its florid generalized form. The rash consists of fine scaling redness in the following characteristic areas: scalp, where it may produce nothing more than scurf or dandruff, nasolabial folds, eyelids, eyebrows, behind the ears (*Plate 5.4*); in the shaved area it may produce folliculitis. On the body the eruption

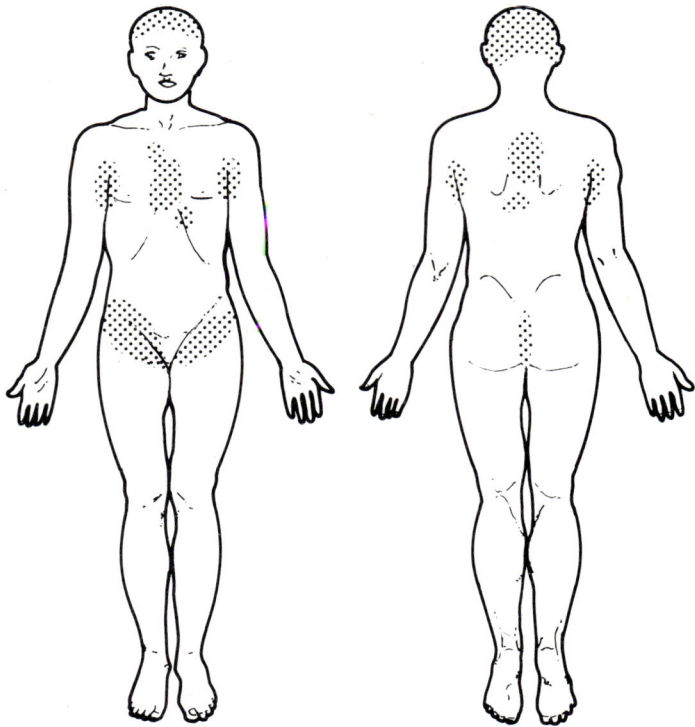

Figure 5.2 *Serborrhoeic dermatitis: the flexures are affected with acute (sometimes infected) or chronic scaly eczema midline of chest. Intertrigo, folliculitis, blepharitis and pompholyx may coexist*

typically occurs on the sternal and interscapular areas. It sometimes occurs as a diffuse small folliculitis or as circular red scaling areas. The severe cases may involve the trunk, upper arms and thighs. The intertriginous form involves the body folds. The retroauricular folds, axillary and submammary area, groins, perineum, natal cleft and umbilicus may exhibit glazed and red marginated patches which later become fissured, infected and moist. This flexural involvement may be part of a more generalized dermatitis with associated pompholyx of the hands and feet.

For Differential Diagnosis *see Table 5.2.*

Napkin dermatitis *(Plates 5.14 and 5.15)*

Napkin dermatitis is most usually a localised form of seborrhoeic eczema. Seborrhoeic eczema tends to occur in the fold areas of skin which are damp; hence if there is any tendency to seborrhoeic eczema in an infant the napkin area will be involved. However, cases of contact dermatitis can occur due to the irritating effect of urine or

Table 5.2   Differential diagnosis

	Seborrhoeic dermatitis	Psoriasis	Pityriasis rosea	Ringworm
Scalp	Diffuse dry or greasy scaling	Heaped up palpable scaly patches sharply demarcated	Unaffected	Patchy hair loss with inflammation. 'Kerion' in cattle ringworm
Face	Blepharitis; scaly nasolabial folds; folliculitis barbae	Rarely involved	Rarely involved	Demarcated circinate lesions with scaly or vesicular margins. Resolution towards centre. Microscopy positive
Trunk and limbs	Figurate lesions sternal and interscapular areas, or follicular papules; eczematous patches limbs; moist red intertrigo of body folds	Infiltrated silvery scaly patches especially over knees and elbows; punctate bleeding on scratching; glazed intertrigo	Vest and pants distribution. Oval medallions with collarette of scales	As for face

faeces in the napkin, chafing of the wet napkin aggravated by occlusive plastic pants, or soap and detergent residues after laundering. Clinically there is a marginated red or glazed dermatitis involving the convex surface of the buttocks, thighs, external genitalia, pubic areas and lower abdomen—those areas most in contact with a wet napkin. This is in contrast with the seborrhoeic eczema which tends to be maximum in folds. Papules, vesicles and pustules are occasionally seen as a manifestation of miliaria (prickly heat) and occasionally sparse papulo-erosive lesions are seen which simulate congenital syphilis.

Recalcitrant pustular eruptions of hands and feet *(Plate 5.16)*

In the absence of focal infection or psoriasis, the term 'acrodermatitis pustulosa perstans' is used. The term 'pustular bacterid' is used in those rare instances where there is demonstrable focal infection, and 'pustular psoriasis' when psoriatic lesions are present.

These conditions are characterized by pustules without much

secondary erythema of palms and soles. The pustules are sterile and they tend to dry to a thin scale forming a discrete brownish macule. When the condition becomes chronic, fissuring and hyperkeratosis may be seen.

This group of conditions is unrewarding to treat. Fluorinated steroid creams used under polythene may produce temporary amelioration, though they can cause a rebound effect with eventual worsening.

Very occasionally dapsone effects remission. When the patient is incapacitated a small maintenance dose of systemic steroid may be required. In difficult cases 10% crude tar in zinc paste or 1% dithranol in Lassar's paste can be tried and PUVA helps some cases.

Exfoliative dermatitis *(Plate 6.3)*

Generalized erythema and scaling involving over 80 per cent of the body is designated as exfoliative dermatitis or generalized erythroderma.

Aetiology

Five main groups are recognized:

(1) Progression of pre-existing dermatoses, including psoriasis, contact, atopic and seborrhoeic dermatitis. In these conditions overtreatment is a common precipitating factor. Similarly the withdrawal of systemic steroids is an increasingly common cause of generalized exfoliative dermatitis; the current misuse and overuse of systemic or topical steroids in psoriasis is the main factor.
(2) Certain drugs such as penicillin and sulphonamides. An acute streptococcal infection and other acute infections may have the same effect.
(3) Mycosis fungoides, leukaemic and other lymphomas sometimes present with exfoliative dermatitis.
(4) Rare idiopathic forms, e.g. congenital ichthyosiform erythroderma and pityriasis rubra pilaris.
(5) Idiopathic. Cases are seen quite frequently which do not fit into any of the above patterns and no underlying or precipitating cause can be found.

Clinical features

The generalized erythema and scaling may be of sudden onset. Constitutional symptoms may be slight, although thirst and oliguria occur during the development of the acute phase and thermoregulatory disturbances are common. In the later stages of the disease hair and nails may be shed and lymph nodes become enlarged (dermatopathic lymphadenopathy or lipomelanic reticulosis). This is a non-specific lymphadenopathy occurring in erythroderma from any cause. At this stage weight loss is often apparent due to the excessive desquamation and consequent protein loss. Haemodynamic complications, including high output cardiac failure, reduction of blood flow to other organs, hypervolaemia and increased capillary permeability can occur. Thermoregulation may also be a problem.

It has been demonstrated that widespread skin disease can cause malabsorption. Shuster and Marks have called this intestinal dysfunction dermatogenic enteropathy and have shown that patients with generalized eczema and psoriasis have a modest increase in faecal fat excretion (usually less than 20 g/day) and malabsorption of iron, folate, calcium, lactose and D-xylose. There may be associated protein-losing enteropathy. The intestinal malfunction responds to treatment of the skin alone. The characteristic feature is the mildness of the absorptive defect together with the rash and normal jejunal biopsy.

Chronic superficial dermatitis

This is a rare dermatosis which presents with oval superficial scaly red patches on the trunk, often with a yellowish tint. The characteristic feature of this condition is that it lasts for many years and is particularly unresponsive to any form of treatment.

Asteatotic eczema

This condition occurs in elderly patients whose skin tends to dry with age. It produces a dry scaly rash with reticulate cracks producing a 'crazy paving' appearance.

Prurigo nodularis *(Plate 5.17)*

A very rare disorder with characteristic itchy nodules about 10–15 mm scattered all over the skin. It is often a manifestation of atopic eczema.

Neurodermatitis

Synonym: Lichen simplex chronicus (*see* Chapter 20).

Hypostatic eczema (Varicose eczema)

Aetiology

Incompetence of veins leads to diminished blood supply and oedema.

57

The devitalized skin has a propensity to develop eczema and is more vulnerable to irritants and trauma.

Clinical picture

The characteristic distribution is the inside of the ankle and lower leg. When severe the eczema can become generalized, spreading up the legs and even the arms. In long-standing cases the inside of the legs may become slightly pigmented.

Treatment

Treatment depends on the stage and extent of the eczema.

Mild eczema

A bland cream such as Aquosum ointment BP may be all that is required in a mild case of infantile eczema, but most cases will respond to a low potency steroid such as 1% hydrocortisone cream. With an associated dry skin an emollient oil added to the bath is helpful.

Acute eczema

Antihistamines orally often help to relieve itch. Corticosteroid lotions or creams or varying strengths, depending on the acuteness and extent of the eczema will usually control the condition quickly. A potent local steroid may be used for a few days or at the most two to three weeks; once the condition has settled, a milder steroid such as 1% hydrocortisone cream should be sufficient. In acute widespread eczemas, a course of oral steroid is occasionally necessary to control the eruption, starting with 30 mg daily and tailing off over ten days. When there is infection a local antibiotic should be given. Neomycin preparations can be used but there is the risk of sensitization with frequent use on broken skin; it should not be used over prolonged or frequent periods. With severe infection an oral antibiotic such as erythromycin should be given as well as a local antibiotic. Iodoquinoline is frequently added to steroid preparations but sensitization can occur with this antibacterial agent. In the acute phase potassium permanganate soaks 1:10 000 in water are useful.

Chronic eczema

Again the treatment is primarily local steroids of varying strength depending on the severity and extent of the eczema. Oral antihistamines are useful. If itching is particularly troublesome and causes considerable scratching, medicated bandages can be applied. They have a soothing effect and prevent scratching. In chronic eczema ointments are probably more helpful than creams or lotions but the patient's preference may override this advice. It is essential to warn patients about the side effects of local steroids and it it often best to give them two preparations: a potent one to apply when the dermatosis is active and a less potent one such as 1% hydrocortisone cream to apply when the disorder is quiescent. No patient should be given a steroid more potent than 1% hydrocortisone cream without follow-up. As with acute eczema, local treatment with antibiotic ointment is necessary for secondary infection and in severe cases a systemic antibiotic such as erythromycin should be given.

Some recalcitrant cases may respond to a steroid-clioquinol combination or 1–3% coal tar in zinc or Lassar's paste. Proprietary tar-containing preparations are sometimes more acceptable to the patient though they may prove less effective.

Atopic eczema

Very often this condition is associated with dry skin and therefore tends to do better with ointments rather than creams. It may do particularly well with steroid/urea preparations which improve the dry skin as well. Emollient preparations added to the bath help to hydrate the skin. Children often find wool next the skin adds to their discomfort. Atopic eczema responds remarkably well to a spell of inpatient treatment and many intractable cases respond in a hospital environment to the same treatment which has been found ineffective as an outpatient. Once the condition has settled it will be much easier to manage. Tar preparations used to be the standard treatment but are little used now because of their messiness and inferiority to local steroids but there is a place for the use of 3% crude tar in zinc paste as an inpatient.

Seborrhoeic eczema

In intractable cases of seborrhoeic folliculitis systemic tetracyclines given over a period of some months often produce considerable improvement. This eczema often responds to 2% sulphur, 2% salicylic acid in emulsifying ointment and may avoid the need for local steroids indefinitely. Intertriginous cases may require local nystatin or clotrimazole. For the scalp a tar shampoo and salicylic acid lotion BPC is usually sufficient but intractable cases may need overnight application of a preparation such as 2% salicylic acid, 2% sulphur in emulsifying ointment.

Discoid eczema

See treatment of chronic eczema.

Varicose eczema (*See* Chapter 19)

Hypostatic oedema is one of the major factors in causing this condition and therefore prevention or removal of oedema is essential. In severe conditions bed-rest for a period of a week or two may be necessary. Firm elastic bandages, after the eczema is controlled by topical steroids, will prevent oedema developing during the day.

Pityriasis rosea (*Plate 5.18*)

A self-limiting eruption characterized by annulosquamous discs on the trunk and proximal parts of the limbs.

Aetiology

The cause is unknown although viral infection is suspected. Epidemics occur particularly in the spring and autumn. Children and adults are equally affected.

Histopathology

The changes in the skin are those of a subacute dermatitis.

Clinical features

Usually a herald patch is present. It is an erythematous disc 1–3 cm in diameter which is usually found on the chest. After a week or ten days small satellite lesions appear. These enlarge and other discoid lesions suddenly appear covering most ot the trunk. They are often oval in shape lying parallel to the skin creases. Scaling begins in the centre of these discs and when first seen this central scale drops off leaving a characteristic collarette of scales around a periphery. When the lesions begin to fade on the trunk further lesions may still be appearing on the limbs and, in severe cases, even the hands and feet may be affected. The total duration is six to eight weeks. Moderate to severe pruritus usually follows bathing.

Prognosis

Spontaneous involution is the rule although scratching and secondary eczematization may delay healing.

Differential diagnosis

Discoid seborrhoeic eczema. This does not show the characteristic evolution of pityriasis rosea. Seborrhoeic stigmata are usually present. Lesions of ringworm are more inflammatory and may show vesiculation at the edges, and scrapings are positive for fungus.

Treatment

Itching is often severe and antipruritic lotions are helpful. Both bathing and rough underclothing may aggravate the pruritus. Ultraviolet light in small doses appears to abort the attack in some instances.

Otitis externa

Inflammation of the external auditory canal may result from a number of causes. Excessive production of cerumen, the seborrhoeic and atopic diathesis, psoriasis, or anatomical anomalies of the canal may predispose, but the commonest cause is self trauma. Fungal infections are rare.

Clinical features include itching, scaling, redness and oedema of the external meatus. Furunculosis may be present; if so, gentle traction of the pinna will cause exquisite pain.

Treatment

(1) Avoidance of self trauma and contact dermatitis from external irritants.
(2) When the external auditory canal is oedematous and obstructed, an aural surgeon should be consulted.
(3) Antibiotic-steroid ointments—e.g. Betnovate-A or Genticin HC—sometimes effect a dramatic response, although relapse is common. Good results have been obtained from a simple ointment such as white soft paraffin.
(4) Combined systemic antibiotic-steroid therapy is indicated in cases complicated by acute inflammation and impaction.

6 Psoriasis, pityriasis rubra pilaris and lichen planus

A. P. Warin
Andrew Griffiths
Anthony du Vivier

Psoriasis

A. P. Warin

Psoriasis is a common condition of the skin affecting 1–2 per cent of the population. It is characterized by red, scaly plaques which may be limited to the elbows and knees and the scalp, but is often much more widespread. The condition is unpredictable in its course but is usually chronic. Many atypical forms are seen and will be described.

Aetiology and pathogenesis

The cause of psoriasis is not known. There is an undoubted genetic predisposition and many trigger factors seem to precipitate psoriasis in such genetically primed individuals. The trigger factors include streptococcal infections, trauma, drug eruptions, endocrine factors and severe emotional upset.

Genetic marker in psoriasis

There is a strong positive association with HLA B13, B17, CT7 and DMA in plaque psoriasis, and also a negative association with B7 and B8. In the Lewis red cell system there is a positive association with Le (a–b–). In the MNSs system there is a positive association with SS (homozygotes) and a negative association with Ss (i.e. heterozygotes). In the ABO system there is a positive association with group A (only at the 5 per cent level of significance).

It has been calculated that HLA B13/B17 confers a 14-fold increased risk of developing psoriasis compared with a subject without these antigens. A combination of four positively associated antigens, i.e. B13 or B17/A/SS/Le (a–b–), increases the risk of developing psoriasis 200-fold. The D locus antigen (DMA) has the strongest association of all with plaque psoriasis.

Epidermal cell kinetics and cyclic AMP

There is an increase in the germinative cell population of the epidermis in psoriasis. It is increased by a factor of 20–30 by infolding of the epidermis and by the presence of two to three layers of germinative cells in psoriatic epidermis. Using tritiated thymidine, increased labelling of the epidermis is seen. Calculations of the epidermal cell cycle time in psoriasis have varied from 32 to 91 hours. However, to arrive at these figures, many assumptions were made, and recent work suggests that the cell cycle time may be normal.

However, more epidermal cells are undergoing DNA synthesis at any one time in psoriatic epidermis, and the turnover time is faster. This has led to the suggestion of an inhibitor of mitosis being present in normal skin and being lost in psoriatic epidermis. In support of this, cyclic AMP has been shown to be necessary to control cell growth and has been shown to inhibit mitosis in the G2 phase of cell cycle in the normal epidermis. Evidence has been presented that cAMP is reduced in psoriatic epidermis. It is possible that the absence or reduction of cAMP leads to an increase in proliferation of cells. However, it is likely that the decrease in cAMP in psoriatic epidermis is only a link in a chain and not a primary event.

Polymorphonuclear leukocytes (PMNL)

The role of the PMNL remains unknown in the pathogenesis of psoriasis. Histologically PMNLs can be seen migrating from the dilated and tortuous upper dermal capillaries into the epidermis and sometimes forming small microabscesses (Munro abscesses). It has been shown that psoriatic scale is chemotactic to PMNL. This factor is probably derived from complement binding immune complexes in the stratum corneum.

Immunology

The following abnormalities have been found in psoriasis: IgA is raised, and probably IgG also. Circulating lymphocytes and PMNL have specific immunoglobulin receptors on their surfaces. Antibodies can be eluted from these receptors and can be shown to be directed against the nuclei of basal epidermal cells of clinically uninvolved skin, but not in psoriatic skin. It is not present in healthy controls.

Normal human serum contains antibody to stratum corneum (scab). It is mainly IgG, but some are IgM. Scab does not bind to normal skin *in vivo*, but does bind to psoriatic skin *in vitro* and *in vivo*. The titre of scab in psoriatic serum is not higher than normal. In psoriatic epidermis, stratum corneum antigens (scag) appear to bind to scab *in vivo*. The scag/scab complexes bind complement and this is probably chemotactic to PMNL.

It has also been shown that the circulating T lymphocytes are decreased in number, although the B lymphocyte population is normal. At present it is not possible to state whether or not any of these findings are primary or merely secondary events. However, it is possible to suggest a pathogenesis along the following lines. A gene defect leads to malfunction of a clone of 'suppressor' T cells, and thus antigenic epidermal nuclear material becomes 'recognized' by the immune system, leading to the formation of cell-bound anti-basal nuclear antibodies. The subsequent immune response disturbs the basal cell layer and prevents maturation, and leads to the psoriatic process being initiated. The formation of scag/scab complexes is probably a secondary event and leads to complement fixation. These complexes diffuse through the epidermis and attract more PMNL into the epidermis and may themselves stimulate epidermopoeisis. Although this is merely a hypothesis, it suggests existing research possibilities which promise to help unravel the mystery of the pathogenesis of psoriasis.

Histopathology *(Figure 6.1)*

The epidermis shows acanthosis and parakeratosis, with absence of the stratum granulosum. The rete ridges are elongated. There is thinning of the suprapapillary epidermis. The dermis is oedematous with dilated capillaries. Polymorphonuclear cells can often be seen migrating between the dilated vessels and the epidermis. In pustular psoriasis, polymorphs collect in the epidermis to form microabscesses, although these may also be seen in acute plaque lesions.

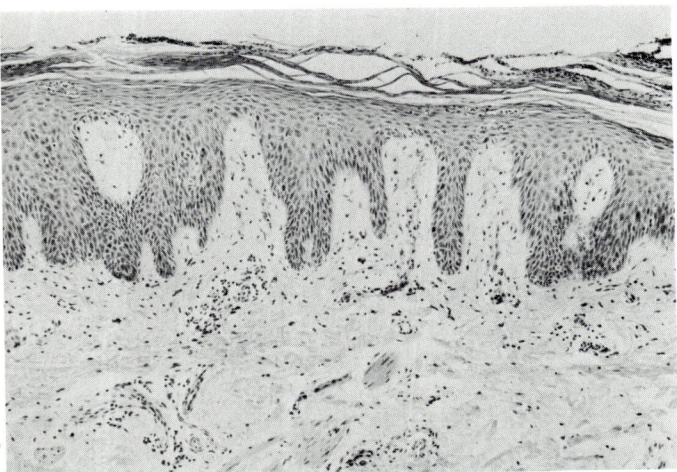

Figure 6.1   *Histopathology of psoriasis. There is parakeratosis, absence of stratum granulosum, Munro abscesses, elongated rete ridges and dilated capillaries in papillary tips*

Clinical features

Psoriasis may present at any age but most commonly starts in the second and third decades of life.

Plaque *(Figures 6.2 and 6.3)*

This is the most common pattern and varies from a few lesions on the

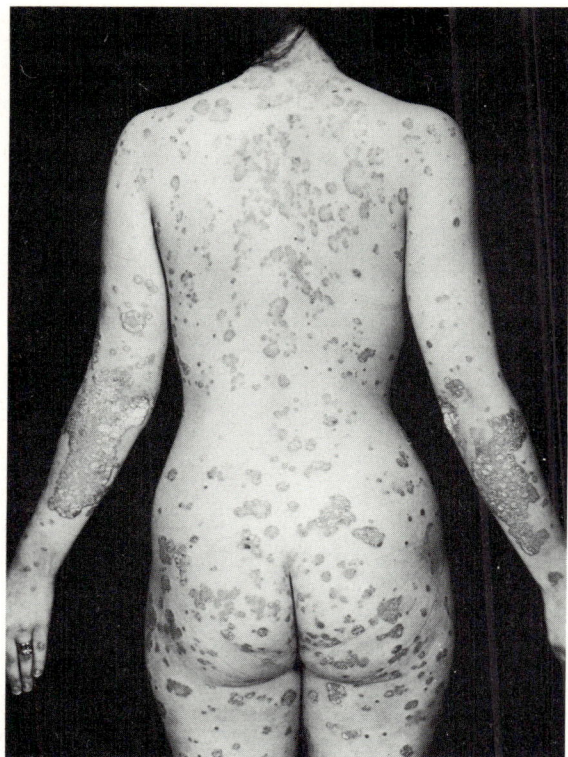

Figure 6.2 *Plaque psoriasis*

elbows and knees to involvement of virtually the whole body surface, but with extensor surfaces of the limbs and back of trunk mainly involved. The plaques are pink or red and are surmounted by silvery scales. If these scales are scratched away, more scales appear until eventually tiny bleeding points appear, as the thinned suprapapillary epidermis is breached. The scalp is commonly involved too, and the plaques are usually palpable and can be seen to extend beyond the hair margin. It is rare for the hair to be lost and scarring alopecia practically never occurs. It is unusual for the face to be badly affected.

Guttate *(Plate 6.1)*

This type of psoriasis occurs mainly in children and adolescents and is characterized by a sudden onset of small lesions all over the body. It is sometimes preceded by a streptococcal sore throat. There is a tendency for guttate psoriasis to heal in one to two months, but many patients go on to the more typical plaque psoriasis. In children who have recurrent streptococcal tonsillitis followed by an attack of guttate psoriasis, the tonsils may be removed. However, in the author's experience, this procedure has not often been helpful.

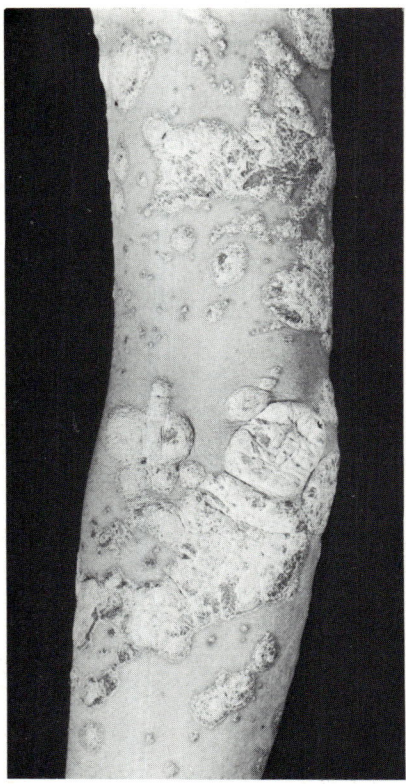

Figure 6.3 *Plaque psoriasis*

Flexural *(Plate 6.2)*

Because of the moist nature of the flexures, the usual silvery scales are not present in flexural psoriasis. However, the pink-red colour is still present and the sharp margin of the plaque is characteristic, though it will occasionally be necessary to exclude tinea infection or contact dermatitis.

Nails *(Figure 6.4)*

Nail involvement is seen in all types of psoriasis and in up to half of all cases. Pitting is the most frequent sign, but onycholysis, subungual hyperkeratosis and salmon-pink patches under the nails are all common. The nails are occasionally lost in erythrodermic psoriasis or in some forms of pustular psoriasis.

'Seborrhoeic'

Psoriasis often involves the 'seborrhoeic' areas of the body preferentially, i.e. the scalp, face, chest, back and around the umbilicus. Often at these sites it forms the typical plaques of psoriasis.

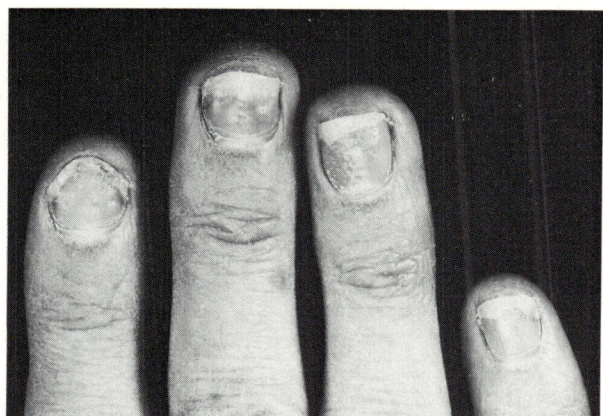

Figure 6.4   *Nail psoriasis: oncholysis pitting*

Occasionally the rash is more eczematous and difficulty can be encountered with 'seborrhoeic' dermatitis. It should be noted that 'seborrheoic' is a misnomer, as there is no evidence of seborrhoea in patients with seborrhoeic dermatitis.

Photosensitive

The face is usually relatively spared in psoriasis. Indeed most patients derive great benefit from sunlight. Occasionally, however, patients are definitely flared by sunlight, and then the face and back of hands are affected preferentially.

Tongue

A geographical tongue is commonly seen in generalized pustular psoriasis. It is of interest that geographical tongue is a common finding in otherwise normal people, and the histology of the lesion is that of pustular psoriasis. A study of genetic markers in patients with geographical tongue would be of interest.

Erythroderma *(Plate 6.3)*

This may occur in one of two ways. Firstly, chronic plaque psoriasis may go into an exfoliative phase. Occasionally this is due to the excessive use of topical potent corticosteroids, or by systemic corticosteroids. Secondly, erythroderma may be the initial presenting feature of psoriasis. Alternatively, generalized pustular psoriasis may revert to an erythrodermic state.

Pustular psoriasis

This occurs in four distinct forms, although one form can sometimes lead to another, especially if injudicious use is made of corticosteroids.

(1) *Pustular psoriasis of the palms and soles (Plate 6.4 and Figure 6.5)*

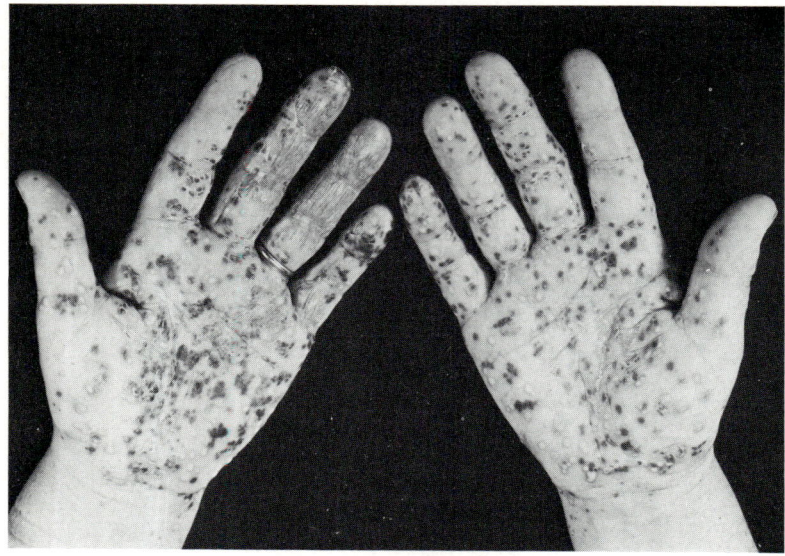

Figure 6.5 *Pustular psoriasis of palms*

consists of yellowish or green sterile pustules occurring on the palms and the soles. It may be symmetrical or asymmetrical. As the active pustules recede, they leave a brown scale. Not all patients with this condition have psoriasis elsewhere, but many do so or develop it later, so that it suggests an association with psoriasis. This variety of pustular psoriasis does not tend to lead to pustular psoriasis on the trunk.

(2) *Acrodermatitis continua of Hallopeau* is a sterile pustular eruption that affects the distal phalanges of the fingers and/or toes. The nails are often lost. It may extend locally and occasionally develops into a generalized pustular psoriasis with a bad prognosis.

(3) *Pustular change in plaque psoriasis*: An ordinary plaque of psoriasis may become pustular spontaneously, or more commonly after over-enthusiastic treatment with tar, dithranol or topical corticosteroids, especially if polythene occlusion has been used.

(4) *Generalized pustular psoriasis of Von Zumbusch (Figure 6.6)* is an acute, generalized pustular psoriasis associated with high fever, and the patient is often severely ill. The pustules are sterile and appear in waves, each wave being accompanied by a rise in fever. There is no doubt that at least some of these cases are caused by systemic or potent topical corticosteroids given for plaque or erythrodermic psoriasis. There is an appreciable mortality in this form of pustular psoriasis.

Unstable psoriasis

This terms implies a stage of psoriasis in which there is marked activity and the course that it is going to take is uncertain, e.g. it

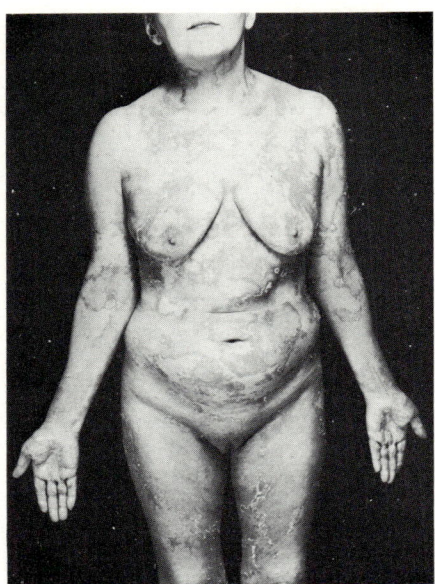

Figure *6.6 Generalized pustular psoriasis*

may become pustular or exfoliative. The use of potent topical corticosteroids is the commonest cause of this phase of psoriasis and great care is required in treatment to prevent the instability from progressing to dangerous forms of psoriasis.

Koebner

Several diseases show this phenomenon whereby the condition is precipitated at the site of trauma. This may be induced in many ways, e.g. scratch, operation wound, sunburn or drug eruption.

Arthritis

Approximately 5–7 per cent of psoriatics have an associated arthritis. There are three main patterns.

(1) *Distal arthritis.* This predominantly involves the terminal interphalangeal joints of the hands and feet, with associated nail involvement. It tends to be less painful than rheumatoid arthritis.
(2) *Rheumatoid pattern.* A typically rheumatoid pattern of arthritis may occur, but the Rose–Waaler and Latex tests are usually negative.
(3) *Arthritis mutilans.* In this type there is severe deformity from the arthritis, which especially involves the small joints of the hands and feet, but also the spine. The arthritis often burns itself out but leaves gross deformity.

Prognosis

It is very difficult to give a prognosis in any individual case. It is possible to induce a remission with treatment, and spontaneous remissions do occur, but the relapse rate is high. The earlier the onset and the more extensive the condition, the more likely the patient is to follow a chronic course. Erythrodermic psoriasis and generalized pustular psoriasis carry an appreciable mortality.

Management

General

It is important to be optimistic about therapy and prognosis. Often doctors only compound the patient's misery by being negative and pessimistic. It is important for the doctor to voice some of the problems that he knows his patient is having, or at least to give the patient a chance to do so. These problems will include the difficulty of using often messy ointments; the embarrassment of leaving scales on a friend's carpet; of being unable to go swimming, and the problems for his or her partner. Genetic counselling will often be requested. Special diets are not relevant, but obese patients will benefit from weight reduction, especially if they have flexural psoriasis.

Specific

Topical

Dithranol 0.05–0.5% in zinc and salicylic acid paste BP, i.e. Lassar's paste, or in a mixture of hard and soft paraffin, is the standard topical treatment used in Britain for plaque psoriasis. The patient is often admitted to hospital, although outpatient treatment is very effective; it is less likely to be effective if the patient treats himself. Care is needed to avoid burning. The face and flexures should be treated with care. Dithranol will stain the skin and sheets or clothing. Treatment can be combined with tar baths and ultraviolet (i.e. Ingram technique). It is possible to clear most patients in two to three weeks and remission of many months can often be achieved. The treatment is not suitable for unstable psoriasis, erythroderma or generalized pustular psoriasis.

Ingram technique

(1) Tar bath: daily: 120 ml coal tar BPC is added to 90 l of water; or polytar emollient (Stiefel) 10–20 ml added to the bath.
(2) Ultraviolet light: three times per week after the tar bath, using SF 40 sunlamp fluorescent tubes (Westinghouse); or Hanua ALQ 600 mercury quartz bulb or Theraktin lamps. Initial exposure of 30 seconds is increased gradually up to a maximum of 10 minutes, to induce a faint pink erythema.

(3) Dithranol in Lassar's paste or a mixture of paraffin is applied, starting with 0.05%, and the patient is covered with tubinette. The dithranol is left on for 24 hours and is then removed with liquid paraffin or arachis oil.

Newer dithranol preparations are now available and are more suitable for outpatient treatment by the patient. They include Dithrolan (Dermal); Dithrocream (Dermal); Psoradrate (Eaton); Stie-Lasan (Stiefel).

Tar preparations. These are usually less effective than dithranol, but are often suitable for outpatient treatment. They are especially useful in the scalp (*Plate 6.5*). A suitable preparation is coal tar and salicylic acid ointment BPC. Tar preparations can also be combined with ultraviolet light (i.e. Goeckerman technique).

Topical corticosteroids. The potent fluorinated corticosteroids will certainly clear psoriasis, especially if polythene occlusion is used. However, the lesions tend to rebound quickly and become more severe than before. There is also a risk of converting the psoriasis into an unstable form. If a large area of the body is treated, enough steroid can be absorbed to produce adrenal suppression and Cushing's syndrome. Because of these side effects, it is now felt that full strength potent steroids used topically have little place in the treatment of psoriasis. Hydrocortisone or a dilute fluorinated preparation may be used on the face or in the flexures.

Systemic

(1) *Corticosteroids:* There was a vogue for using triamcinolone but this has now been discontinued. Initially, systemic corticosteroids are effective, but the psoriasis will break through with a severe rebound, and even an erythroderma or generalized pustular psoriasis may develop.

(2) *Methotrexate (MTX)* is a folic acid antagonist and is a highly effective form of treatment for most types of psoriasis, and it is certainly indicated in severe cases. It is given in a dose of 0.2–0.4 mg/kg body weight each week. It is usually given orally, and the week's dose should be given all at once or divided up over a 24 hour period. There is a definite risk of inducing liver fibrosis and cirrhosis, but by giving MTX as a single weekly dose, the risk is small. It should only be used after careful consideration in women of child-bearing age, and effective contraception must be used. As much care is required when using MTX for psoriasis as is exercised when using antimetabolites or cytotoxic agents in malignant disease. Hydroxyurea and azathioprine are also used, but are not as effective as MTX. A new anti-cancer drug, Razoxane (ICRF 159) shows great promise and is at present under detailed evaluation, but has not yet been approved by the Committee on Safety of Medicines in the UK.

Photochemotherapy (PUVA)

This is a new and exciting development in the treatment of psoriasis.

Psoralens are furocoumarin compounds, some of which can be synthesized and others extracted from plants. 8-Methoxypsoralen (8-MOP) is extracted from the *Ammi majus* L of the Umbilliferae family. 8-MOP is a photo-sensitizing compound and is photo-activated by long-wave ultraviolet light (UVA, 365 nm). In this photochemical reaction, photo-adducts are formed with DNA thymine bases. The inhibition of DNA synthesis and cell division that results from this interaction of DNA and psoralens is thought to be the mode of action of PUVA in the treatment of psoriasis.

8-Methoxypsoralen is usually taken by mouth (10–60 mg depending on body weight). Two hours later, when the blood level of 8-MOP is at its maximum, the patient is exposed to UVA from a high-energy source. The lengths of exposure to UVA depends on the degree of pigmentation of the patient's skin and also the output of the fluorescent tubes. Patients are treated two to four times per week until they are cleared of psoriasis; this is usually achieved after about 15 treatments, although occasionally it may take many more. A majority of patients can be kept clear by once a week maintenance, although some patients will need it twice a week, while some patients can cut down even to once in two or three weeks.

Most types of psoriasis will respond, although the chronic plaque type and the pustular psoriasis of the palms and soles are the most responsive to treatment. PUVA has many advantages. It is an outpatient treatment, it is highly effective, it avoids the need for messy and unpleasant ointments, and a cosmetically pleasing tan develops. However, the UVA light sources are expensive and the long-term side effects of PUVA are not known. Psoralen itself is probably safe, but there are now reports of frameshift mutations in bacteria and cultured mammalian cells produced by psoralen in the dark. However, psoralen is a weak mutant and the risk of systemic cancers is probably very small indeed, though in the presence of UVA, psoralen is highly mutagenic. It is possible that after many years of treatment, skin cancers may develop, and this has been shown to be possible in experimental animals. It is also possible that premature ageing of the skin may occur.

Because of these possible hazards the enthusiasm for PUVA has been tempered with caution. Many treatments for psoriasis have in the past been hailed as dramatic advances, only to be found wanting in subsequent use because of side effects.

Aromatic retinoid (RO–109359, Tigason)

This is a derivative of vitamin A and has a very low toxicity. It is moderately effective in the treatment of psoriasis when used on its own. However, its main advantage is in combination with photo-chemotherapy. If small doses of Tigason are combined with PUVA, only half the dose of UVA is required to clear a patient with plaque psoriasis. Furthermore, if a patient cannot be cleared with PUVA alone, the addition of Tigason can lead to final clearance.

In conclusion, much can be done for patients with psoriasis by employing general measures and a combination of topical and systemic treatments. There is no doubt that PUVA is an exciting development, and it is hoped that it will find a useful place in the long-term treatment of psoriasis.

Pityriasis rubra pilaris (PRP)*(Plate 6.6)*
Andrew Griffiths

The appearance of pityriasis rubra pilaris is quite distinctive. The name describes the cardinal features which are (1) erythema, (2) fine scaling, and (3) keratin plugs in the pilosebaceous orifices; to these should be added (4) gross thickening of the palms and soles.

Incidence

The disease is rare, affecting not more than 1/500 000 of the population. It is found in people of all races and skin colour. The sex incidence is equal.

The age at onset of PRP shows a peak in the first decade and a second peak in the fifth decade. Adult PRP is three times as common as juvenile PRP.

Aetiology

The aetiology is unknown. Recent studies suggest that it may differ in the juvenile and adult types. The skin and nails have an accelerated rate of growth but this is probably a secondary phenomenon related to the intense erythema.

Clinical features

The disease is usually more acute in adults and the cardinal signs are more pronounced. It starts with a red, scaly patch on the upper part of the body, followed within weeks by diffuse facial erythema, heavy dandruff (pityriasis capitis) and yellowish thickening over the palms and soles ('PRP sandal'). Over the succeeding months the disease extends downwards to involve the lower limbs. At this stage the pilosebaceous follicles become red and excess keratin formation results in prominent follicular plugs, imparting a nutmeg-grater feel to the skin (*Figures 6.7* and *6.8*). With further extension the follicular component is lost in sheets of erythema and fine bran-like scaling. The follicular lesions are retained longest on the backs of the fingers.

In 10 per cent of patients this disease progresses to total erythroderma. Itching is a prominent symptom only in the eruptive stage; thereafter it is only intermittent.

Juvenile PRP starts after the age of two or three. It is never present at birth, in contrast to severe types of ichthyosis. The onset

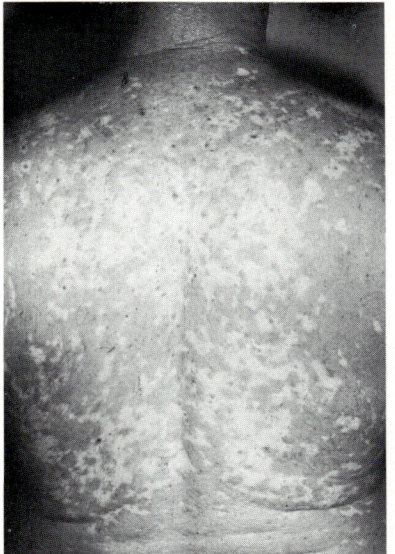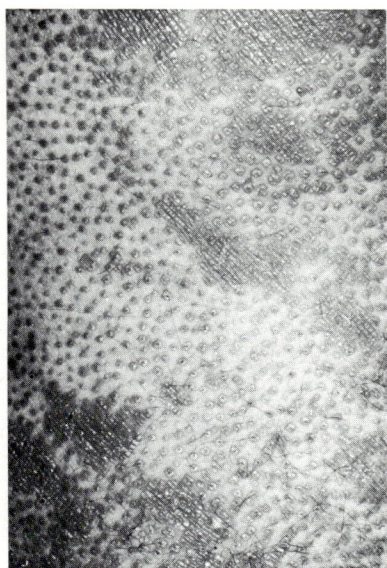

Figures 6.7 and 6.8 *Pityriasis rubra pilaris*

is usually gradual, with thickening of the palms and soles, areas of fine scaling in the scalp and follicular plugging on the body. Erythema is visible but is less marked than in adult cases and shows no tendency to progress to erythroderma. Abouth one-third of juvenile cases have a positive family history with mode of inheritance suggesting autosomal dominant with incomplete penetrance.

Incomplete and atypical forms of PRP have been recognized in adults and juveniles. A local variant affects children in the first and second decades. The prominent feature of this type is well-demarcated plaques of follicular plugging on the knees and elbows.

Diagnosis

Fully developed cases show three signs that are very suggestive of the diagnosis: (1) thickened yellow palms and soles; (2) the erythema has a curious orange tinge; (3) small islands of unaffected skin remain in the middle of the erythematous sheets.

Systemic investigations are normal.

Histopathology

The histological changes consist of mild epidermal thickening with hyperkeratosis showing scattered foci of retained nuclei (parakeratosis). When present these changes help to distinguish PRP from psoriasis, with which it is often confused.

Complications

In extensive cases heat regulation is grossly disturbed from impaired ability to sweat and from excessive heat loss through the erythematous skin. Transepidermal water loss is pronounced and may lead to dehydration. Prolonged erythroderma may produce further complications.

Differential diagnosis

Seborrhoeic eczema, psoriasis, and drug eruption.

Treatment

Simple emollients, such as vaseline, give the patient most comfort. Topical and systemic steroids are not effective. A few patients respond to cytotoxic drugs, but the results are less impressive than in psoriasis. Anti-keratinizing analogues of vitamin A hold some promise for the future (Tigason).

Lichen planus

Anthony du Vivier

Lichen planus is a pruritic, non-infectious disease of the skin and mucous membranes, usually seen in adult life and having a limited course. The morphology and distribution of the eruption are so characteristic that diagnosis is usually easy (*Plate 6.7*). It is relatively common, accounting for about 1 per cent of dermatological consultations. Distribution is world-wide but there is a curious and unexplained increased incidence in Nigeria.

Aetiology

The aetiology is obscure in most cases but there are enough indications from known causes to suggest that antigenic stimulation results in an immunological reaction in the skin. A viral antigen has been suggested but there is no convincing evidence for this at present. An increased association with diabetes mellitus has been reported from some investigations.

There are a number of situations in which lesions morphologically and histologically identical to lichen planus occur.

Graft versus host reactions

About one-third of patients undergoing bone marrow transplantations have been reported as developing lichen planus-like eruptions with clinical, histological and direct immunofluorescent findings very similar to those of idiopathic lichen planus. All the patients had oral lesions.

Graft versus host disease is an immunological reaction between donor immunocompetent cells and host tissues. In these cutaneous eruptions it has been shown that the basal cell layer of the epidermis is the first to be damaged. These observations have led to speculation that lichen planus is a reaction between primed lymphocytes and epidermal antigens.

Drugs

Mepacrine is perhaps the best documented offender. Troops were given this drug as an antimalarial during the Second World War, and a large number developed skin eruptions. The condition appears to be identical in every respect to lichen planus, though it may persist longer and produce more scarring.

Heavy metals, antidiabetic drugs, phenothiazines, beta blockers, quinidine and antituberculous drugs have all been documented as causing the eruption.

Colour developer

A remarkable contact dermatitis occurs on the lower forearms and backs of the hands due to immersion of these areas in colour developer. Contact dermatitis is normally, as the name implies, an eczematous eruption and is due to a delayed hypersensitivity reaction to an external allergen; although eczema can occur from colour developer, an eruption identical to lichen planus is well recognized. This picture is not seen with other commonly encountered allergens such as nickel and rubber.

Histopathology *(Figure 3.1*, p. 24)

The histology of lichen planus is characteristic. A superficial band-like, dense lymphocytic infiltrate is situated immediately beneath the epidermis, which it pushes up, thus forming a papule. The basement membrane and basal cell layer of the epidermis is destroyed and liquefaction degeneration of the cells is seen. Some degenerating cells collect to form eosinophilic 'colloid bodies'. Other changes in the epidermis are thickening of the stratum corneum and granular layer, some acanthosis and a flattening of the rete pegs giving a saw-tooth appearance. Immunofluorescent studies have demonstrated that the infiltrate is essentially composed of thymus-derived lymphocytes and that the colloid bodies represent deposits of immunoglobulin, particularly IgM.

Clinical features

Lichen planus is easily recognized once the physical signs have been demonstrated. Careful study of the morphology and distribution of skin eruptions are two cardinal observations to be made in dermatological diagnosis and lichen planus illustrates the wisdom of this principle. Study reveals a small papule, polygonal in shape, with a flat and shiny surface. Sometimes a white reticulate appearance is seen on this surface, known as Wickham's striae. The purple or violaceous colour of the papule is striking and points to the diagnosis. As the condition subsides the colour turns brown as a result of post-inflammatory hyperpigmentation; this fades in time. The distribution is also characteristic. A symmetrical eruption is found usually on the flexor surfaces of the wrists, ankles, forearms and legs and on the lumbar region, but it may extend to other parts. Lesions may be seen also in areas damaged by trauma, a phenomenon described by Koebner, and which also occurs in psoriasis and plane warts. Thus lesions made up of many individual papules are seen in skin damaged by scratching. The finding of lesions in the mouth may be confirmatory. A delicate white lace-like patterning occurs most often on the buccal mucosae and also on the tongue, gums and lips. In isolation these lesions may be mistaken for premalignant change (leukoplakia) but careful examination may reveal characteristic changes elsewhere, or biopsy of the oral lesions will differentiate the condition. Rarely malignant change may occur in oral lesions. Genital lesions are common, especially in males, and if they occur alone may lead the patient to believe that he has venereal disease. However, the papules are identical to those elsewhere on the skin although sometimes grouped to give an annular appearance and usually lesions are also present in the mouth.

Less common features are nail and scalp involvement, and the development of hypertrophic lesions on the shins and ankles. The nails may be thinned in such a way that longitudinal ridges appear along the length of the nail. A characteristic feature of nail involvement is pterygium formation, which is an adhesion between the epidermis of the dorsal nail fold and the nail plate. This results in partial destruction of the nail. Rarely nails are shed permanently. If the scalp is involved, permanent hair loss may result due to scarring, which is an unusual feature of lichen planus elsewhere. Finally, greatly thickened lesions may develop on the lower legs; these retain their characteristic purple colour. This hypertrophic variety may occur in association with typical widespread lesions or as the sole manifestation of the disease. These lesions differ in that they persist for many years.

Differential diagnosis

Lichen means a collection of papules, and chronic scratching or rubbing of the skin will produce this appearance. In atopic eczema lichenification occurs in skin flexures and is easily distinguished from lichen planus because the patches are larger. However, in other endogenous eczemas and prurigos small localized areas of lichenification may occur and these, particularly on the legs and in coloured races, may cause confusion. Psoriasis must be considered, especially on the legs, if the characteristic silvery scale is absent after partial treatment. Scabies bears some resemblance to lichen planus in terms of distribution, but the papules are neither purple nor flat-topped and shiny, and usually burrows are present. If itching is absent syphilis should be considered. If the diagnosis remains in doubt, the specificity of the histopathology will confirm.

Treatment

The condition in the vast majority of patients is self-limiting, resolution occurring between nine and 18 months, and the patient should be made aware of this. It is a glucocorticosteroid responsive disease; although these drugs probably do not alter the course of the disease, they suppress the manifestations. Usually topical steroid therapy is adequate. The choice of steroid depends on the site of skin affected, since the thickness of the stratum corneum is the rate-limiting factor for the penetration of the drug. Betamethasone-17-valerate ointment (Betnovate) or its equivalent, or the most potent available steroid clobetasol propionate ointment (Dermovate) are the most helpful. Occlusive techniques or intralesional steroid may be required for resistant areas, especially hypertrophic lesions occurring on the legs. Oral antihistamines are sometimes required for their sedative effect and there is an undoubted place for a short course of systemic steroids in severe cases.

7 Acne, rosacea and perioral dermatitis

Keith Liddell

Acne

Acne is a disorder of the pilosebaceous unit and usually manifests itself in adolescence. It is generally characterized by seborrhoea and comedone formation, and inflammatory lesions such as papules, pustules, nodules and cysts may develop.

Aetiology

Acne is probably the result of four main interactions, namely:

(1) sebaceous gland hyperplasia producing seborrhoea;
(2) pilosebaceous canal obstruction;
(3) bacterial enzyme activity;
(4) biochemical change in lipids.

Androgens stimulate the sebaceous glands and, while plasma testosterone levels are usually normal in males with acne, recent work has suggested that half of female acne patients have raised plasma testosterone levels. However, increased end-organ sensitivity may be a factor. It has been found that the tissue-active androgen 5-alpha-dihydrotestosterone (derived from the transport androgen testosterone) is increased in acne subjects, and this could be significant.

Androgens as well as bacterial enzymes and free fatty acids probably play a part in the abnormal hyperkeratosis which occurs in the pilosebaceous canal. The follicular canal is lined with stratified keratinizing epithelium and in the normal course of events the top layers of cells separate and pass out with the sebum. In acne the normal secretion of sebum is disrupted by narrowing of the follicular canal due to thickening of the walls resulting from the keratinized cells not being shed. The resulting obstruction originates in the mid and lower part of the duct and is not merely a plug at the distal end.

Free fatty acids are mainly derived from hydrolysis of the triglycerides in sebum by hydrolysis with bacterial esterases, principally from *Propionibacterium acnes* (C. acnes) and *Staphylo-*

coccus epidermidis to a lesser degree. Fatty acids diffuse through the follicular walls and cause inflammation, and liberated keratin from the injured follicles causes a granulomatous reaction in the dermis. Fatty acids and squalene (another constituent of sebum) may be comedogenic in man. Increased sebum viscosity and the inability of an inadequate or lanugo hair to keep open the pilosebaceous orifice and permit drainage of sebum are probably contributory causes.

The underlying factor in these hormonal, mechanical and biochemical changes is probably genetic. Polygenic mode of inheritance has been suggested and acne is also influenced by external agents. There have been few detailed family studies but a dominant inheritance has been demonstrated in a personal study.

Some relationship between the acne and diet has long been suspected, with greasy foods, pork and chocolate especially incriminated, but there is no scientific evidence for this belief. Certain drugs are known to cause or aggravate acne, notably iodides and bromides; these were often contained in cough medicines in the past but are rarely used today. Anti-epileptic drugs such as phenobarbitone and troxidone provoke acne and may account for an apparent increase in the incidence of the condition in epileptic subjects. Corticosteroids, testosterone and isoniazid can all exacerbate acne. Industrial agents may cause a type of acne, e.g. chloracne, from chlorinated hydrocarbons.

Clinical features

Acne manifests itself at puberty and can persist into the twenties or even later. Mature onset acne occurs more commonly in females. Acne characteristically affects the areas of skin which contain the most sebaceous glands, i.e. the face, back and chest, and in severe cases the upper arms may be affected.

The fundamental lesion is the blackhead or open comedone; the colour is due to melanin accumulating at the blocked orifice. Whiteheads represent closed comedones, i.e. blocked pilosebaceous follicles, and are often imperceptible to the naked eye. Inflammatory lesions may then develop, i.e. papules, pustules and, in the progressively severer forms, deeper pustules, nodules and cystic lesions appear. The term 'acne conglobata' is reserved for severe cystic acne with cysts coalescing, sinus formation and the tendency to secondary infection. Scarring is often the unhappy legacy of acne, with pits or pock-marks and occasionally keloid formation.

Acne *per se* is not a psychosomatic condition, but it may be exacerbated by stress and, because of the anguish it causes, it may in some cases be self-perpetuating.

About 60 per cent of female patients report premenstrual aggravation of their acne, and this may be associated with fluid retention causing overhydration of the keratin layer and so adding to the obstruction of the pilosebaceous canal.

Treatment

Since acne is a chronic relapsing condition with spontaneous remissions and unexplained relapses, it is difficult to assess the long-term efficacy of treatment. However, the importance of early treatment cannot be overemphasized, both for the prevention of scarring and of psychological damage.

Many mild cases clear spontaneously.

Local treatment

Though topical therapy is time-consuming and sometimes unwelcome, it is the first line of treatment and often satisfies a psychological need of the patient to touch the lesions.

Thorough cleansing of the skin with cetrimide solution or washing with water and a suitable anti-acne soap serves to degrease the skin besides removing some of the bacteria, scales and comedones.

Careful removal of comedones with a blackhead extractor after hot soaks can be helpful, but squeezing or picking of other lesions is ill-advised. Many patients find that their spots are improved by natural sunlight, though some shrink from exposing their lesions and resort to ultraviolet lamps. Mild peeling promotes drainage through the obstructed canals. Ultraviolet light may also have a mild antibacterial effect, while the resulting suntan helps to mask the lesions and thus improves morale.

Desquamative agents help to unblock the pilosebaceous canals. Sulphur application was employed to induce exfoliation, but in recent years doubt has been cast on the use of elemental sulphur as it may be comedogenic. Benzoylperoxide, with powerful oxidizing and antibacterial properties, is a good desquamating agent, particularly in the gel form, as this probably penetrates the follicles. Retinoic acid has given good results in treating comedones and it has been suggested that there is a synergistic effect between benzoylperoxide gel and retinoic acid, but they should be applied at different times of the day.

Topical antibiotics have been disappointing in the treatment of acne and sensitization is a potential risk. However, studies on new presentation of topical antibiotics, particularly erythromycin and clindamycin, are encouraging. Applied locally, steroids do not affect the basic aetiological factors in acne. The stronger fluorinated steroid preparations are contraindicated, particularly on the face.

Intralesional steroids are helpful in cystic acne, but a small amount only must be used to avoid atrophy. The cysts should not be incised or excised, or scarring will result. Brasivol, an aluminium oxide abrasive cleanser may prove useful in superficial scarring. Dermabrasion may reduce severe scarring. X-ray therapy should only be used as a last resort, and never in patients under 18 years.

Systemic treatment

Oral tetracycline is of considerable value in the treatment of acne which is resistant to local measures. Tetracycline is selectively

81

concentrated in the acne lesions and though its exact mode of action is not fully understood, it may, by reducing the lipolytic bacteria have a direct effect on the sebaceous unit and its metabolism. Initially 250 mg of tetracycline twice daily, before food, is usually sufficient and this dosage should be maintained for about a month. If improvement is satisfactory it can be reduced to a daily dose for another one or two months as necessary. In severe cases a longer course or larger doses of tetracycline may be required. Minocycline is a valuable reserve treatment for resistant cases but its cost precludes routine usage. Septrin or Bactrim and erythromycin are other antibiotics useful in acne.

Oestrogens reduce sebaceous gland activity, but only if taken in unphysiological dosage. This makes them unsuitable for male patients because they may cause gynaecomastia. High dosage oestrogen contraceptive pills containing a non-androgenic progesterone have proved helpful in female acne patients, and if contraception is also required this line of treatment should be considered. Low dose oestrogen contraceptive pills are of little benefit in acne and a pill containing a progesterone which is converted to androgen may even aggravate the condition. Some patients with premenstrual flare-up acne have responded to a diuretic taken each morning in the two weeks prior to menstruation.

The effect of antiandrogens is being studied, and in particular that of cyproterone acetate, together with its contraceptive value when combined with a low dose oestrogen. This work is in an experimental stage. The probable feminizing effect on a male fetus is a potential danger, and antiandrogens have not been approved by the Committee on Safety of Medicines, in the UK, for the treatment of acne. Recently publicized claims of a breakthrough in the treatment of acne with 13-*cis*-retinoic acid should also be treated with reserve. The series studied have been small; comparison with control groups is lacking, and present side effects are unacceptable.

Atypical acne

It is well to remember that acne may be a manifestation of some internal condition such as a virilizing tumour, Cushing's syndrome or Stein–Leventhal syndrome. When acne is associated with hirsutism and menstrual irregularities it is advisable to carry out hormonal investigations.

Infantile acne

This usually occurs on the cheeks of infants and consists of comedones and papules, but pustules are rare and cysts even rarer. The condition used to be attributed to a carry-over of maternal hormones but current thinking favours a genetic factor link with the possibility of contributory influence by the endocrine environment of the fetus. This may explain the greater incidence of infantile acne in males. Although the condition usually clears by the age of three, it may indicate a predisposition to acne in adolescence.

Acne excoriée

Excoriated acne generally occurs in females. There are few acne lesions present and the condition is principally caused by the patient picking at small lesions, producing unsightly scars and so inducing a type of dermatitis artefacta. The condition is often associated with nervous tension.

Acne necrotica

Some authorities attribute acne necrotica to energetic picking of acne lesions, but others doubt whether it is related to ordinary acne at all. While it is generally agreed that anxiety and emotional stress help to precipitate the condition, it is a fact that *Staphylococcus aureus* is usually found in the early lesions. The major form is called acne necrotica varioliformis because it leaves large varioliform scars, and the minor form is entitled acne necrotica miliaris because there are many small lesions. In both types the typical lesion is a conical pink round papule which is later surmounted by a pustule, and eventually a scab forms. The hair margin, scalp, nape of the neck and nose are affected, but only very rarely do the sternal and interscapular areas suffer. The lesions often irritate. Treatment is with antibiotic-hydrocortisone application and systemic tetracycline.

Differential diagnosis

Acne is easily diagnosed, but occasionally it may be confused with rosacea, perioral dermatitis, acne agminata, papulonecrotic tuberculide, milia, sarcoid, flat warts and secondary syphilis in the nasolabial grooves. Adenoma sebaceum may be misdiagnosed as infantile acne, and if the child is epileptic or mentally retarded tuberous sclerosis must be considered.

Rosacea *(Plate 7.1)*

Rosacea predominantly affects the face. It is characterized by a persistent, blotchy erythematous rash, associated with telangiectasis and swelling; papules and pustules are sometimes superimposed. It is usually seen on the forehead, nose, cheeks and chin, but it can affect the neck and rarely the limbs. Occasionally there is unilateral involvement, or one side is more severely affected than the other. The periorbital and perioral areas are usually spared. Pruritus is uncommon and the lesions are not tender, but the patient is troubled by the cosmetic effect.

The aetiology of rosacea is not known, but it is probably associated with a persistently dilated sub-papillary venous plexus, and sufferers are often vasomotor labile. The mite *Demodex folliculorum* may be increased in rosacea, but the mite is frequently seen in normal skin and other disorders of the facial skin. Despite a tendency to blushing, there is no sound basis for attributing rosacea to psychological stress. Many patients find that exposure to sunlight or a cold wind, hot beverages, spicy or curried food, or alcohol may cause a temporary exacerbation.

Rosacea is frequently complicated by conjunctivitis, and kerato-conjunctivitis leading to corneal ulceration and opacity can be a serious complication.

Rosacea is most commonly seen in females in the fourth and fifth decades, but rhinophyma, which is a common complication of rosacea, is generally seen in men (*Plate 7.2*). It is characterized by swelling and redness of the nose due to irregular hypertrophy of soft tissues, and this appearance has led to the misconception that alcohol causes rosacea.

Differential diagnosis

Seborrhoeic dermatitis, acne vulgaris, perioral dermatitis and polymorphic light eruptions may be confused with rosacea. Rarer and more serious conditions that must also be distinguished from rosacea include lupus erythematosus, dermatomyositis, sarcoidosis and the malar flush of mitral stenosis.

Treatment

Avoidance of extremes of temperature and abstinence from alcohol and hot beverages is generally helpful, while discussion of emotional problems, together with a mild tranquillizer may benefit some patients. Local applications are of limited value. Aqueous creams can be used to cleanse the skin but sulphur-containing preparations should be avoided because of likely sensitivity.

Hydrocortisone cream may improve the inflammatory aspects, but potent fluorinated topical steroids should be avoided; they may bring about initial improvement but prolonged use tends to increase the erythema and telangiectasis (*Plate 7.3*). Systemic tetracycline in a dosage of 250 mg twice daily before food is effective in the treatment of papules and pustules, and it is probable that its effect is not purely antibiotic. Rhinophyma once established does not respond to systemic tetracycline and plastic surgery may be necessary. Metronidazole has been found beneficial in the treatment of keratoconjunctivitis and in those patients with rosacea who cannot tolerate tetracycline.

Perioral dermatitis

Perioral dermatitis is characterized by patches of closely packed papules, papulovesicles and superficial pustules on a pinkish background, appearing on the chin and sometimes the nasolabial folds (*Plate 7.4*); there is sometimes a band of uninvolved skin immediately adjacent to the lips. The condition occurs most commonly in females in the third and fourth decades. The eruption may be sore and may be mildly irritating.

The condition is regarded by many authorities as a *forme fruste* of rosacea but it was originally labelled 'light sensitive seborrhoeide' in 1957. It has been diagnosed with increasing frequency in the last two decades. The aetiology is in doubt. There is no convincing evidence of infection, hormonal imbalance, light sensitivity, emotional stress or disorder of the general health. Some authorities have suspected *Candida* as a possible cause. Biopsies have shown eczematous changes, and allergic contact and primary irritant dermatitis have been considered as possible causes, but there is little supporting evidence. Although perioral dermatitis may be seen in patients who have never applied fluorinated steroid preparations, it is agreed by dermatologists that potent steroids aggravate the condition and in most cases are the cause.

Several factors differentiate perioral dermatitis from rosacea: the histopathology is different, ocular changes are absent, and it occurs in a younger age group.

Treatment

Cleansing the affected area with aqueous creams and local applications of hydrocortisone may be marginally beneficial, but a good response is generally obtained with systemic tetracycline in a similar dosage as that recommended in acne and rosacea. It is important to warn the patient that withdrawal of the potent steroid cream will lead to a rebound exacerbation of the condition initially.

8　Bacterial infections and syphilis

Patrick Hall-Smith
R. J. Cairns
W. F. Felton

Bacterial infections

The commonest organisms in skin infections are staphylococci and streptococci. However, the mere presence of pathogenic staphylococci or streptococci does not mean that the organisms are actively concerned in the production of lesions of the skin. Apart from trauma there is a variation in the susceptibility of individuals to infection. Seborrhoeic subjects may be more prone to pyococcal infection (pyoderma) than those with a normal skin.

Boils (furunculosis)

A boil is a deep-seated folliculitis by infection of the hair follicles with *Staphylococcus pyogenes* and can lead to perifollicular cellulitis, suppuration and necrosis.

Boils may be single or multiple; they can occur anywhere on the body surface, but most commonly over sites subject to friction and which can easily be rubbed and scratched by the patient. The back of the neck, face, buttocks and axillae are common sites. The boil appears as a red, tender nodule which points after about three days, discharging pus and necrotic core. The same phage type staphylococcus may be isolated from the boil, nose, or perineum.

A carbuncle is an aggregate of boils which discharge through several openings; the patient may complain of pain; malaise and fever are common.

Treatment

A solitary painful boil may be splinted and protected by a boil plaster; where it is fluctuant, or about to point, the surface should be opened by a needle and the contents very gently expressed; violent manipulation and squeezing must be avoided.

Spread of the infection to the surrounding skin may be prevented by repeated application of povidone–iodine (Betadine skin cleanser) or hibitane 0.5% in isopropyl alcohol. Systemic antibiotic therapy is not justified with solitary lesions unless there is surrounding cellulitis, when erythromycin, a synthetic penicillin (flucloxacillin) or cephalexin should be prescribed.

Recurrent boils are a difficult problem. It should be explained to the patient that the causative germ, the staphylococcus, lives in the nostrils, and sometimes the anal and vulval area, and is conveyed from these sites to the skin elsewhere by the fingers. The antibiotic sensitivity of the organism should be determined prior to beginning treatment, and urine testing for sugar must be routine in these cases.

The patient should be instructed to keep exploring fingers away from his nose and other orifices, and any associated anal or vulval pruritus should be treated with an antibiotic–hydrocortisone cream. The application of a neomycin–hibitane ointment to the nasal vestibule twice daily may help to rid the nose of the staphylococcus, and to control skin staphylococci a povidone–iodine skin cleanser is of value. The staphylococcus is ubiquitous and it may be necessary to treat the patient's family in the same way. A course of general ultraviolet light is useful. Any obvious infection in the nose or sinuses should be eliminated and the general physical state of the patient assessed.

Hidradenitis suppurativa *(Plate 8.1)*

A chronic infection of apocrine glands that most commonly occurs in the axillae, though the groins and perianal areas are sometimes involved. It occurs only in adolescents and adults as the apocrine glands are not fully developed before puberty.

The condition is commonly confused with boils but the chronicity, resistance to treatment and the development of sinuses is characteristic.

Treatment

Response to topical and systemic antibiotic therapy is disappointing. X-ray therapy may produce transient benefit but severe cases may require plastic surgery.

Impetigo *(Plates 8.2 and 8.3)*

Impetigo is a contagious, superficial skin disease usually of both staphylococcal and streptococcal origin.

Aetiology

Staphylococcus aureus of phage types 71 and 80/81 penetrates the stratum corneum and causes an acute inflammation. Haemolytic streptococci may act as secondary invaders; both streptococci and nephritogenic staphylococci may be responsible for a subsequent acute glomerulonephritis. This is rare though more common in children than in adults, and usually seen in the tropics.

Clinical features

The nostrils, chin and cheeks are frequently involved but no part of the body is exempt. The primary lesion is a vesicle which extends; polycyclic or circinate lesions may occur 3–5 cm in diameter. Rupture of the vesicles produces seropurulent 'stuck on' honey-coloured crusts which, if untreated, may become very thick.

Bullous impetigo of the newborn (pemphigus neonatorum) used to occur in epidemic form in nurseries; if severe, large areas of the body may be denuded of epidermis (Ritter–Lyell syndrome). Bullous lesions are occasionally seen in older children and adults.

Investigations

Cultural studies should be undertaken though the results are not always rewarding. Bacterial investigations should be made when infection is not responding in 48 hours to antibiotic therapy, when symptoms are present or when infection follows surgery.

Treatment

(1) Gentle removal of crusts with soap and water or 1% cetrimide.
(2) The application of topical antibiotics need be continued for a week or less, so the sensitizing potential of neomycin need not be an anxiety. Fucidin cream is also effective. The widespread use of tetracycline has given rise to resistant strains, so they may not be as effective topically as formerly.
(3) A systemic antibiotic should be used in extensive cases, and especially so in children; a seven-day course of erythromycin or flucloxacillin is the antibiotic treatment of choice.

Sycosis barbae *(Plate 8.4)*

Sycosis barbae was at one time a relatively common disease in adult males; it is now seen infrequently. Sycosis is a subacute or chronic folliculitis of the beard area due to *Staphylococcus pyogenes*. Sufferers are often seborrhoeic with an associated blepharitis, and staphylococci of the same phage type as that which causes the folliculitis may be isolated from the nose.

Clinical features

The chin and upper lip may exhibit follicular-papular pustules. These papulo-pustules with a central hair may remain discrete, though some subacute and chronic cases may give rise to a pustular boggy plaque which the ancients thought resembled a ripe fig: hence the label 'sycosis'.

Pseudofolliculitis barbae may be mistaken for sycosis barbae. This inflammatory reaction in the hair follicle commonly occurs over the shave areas of the neck and angle of jaw. It is seen in men with tightly curled shave hair which tends to grow back into the skin. Shaving may remove the exposed curly arc of the hair leaving the distal end buried in the skin, with a resultant inflammation and secondary infection. Negroes are especially prone to this condition.

Treatment

Chronic sycosis barbae requires systemic treatment with erythromycin or flucloxacillin. Tetracycline-resistant staphylococci are now common. Less severe cases may respond to topical antibiotics such as gentamicin sulphate cream (Genticin, Cidomycin) or sodium fusidate ointment (Fucidin).

Pseudofolliculitis barbae may require cessation of shaving, though a trial may be made of an antibiotic-steroid cream.

Acne keloid (Folliculitis cheloidalis, Dermatitis papillaris capillitii) *(Plate 8.5)*

This occurs only in post-pubertal males. The pathologic mechanism may be similar to pseudofolliculitis barbae. Clinically there is a clustering of follicular papules and pustules on the nape of the neck just below the hairline. Later keloidal papules develop and can coalesce into a linear keloidal band which may be infected and crusted. Severe cases exhibit discharging sinuses.

Treatment

Long-term topical and systemic antibiotic therapy and intralesional corticosteroids. Very severe cases require plastic surgical excision.

Toxic epidermal necrolysis (Lyell's syndrome) *(Plate 8.6)* *(See* Chapter 13)

Erysipelas

Erysipelas is an acute superficial infection of the skin due to *Staphylococcus pyogenes*. The site affected, often the scalp, face or limb, becomes red, tender, hot and swollen. There may be a barely discernible adjacent fissure which allow access to the streptococcus. The patient is pyrexial. Recurrent attacks may give rise to lymphoedema.

Cellulitis *(Plate 8.7)*

Cellulitis is a diffuse inflammation of the subcutaneous tissues and may be acute or chronic. Like erysipelas, it is due to the streptococcus, which invades the loose connective tissue through a breach in the skin or an ulcer. Some acute cases, as with erysipelas, may show vesicles or be haemorrhagic, and the separation of erysipelas and cellulitis can be blurred. Erysipelas is more superficial, with a better defined edge.

Treatment

Both conditions require penicillin in full dosage for five to seven days. Recurrent and chronic cases demand full investigation.

Ecthyma *(Plate 8.8)*

Ecthyma is a rare form of infection that begins with a small vesicle and forms a crusted ulcer by extending into the superficial dermis. Adherent crusting occurs on the surface; due to involvement of the dermis permanent scarring results. The legs are most frequently involved. In common with impetigo, it is usually a mixed infection of both streptococcal and staphylococcal origin.

Treatment

Local and systemic antibiotic therapy and a general assessment of the physical state of the patient should be undertaken.

Bockhart's impetigo

A superficial pustular folliculitis occurring on any hairy area; the hairy legs of men of poor hygiene sometimes show this condition.

Treatment

As in ecthyma, systemic antibiotic therapy in addition to topical antibiotic ointments or lotions is usually necessary, though soap and water are equally important.

Erysipeloid

This condition, due to *Erysipelothrix rhusiopathiae*, and not to be confused with erysipelas, follows a prick in the finger or hand from a fish or meat bone. It occurs as an occupational disease of fish and meat handlers and housewives. The involved finger or hand is swollen, tender and of a red-violet hue. The infection shows a tendency to spread to other fingers and does not respond as readily to penicillin as erysipelas.

Gram-negative infections

Gram-negative infections are of increasing importance. Broad spectrum antibiotics, immunosuppresive drugs and local hydration of the skin from poor evaporative conditions predispose and the clinician should be alerted to the possibility of Gram-negative infection in such circumstances. Clues to the diagnosis are the appearance of greenish pus with a distinctive green staining of the dressings and a 'mousy' or 'new mown hay' odour. Ulcerated and denuded areas and exudative dermatitis are particularly prone to such infection. On widely damaged areas, such as burns, the Wood's light examination may show areas of blue-green fluorescence due to the pigment pyocyanin produced by *Pseudomonas pyocyaneus*. Smears from the fluorescent areas should be examined for Gram-negative rods and cultured. It should be remembered that any occluded or ulcerated area is liable to produce overgrowth of Gram-negative organisms. Under occlusive dressings which are commonly used for pressure bandaging of varicose ulcers the presence of satellite pustules is sometimes an early sign of Gram-negative infection. If the ulcers are only re-dressed once weekly or every few days, then gentian violet or carbol-fuchsin paint should be used as they are the only antimicrobic agents which retain their effect for more than a few hours. With inpatients and where home nursing is practical, leg ulcers can be treated with four-hourly wet dressings of saline, eusol, aluminium acetate solution (BNF) and 0.25–0.5% aqueous silver nitrate compresses. A povidone dry powder spray is a useful application for moist, infected ulcers; it is unlikely to sensitize and will not produce bacterial resistance.

Transmission of Gram-negative organisms is by direct contact as the result of contaminated hands or by damp substances. Airborne dispersal is probably not an important factor.

A serious bacteraemia with Gram-negative organisms produces disseminated suppurative 'mycotic' aneurysms of small arteries of both the viscera and the skin, and a characteristic cutaneous lesion termed ecthyma gangrenosum. The renal excretion of pyocyanin results in a green urine that fluoresces under ultraviolet light. Gram-negative bacteraemia is sometimes associated with serious underlying disease and the high mortality rate is due to the underlying disease rather than the bacteraemia.

Pseudomonas pyocyaneus is usually sensitive to polymyxin B and gentamicin. Gentamicin or colomycin by injection is indicated for systemic infections.

Tuberculosis of the skin

Cutaneous tuberculosis is now relatively rare; this parallels the decreasing incidence of both pulmonary and non-pulmonary forms of the disease. The morphological type of lesion following infection with *M. tuberculosis* depends on the source of the infection and the age and immunologic state of the patient. Histologically the dermal lesions of tuberculous origin usually show a granulomatous type reaction and, again on histological grounds, skin tuberculosis can be divided into two main groups:

(1) eruptions in which tubercle bacilli can be demonstrated in the lesions, and
(2) tuberculides—an allergic or 'id' eruption due to a primary focus elsewhere; no tubercle bacilli are found in the lesion.

Classification (modified from Lever)

(1) Primary tuberculosis
    (a) Local inoculation. The rare tuberculous chancre is mainly seen in children who are Mantoux negative, i.e. those who have contracted no previous tuberculous infection. The lesion may occur as a small persistent sore, sometimes originating at the site of an abrasion; there is an associated lymphadenitis. Lupus vulgaris may develop at the site of the lesion. The face, hand, knee, foot or other sites vulnerable to trauma are the commonest location for a primary tuberculous chancre.
    (b) Haematogenous infection. The rare generalized miliary tuberculosis produces embolic lesions manifested by papules, vesicles and pustules leading to small ulcers.
(2) Reinfection tuberculosis
This occurs in those already sensitized by earlier exposure to the tubercle bacillus. The infection may be local or haematogenous.
    (a) Local infection
        (i) Lupus vulgaris—due to dermal deposition of tubercle bacilli from without or within, i.e. lymphatic or haematogenous spread from a focus in bone, joint or lymph node. The lesions consist of reddish-brown, tumid and demarcated patches containing pin-head, deep-seated nodules. When the vessels are compressed with a glass slide (diascopy) the nodules appear as translucent 'apple jelly' nodules (*Plate 8.9*). Later the overlying epidermis becomes atrophic with contraction of the tissue. Superficial ulceration and verrucose thickening may occur; rarely squamous cell epitheliomata develop.
        (ii) Tuberculosis verrucosa cutis. Warty lupus is seen in individuals with a high degree of immunity from previous pulmonary or alimentary infection. The tubercle bacillus gains access through a breach in the skin. Infection may be contracted from an infected human or animal source (butcher's wart). The lesions may be single or multiple, and consist of hyperkeratotic verrucose patches, with a tendency to annular formation and central scarring. Pus containing tubercle bacilli may be expressed from the lesions.
        (iii) Scrofuloderma ('King's Evil') is usually seen on the side of the neck or supraclavicular area as a fluctuant violaceous

swelling which suppurates, forming an ulcer with irregular undermined edges. The underlying tuberculous focus is in the lymph node or bone and extends to the skin by lymphatic spread.

(iv) Tuberculosis cutis orificialis. Shallow irregular superficial ulcers involving mucous membrane and skin resulting from advanced visceral tuberculosis, e.g. lung, kidney, bladder, the organisms having gained access through the mucocutaneous region.

(b) Haematogenous infection—tuberculide

An allergic reaction in those already sensitized to tuberculin; no tubercle bacilli are demonstrable in the lesions.

(i) Erythema nodosum (*Plate 19.8*) can occur as a sensitivity reaction to the tubercle bacillus. The onset of the eruption may be heralded by fever, malaise, joint pains, or gastrointestinal disturbance. The eruption is symmetrical and appears suddenly, most often on the shins, occasionally on the extensor aspect of the forearms and more rarely on the thighs and upper arms.

In their early stages the lesions are red, hot, swollen and exquisitely tender, but almost never go on to ulceration. Streptococcal and meningococcal infection, sarcoidosis, and sulphathiazole can also give rise to erythema nodosum.

(ii) Erythema induratum (Bazin's disease) (*Plate 8.10*). The lesions of erythema induratum usually affect the calves rather than the lower part of the legs, ankles and feet. This helps to differentiate it from chronic chilblains. It may progress to deep ulceration.

(iii) Papulonecrotic tuberculide. The extremities and the trunk may be affected with crops of inflammatory indolent papules which undergo central necrosis. It can occur simultaneously with erythema induratum.

Other rare tuberculides are lichen scrofulosorum in children and varieties affecting the face known as lupus miliaris faciei and acne agminata.

Lever, however, maintains that there is no convincing evidence in favour of a tuberculous genesis of erythema induratum and papulonecrotic tuberculide and thinks they could represent a form of vasculitis; lichen scrofulosorum could be a lichenoid form of sarcoidosis.

Treatment

A patient with skin tuberculosis requires complete clinical examination and investigation for possible tuberculosis elsewhere. Chemotherapy with isoniazid, streptomycin, PAS and rifampicin has revolutionized the management and prognosis of these conditions. Both lupus vulgaris and tuberculosis verrucosa cutis respond extremely well to isoniazid alone in a dose of 4 mg/kg of body weight. The usual adult dose is 300 mg daily, which must be continued for at least 12 months. Some authorities might prefer to use isoniazid in combination with PAS 12–16 g daily or streptomycin, which combination is the treatment of choice in scrofuloderma and erythema induratum. Children with primary tuberculosis are best treated in collaboration with a paediatrician.

Syphilis

This is a chronic systemic infection with *Treponema pallidum*. The disease normally passes through several definable stages: primary, secondary, latent and tertiary. Only the primary and secondary stages are infectious. The diverse clinical manifestations and the course of the infection are determined by immunological response provoked by the organism, the size of the inoculum and the route by which the organism reaches the host tissues. An effective defence mechanism may lead to self-cure or the organism may exist a lifetime without clinical evidence of the disease. Furthermore, atypical or *forme fruste* variants of the disease are seen in inadequately treated patients (*see* p. 99).

Incidence

The eight-year decline in early syphilis followed the ending of the Second World War but in the subsequent decade early infectious cases were reported in increasing numbers among all social groups from many countries. The incidence now remains stationary in the UK where the majority of new cases are seen in male homosexuals.

Mode of infection

The disease is transmitted by sexual contact. Nevertheless non-venereal infection of doctors, dentists and midwives occasionally arises accidentally from an infective patient. Some individuals acquire the disease from early mucosal lesions (e.g. kissing), from contagious secretions on drinking utensils and from infected needles used to vaccinate, tattoo, etc. Occasionally, syphilis results from transfusion with infected blood and congenital syphilis is acquired by transplacental spread of the maternal infection. Non-venereal transmission is occasionally found with overcrowding; in these conditions of endemic syphilis primary lesions are rare.

Clinical features

The primary lesion or chancre appears at the site of inoculation where most of the spirochetes remain. It is found most frequently on the ano-genital region, but may occur elsewhere (e.g. lips, tongue, tonsil, rectum) as a painless, indurated, eroded papule up to 1 cm across. The clean base oozes highly infective serum which contains abundant spirochetes. Regional lymph nodes are enlarged, painless and rubbery. Multiple chancres are rare.

Although the infection is acquired immediately on exposure and spirochetaemia appears within hours or days, the chancre appears only some three weeks (ten to 90 days) after first contact with the disease. Spontaneous healing after four to 12 weeks sometimes leaves the tell-tale atrophic scar.

Absolute diagnosis is by positive dark-field examination from either the chancre or satellite lymph nodes. Serological tests only become positive five to eight weeks after initial exposure and are, therefore, unreliable for the diagnosis of early syphilis.

Secondary syphilis *(Plate 8.11)*

About eight weeks after the appearance of the primary lesion the disease passes into the secondary stage and by this time the serological tests are positive. Individual patients exhibit widely varied clinical manifestations. Some present with no systemic upset and a transient eruption which is easily overlooked or disregarded; others present with fever, malaise, sore throat, hoarseness and slight deafness, and a widespread, symmetrical, non-itchy rash. Iritis with photophobia is sometimes an early symptom, preceding the eruption by several days.

The earliest form of the rash is often the *macular syphilide* (roseolar syphilide) which begins on the flanks. It is sometimes only visible in a good light and is perhaps first noticed by the patient while bathing. The pale pink macules 0.2–1 cm across may fade in a day or two, or extend to the shoulders, back and over the scapulae where they are particularly well-marked.

The *papular exanthem* is usually superimposed on an existing macular syphilide and is seen over the same areas, but with a predilection for the face, palms and soles *(Plate 8.12)*. Papules are infiltrated 3–6 mm across and feel almost 'shotty' when palpated between the thumb and forefinger, and they are tender (Ollendorf's sign). Secondary syphilitic papules are round, shiny, hemispherical and soon evolve from pink to dusky red brown (coppery 'raw ham') and brown lesions which develop an easily abraded central scale. When the central scale has separated a dull red papule remains with a marginal 'collarette' of scales resembling pityriasis rosea. Subsequent cropping is usual and later outbreaks may be confined to the legs—another cause of confusion with pityriasis rosea.

Large lesions may be oval in shape and reach 1–3 cm across with abundant loose self-detaching scales—the psoriasiform syphilide.

Important additional physical signs of secondary syphilis include lymphadenopathy, alopecia, intertriginous eroded papules (condylomata lata) and characteristic mucosal lesions.

Lymph node enlargement is widespread and includes epitrochlear and mastoid nodes. Enlarged lymph nodes remain discrete, painless, rubbery or 'shotty' and are sometimes palpable several months after the eruption has faded.

Alopecia appears as numerous areas of thinning on the scalp and, less commonly, on the eyebrows and beard area—the so-called 'moth eaten' alopecia. Follicular plugging and atrophy is absent. As with any febrile disease a diffuse telogen defluvium is sometimes seen three to five months after the febrile episode.

Condylomata lata constitute grey-white eroded papules appearing as 'split papules' at the angles of the mouth and flat-topped wart-like lesions in any intertriginous zone. the anogenital, genito-crural, natal cleft and axillary folds are the sites of predilection; the lesions are sometimes encountered under pendulous breasts, in the umbilicus and toe webs. The exuding serum from condylomata contains many treponemata and is highly infectious.

Mucous membrane lesions are common and the typical finding is a mucous patch; this is painless, raised, oval and covered with an easily detached grey-white necrotic membrane. A linear series of such abraded lesions is called a *'snail track ulcer'*. The soft palate, fauces and buccal mucosa are commonly affected. On the tongue they appear as 'bald patches' and sometimes heal leaving superficial scars.

Although secondary syphilides are usually non-pruritic, the *presence of pruritus in no way invalidates the diagnosis*. Syphilides are sometimes pruritic and pruritic dermatoses such as scabies and pediculosis may coexist with syphilis. Furthermore, hepatic disease (viral or syphilitic) is another possible cause of pruritus.

The distribution and density of the secondary eruption is sometimes modified by local factors. Thus seborrhoeic subjects show profuse lesions along the frontal hair margin (crown of Venus), in the presternal and interscapular regions. Similarly the sides of the neck may be severely affected (collar of Venus). Perniotic areas are sometimes spared, but when the rash does affect these areas of poor circulation it may be slow to clear. For reasons unknown there is sometimes unusual persistence of the eruption along the hair line, palms and soles. In some cases only the palms and soles are affected by the papular syphilide; small dull-red palmar and plantar papules with the tell-tale collarette of scales are diagnostic. A rare variant confined to these sites show horny wart-like papules, the so called *syphilitic corns*.

Other uncommon variants are the annular and corymbose syphilides. The rare follicular lues is often marked on the extensor surface of the trunk and limbs; pustular lues on the back, palms and soles; rupial syphilis on the face and scalp. Like all secondary eruptions they show a bilateral and symmetrical distribution.

Further general symptoms that may accompany the eruption are headache, neck stiffness (even rigidity from meningitis) polyarthritis, nocturnal bone pains (osteoscopic pains) from periostitis. In rare instances the liver and kidneys are severely damaged. Anaemia, leucocytosis and a raised ESR are common findings. Without treatment the noticeable signs of secondary lues disappear over weeks or months.

In summary, the important features which characterize the eruption of secondary syphilis are:

(1) a symmetrical eruption which evolves, spreads and shows cropping;
(2) the lesions are infiltrated, dusky red and darken; collarettes are often present;
(3) itching is usually absent;
(4) Systemic symptoms are sometimes marked.

Secondary relapse

If the primary and secondary stages are not diagnosed and the infections runs its course without treatment, the primary chancre will heal, the rash fade, and the other signs disappear. In a proportion—perhaps as many as 25 per cent—of such cases there will be a mucocutaneous relapse during the first two years after infection; however owing to the widespread use of antibiotics for all types of infection the chances of incidental treatment have increased, and relapses are relatively less common.

The lesions are infectious. They are often less marked than in the first attack. They may be livid or violaceous in colour, and assume circinate patterns on the genitalia. They may be limited to lesions of the palms and soles.

Latent syphilis

An asymptomatic infection in which the diagnosis is established only on the basis of positive serological and negative spinal fluid examination. It is often diagnosed in the course of routine serological testing. Latency terminates in spontaneous cure (negative serology) or persistent seropositivity in 75 per cent of patients. However, with clinical progression about 10 per cent will develop cardiovascular lues, 10 per cent neurosyphilis and about 15 per cent benign tertiary syphilis with gummata. Latent syphilis should therefore be treated.

Tertiary syphilis

This non-infectious stage of the disease first appears six to 30 years after the initial infection. It includes cardiovascular, neurological and late benign syphilis with cutaneous, osseous and visceral gummata. Only the mucocutaneous manifestations are mentioned here.

A gumma is a chronic granuloma, often with central necrosis, appearing in the dermis or subcutaneous tissue as a relatively painless torpid nodule.

Dermal gummata erupt as groups of indolent dusky-red nodules in the skin (*Plate 8.13*). They are unilateral or asymmetrically disposed and frequently form grouped, annular, arciform or serpiginous patterns. Individual nodules are pea-sized, firm and indurated; the surface may remain intact, showing scaling, or it may ulcerate. Spontaneous and complete healing of ulcerated gummata proceeds, whilst new gummata continue to appear in the adjoining skin. The scarring leaves characteristic groups of 'tissue paper' scars—atrophic wrinkled skin, patulous follicles and a surrounding band of melanosis.

A particular variant is the *late psoriasiform syphilide* comprising groups of dermal gummata covered with greyish crusts. The unilateral distribution, arciform, horse-shoe or serpiginous pattern, and the nodular infiltration, distinguish the eruption from psoriasis.

Subcutaneous gummata are common lesions of tertiary syphilis. They sometimes appear at the site of trauma as a small subdermal nodule. This slowly enlarges, becomes attached to the overlying skin, which is dusky-red, and breaks down producing a characteristic gummatous ulcer. Individual gummatous ulcers are circular or reniform 'punched out', 5–10 cm across, with a vertical wall and a clean granular floor.

Often the base has a yellow slough—the 'wash leather' base—and the surrounding skin is dark red in colour. When grouped gummata necrose they leave confluent 'punched out' areas of arciform 'broken rings', horse-shoe shaped or serpiginous ulceration. Often within large areas of gummatous ulceration characteristic 'islands' of normal skin persist supplied by end arteries free from syphilitic endarteritis. Satellite nodules which are a feature of other granulomata (lupus vulgaris, lupoid leishmaniasis, tuberculoid leprosy, etc.) are absent. Nodules, unlike those seen in lupus vulgaris and leishmania recidivans, never relapse within the scar tissue. The scars of tertiary syphilis are non-contractile; thus gummata on the cheeks and eyelids heal without causing ectropion.

The sites of predilection are the upper third of the shin, the sternoclavicular region, the face and scalp. Over the ischial region gummata have been mistaken for decubitus ulcers (pressures sores).

The coexistence of nodules, ulcers and scars (Stokes triad) strongly suggests active tertiary syphilis. Following treatment the presence of arciform or polycyclic 'tissue-paper' scars with peripheral melanosis provides indelible evidence of tertiary syphilis.

Juxta-articular nodules are fibrous nodules 1–4 cm in diameter that probably originate in old gummata.

Mucosal gummata may cause destruction of deep tissue including bone. Such gummata are relatively painless except with superimposed infection when extensive contractile scarring and deformity are found.

Chronic interstitial glossitis represents a diffuse gummatous infiltration of the tongue with leukoplakic patches, eroded glazed areas and fissuring; such epithelial changes are precancerous. Collective signs of cardiovascular and neurosyphilis may coexist with tertiary syphilis of the skin. Serology is positive in only 60–70 per cent of patients with tertiary syphilis.

Atypical syphilis

Atypical syphilis is now seen in a high proportion of patients as a result of partial suppression of the disease by antibiotics. It arises from incomplete penicillin therapy, suppression by tetracyclines (e.g. for acne, non-specific urethritis) or penicillin prescribed for gonorrhoea.

The primary lesion may be modified or absent. Atypical chancres may be non-ulcerated or a primary infection may appear as a diffuse syphilitic balanitis without lymphadenopathy. Only a few atypical secondary lesions (syphilis d'emblée) may herald the onset of the disease.

Venereal diseases very often masquerade together, particularly in the sexually promiscuous. Any patient, therefore, with a venereal disease, e.g. scabies, pediculosis pubis, especially if receiving antibiotics, should be carefully checked for syphilis.

Congenital syphilis

Congenital syphilis is now rarely seen in the UK although it is still common in certain parts of the world. The effect of prenatal infection on the developing fetus is determined by the 'antigenic load' and stage of tissue development when the fetus first becomes infected. The stage of maturity of the immunological system when first exposed to foreign antigens determines whether 'tolerance' or immunological reactivity will result. Four distinct syndromes are recognized:

Early fetal infection with *immune tolerance* causes severe and widespread disease, abortion or stillbirth. The stillborn fetal skin shows widespread necrolysis and bullae with abundant spirochetes demonstrable in the blood and many tissues.

Later transplacental infection, again with immunological non-reactivity, produces a live birth with cutaneous signs. Large dusky papules and bullae are most marked on the hands and feet, the so-called 'syphilitic pemphigus neonatorum'. The blister fluid contains many spirochetes.

With fetal infection occurring late in pregnancy the child is born apparently healthy and no signs develop for the first three to six weeks; then weight loss may be an initial sign. In these infants diverse rashes identical with those of secondary lues appear. The palms, soles, napkin and muzzle areas are, however, particularly affected; the trunk is relatively free. In intertriginous zones the skin may be denuded and florid condylomata may be present. As in secondary lues patchy alopecia, mucous patches and painless lymphadenopathy are noted; 'snuffles' (an infectious nasal discharge), if haemorrhagic, is almost diagnostic and a hoarse 'aphonic cry' completes the picture.

Spirochetaemia is accompanied by hepatosplenomegaly and pulmonary infiltration ('white pneumonia' of Virchow). Periostitis, dactylitis and chondroepiphysitis result from damage to osteoblasts in the growing bones. Healing infiltrated papules and fissured lesions around the mouth and anal region leave characteristic scarring (rhagades) which persists as a marker of earlier disease.

Late congenital syphilis

This appears after the second year of life with non-infectious tertiary-like manifestations. Diagnostic difficulties arise because the onset may be delayed to between the ages of seven and 15 years and *skin signs may be absent.* Gummata localize particularly in the nasal septum (producing 'saddle nose') and the palate (producing perforation). Frontal bossing (Parrot's nodes, cranio-tabes) from cranial periostitis and diffuse tibial periostitis produces pseudo-bowing ('sabre tibiae').

Painless joint effusions are rarely seen but when present constitute the characteristic 'Clutton's joints'. The well-known 'bulldog' facies and the Hutchinson triad (interstitial keratitis, nerve deafness, deformed second dentition) characterize late congenital syphilis.

The onset of nerve deafness and keratitis may be delayed to the early twenties and these features are sometimes accompanied by iritis and choroiditis. It should be remembered that about 10 per cent of late congenital syphilitics develop meningovascular syphilis, juvenile tabes or juvenile GPI. Only rarely are skin gummata, ulcers and 'tissue paper' scars found.

An uncommon manifestation of congenital syphilis is *paroxysmal cold haemoglobinuria*; with exposure to cold the patient develops chills, fever, *urticaria* and back pain; the urine becomes dark red or brown.

Differential diagnosis

It is important to think of syphilis even when the history does not immediately suggest this diagnosis; diagnostic difficulties arise for several reasons:

(1) Many practitioners have received their medical training in an era when syphilis was rare.
(2) The signs of early syphilis are masked or suppressed by antibiotics (*see* p. 99).
(3) Syphilis sometimes shows only transient and atypical features; it may only show in sunburn or already inflamed areas, or on palms and soles.
(4) Syphilis imitates many dermatoses; it has been called 'the great pretender' or 'the disease that can wear a hundred disguises'. Olser said 'he who knows syphilis knows medicine'.

Primary syphilis requires differentiation from chancroid, herpes simplex, scabies ('scabetic chancre') and lymphogranuloma venereum. Secondary syphilis has been mistaken for eczema, pityriasis rosea, rubella, drug eruption, guttate psoriasis, pityriasis lichenoides chronica and lichen planus. To add to the diagnostic problem any of these conditions many coexist with syphilis.

Tertiary gummatous syphilides are sometimes confused with halogen granulomas, lupus vulgaris, leprosy, dermal leishmaniasis, arciform mycotic granulomas, glossitis and lingual leukoplakia.

Latent syphilis may first present as a penicillin fever and rash 12–36 hours after the initial dose (Herxheimer reaction).

Congenital syphilis may appear as a napkin rash with granulomata or erosions and may be mistaken for bullous impetigo or Stevens–Johnson syndrome.

Immunology

The primary chancre probably represents a local Arthus phenomenon (Type III) although this point is not proven. Secondary lues, being a systemic infection with bacillaemia, provokes immune complex disease which provides the basis of the widespread cutaneous and visceral pathology. Untreated primary and secondary syphilis shows solid immunity; reinfection from reinoculation does not occur. In tertiary syphilis, however, experimental inoculation produces an extrinsic gumma. Thus when anogenital gummata appear the patient should be questioned for recent exposure. The Herxheimer reaction is probably a general Type III reaction provoked by antigen overload.

Types of serological tests

Two tests are used routinely for diagnosis and screening. The Venereal Disease Research Laboratory (VDRL) test and the Treponema Pallidum Haemagglutination (TPHA) test. Automated techniques are used and quantitative estimations can be made. When one or both of the screening tests give a positive result laboratories may carry out the Fluorescent Treponemal Antibody-Absorption (FTA) test. This is performed individually and the procedure is relatively costly.

VDRL test

The VDRL is a flocculation test employing a standard cardiolipin antigen which detects the presence of an antibody known as reagin. It is found to be positive in 70 per cent of cases of primary syphilis. The titre rises from neat serum to 1 in 40, the highest levels being found at the secondary stage. After treatment it falls rapidly but may remain positive at a low titre for some months. The longer treatment has been delayed the longer it takes for the titre to fall. A rise in titre during the follow-up period or later may give warning of a reinfection.

False positive reactions may be due to technical errors or to diseases other than syphilis—the so-called biological false positive (BFP). BFP reactions are detected by finding that the VDRL is positive while the TPHA and FTA (Abs) are negative. Acute BFPs are associated with a wide variety of infectious diseases or inoculations against them. They persist for no longer than six months. Chronic BFP reactions may persist for life and tend to be associated with autoimmune and collagen-vascular disorders.

TPHA test

The TPHA makes use of an indirect haemagglutination technique. The treponemal antigen is absorbed onto tanned red cells which are mixed with dilute test sera. The test is highly specific and reports of BFPs have been very rare.

The test becomes positive rather later than the VDRL. It is reported in titres of 1 in 80 to 1 in 1280. The former represents only a trace. It has been noted that the TPHA titre may increase immediately following treatment of a primary infection. During the secondary stage and in the untreated latent case the maximum titre of >1 in 1280 may be reported. The rate at which the titre falls depends on the duration of the infection before treatment. If this has been delayed for some years there may be no fall during the period of follow-up. Even when there is a fall during the first months in an early case, positive results at low titres of 1 in 160 may sometimes be reported indefinitely and long after the VDRL has become negative.

FTA (ABS) test

A suspension of dried *T. pallidum* is used as the antigen. This is mixed with the test serum and antihuman globulin conjugated with fluorescin. The treponemes fluoresce when the preparation is examined microscopically using ultraviolet light, if the test is positive. The test serum, which may contain group antibodies to commensal treponemes, is previously treated with sorbent to remove them.

The test is reported as positive or negative, occasionally as a weak positive or trace. As it is not automated, quantitative measurements are not carried out routinely. Unless otherwise specified the test indicates the presence of IgG antibodies. Positive results are found earlier than with the TPHA but there is the same persistence over periods of many years even after satisfactory treatment.

The FTA (Abs) IgM test can be carried out in some laboratories. The IgM antibodies are present in nearly all cases of untreated syphilis. They usually disappear rapidly after treatment while the IgG antibodies persist. Their presence supports the diagnosis of an untreated infection and their reappearance points to the possibility of reinfection.

The persistence of a positive FTA (Abs) IgM sometimes occurs when a test for the rheumatoid factor is also positive. In such a case the IgM test does not necessarily indicate continuing activity of syphilis.

The FTA (Abs) IgM test can be useful in the diagnosis of congenital syphilis in neonates. While reagin and treponemal IgG antibodies can cross the intact placenta, the IgM antibodies cannot do so. Their demonstration in neonatal blood is therefore strong evidence of congenital infection.

Treatment

Early treatment in the primary and secondary stages is curative with penicillin. In primary or secondary disease benzathine penicillin or preferably a benzathine procaine penicillin combination 2.4 mega units is given intramuscularly, followed by 1.2 mega units twice weekly to a total of six injections.

In penicillin sensitive individuals erythromycin or tetracycline 500 mg six-hourly is given for 15 days (total 30 g) and is repeated after six months. The failure rate is higher with this regime than with penicillin.

In tertiary syphilis preliminary tetracycline for seven days prior to penicillin probably diminishes the risk of Herxheimer reaction. Alternatively, prednisone 20 mg daily starting 24 hours before commencing penicillin reduces the chance of this reaction.

All contacts of infective patients should be treated with full courses of penicillin.

Table 8.1 Major features of secondary and tertiary syphilis

	Secondary	*Tertiary*
Onset from initial infection	10–26 weeks	3–30 years
Duration	Up to 2 years	Life-long
Infectivity	Marked	None
Incidence in syphilitics	90%	15%
Immunological mechanism	Type III (immune complex disease)	Type IV (Cell-mediated immunity)
General features	Malaise, nerve deafness, laryngitis, lymphadenopathy	None
Mucosae	'Snail-track' ulcers	Leukoplakia, Gummata
Skin lesions	Often transient, Widespread, Symmetrical, macules, papules	Persistent, Localized, Unilateral, Nodules, ulcers, scars
Occasional features	Hepatitis, Nephritis, Meningitis	Cardiovascular and/or neurological disease
Serology	100% positive	60–70% positive
Histology	Subacute inflammation, (perivascular), Plasma cells: many Slight endarteritis	Granuloma in mid-dermis, Plasma cells: many Marked endarteritis
Treatment	Penicillin im for 10 days	Tetracycline 7 days; then penicillin im for 10 days

NOTE: For Leprosy *see* Chapter 12 on Imported Skin Diseases.

9 Fungal infections

Denis Sharvill

This chapter will deal only with superficial infections of the skin, nails and hair by the dermatophyte fungi and with certain diseases caused by *Candida albicans* and some other yeast-like organisms. Space does not permit inclusion of systemic mycoses, which may have superficial manifestations, exotic mycoses such as tinea nigra, chromoblastomycosis, etc., or with opportunistic infections which are becoming commoner with the increasing use of immunosuppressive and cytotoxic drugs.

Although dermatologists did much pioneering work in mycology, they also introduced nomenclature and classifications based on clinical features which are no longer useful. Mycological jargon will be kept to a minimum, but some understanding of the subject is necessary for the intelligent management of ringworm (tinea). Many conditions which have been regarded as fungal, for example erythrasma, are caused by agents which are no longer classified as fungi but for clinical convenience can be described here.

After corticosteroids, antifungal agents are the most commonly prescribed skin preparations in the UK. Apart from the fact that many of them are of little value, this must represent gross over diagnosis of tinea. The true incidence of fungal infection is not known. Figures based on hospital outpatients must be misleading. Surveys of tinea pedis in specialized populations such as coal-miners, soldiers, or users of swimming baths are interesting. They serve to demonstrate the large numbers of symptomless carriers and the numerous foot disorders in which no fungus can be seen. They also show how readily tinea pedis spreads where people go barefooted on wet floors. On the other hand, the very inadequate clinical trials of new fungicides show how few cases of fungal infections reach even the larger hospital skin departments. In a personal series of 30 000 new skin referrals there were only 170 cases of symptomatic tinea pedis, 102 tinea unguium, 24 tinea capitis, and 435 tinea corporis. This is in a coal-mining area; many patients have tinea pedis of which they are unaware. In a personally operated diagnostic mycology service for local general practitioners and veterinary surgeons, fewer than 10 per cent of specimens submitted are positive for fungi or yeasts.

Tinea pedis *(Plate 9.1)*

Clinical features

When looking at patients who complain of rashes on their feet, think of tinea last of all! Positive features suggesting tinea are:

(1) Scaling confined to the outer toe webs and the under surface of the toes; seldom the dorsa unless spread there by topical steroids.
(2) Scaly rashes on the soles, which are commonly unilateral or at least asymmetrical, more marked anteriorly and accentuated in the natural skin creases.
(3) Blistering which is episodic, often confined to one foot, the vesicles or bullae being quite large, 5–10 mm, and containing glairy fluid, usually scanty, appearing over several weeks or recurring annually.
(4) Evidence of tinea elsewhere, especially in nails or groins.

Involvement of all toe spaces, symmetrical scaly rashes of the whole of both feet, symmetrical small vesicles, or primary pustules on the inner soles or heels are usually due to some other cause.

Diagnosis must be confirmed by the microscopic examination of detached scales or roofs of vesicles in 10 or 20% potassium hydroxide solution, when mycelium should be easily found.

The most commonly isolated dermatophyte fungi in tinea pedis are *Trichophyton rubrum* and *Trichophyton mentagrophytes*. *Epidermophyton floccosum* is now an uncommon cause of tinea pedis.

Differential diagnosis

This includes simple maceration of the toe spaces associated with hyperhidrosis. Psoriasis may also arise as a purely interdigital condition and is, of course, common on the soles, even without any rash elsewhere. Pustular psoriasis and the similar pustular bacterid are common and can be misdiagnosed as fungal infections. Contact dermatitis from rubber or other chemicals in footwear may be suggested by its distribution and must be investigated by patch testing. The increasingly common symmetrical dermatosis of the anterior aspect of the sole and under surfaces of the toes in children in no way resembles tinea, though it may sometimes resemble eczema or psoriasis. Tinea pedis is uncommon before puberty. A soft corn commonly appears in the outer space. It is usually painful and can simulate tinea.

Treatment

Treatment of tinea pedis depends on correct diagnosis. Clinical diagnosis is little better than guesswork. One has to decide whether the fungus is the first object of attack, or whether to concentrate on secondary sepsis and maceration; if the latter, then soaks of 1:8000 potassium permanganate, topical antibiotics, antibacterial agents such as hydroxyquinolines, or systemic antibiotics are indicated. It is increasingly difficult to maintain a place for the classic preparations of Whitfield and Castellani, at any rate as primary treatments. Most of the older proprietary fungicides are of small value and must soon disappear, for example undecanoic acid, phenylmercuric nitrate, chlorphenesin, and many more. The newer imidazoles, clotrimazole (Canesten) and miconazole nitrate (Daktarin, Dermonistat) are more effective and have a useful antimicrobial action as well. They very seldom sensitize. They need to be applied twice daily and continued for six to eight weeks, despite apparent cure. There is a great and understandable temptation to evade diagnosis by treating patients with widely advertised blunderbuss preparations containing mixtures of corticosteroids, broad spectrum antibiotics, especially neomycin, and fungicides, very often nystatin. These may at first appear to produce gratifying results, but they seldom eliminate the infection.

Griseofulvin is of no value in simple interdigital tinea, but should be used for widespread tinea of the soles, in addition to local treatment, in blistering tinea. An adult requires 1 or 2 g daily and it should be kept up for six to eight weeks. Griseofulvin is fungistatic, not fungicidal, and does not produce immediate results. It is of no value against *C. albicans*, which can cause or be associated with typical interdigital 'athlete's foot'.

Tinea manuum *(Plate 9.2)*

Interdigital tinea does not occur on the hands as it does on the feet (*see under C. albicans*). *Trichophyton rubrum*, however, may attack the palms, as it does the soles, causing a similar scaling which emphasises the skin creases, commonly asymmetrically. It may be misdiagnosed as contact dermatitis, especially in coal-miners (in whom 'epidermophytosis' is an industrial disease). Active, inflammatory tinea elsewhere may cause an id eruption, which can be generalized but is often confined to the hands as a vesicular or fine papular rash. Differential diagnosis includes all the many forms of eczema, dermatitis and psoriasis. Erythema multiforme is sometimes misdiagnosed as tinea, simply because the lesions are round. Granuloma annulare bears no resemblance at all to any fungus infection except that the lesions are often circular, but it is most commonly referred to hospital as ringworm after the failure of griseofulvin.

Tinea cruris *(Plate 9.3)*

This is best considered separately from other forms of tinea corporis. It affects one or both groins, nearly always in men, often unilaterally or asymmetrically. The depth of the groin is usually spared. There may be multiple discs or rings on the inner thighs, or simply a long, polycyclic scaly edge, often spreading posteriorly to involve the buttock. The commonest cause of tinea cruris is *T. rubrum*, but *T. mentagrophytes* and *E. floccosum* are also quite frequently isolated.

This must be distinguished from simple intertrigo due to friction in the obese and from *Candida* infections. Flexural psoriasis may be confined to the groins or to the perianal area and is often misdiagnosed. It may have a well defined but usually non-scaly edge, and the characteristic bright red shiny appearance. Erythrasma will be mentioned later. Very acute trichomonal vaginitis in women, when accompanied by profuse discharge, may cause chafing of the inner thighs accompanied by extreme discomfort. Such unfortunate women occasionally spend several weeks on a dermatological waiting list, whereas a few moments in the department of genital medicine could provide a diagnosis and a rapid cure with metronidazole.

Tinea cruris usually clears satisfactorily with a topical fungicide, but the old-fashioned strongly keratolytic applications should be avoided on the thin skin of the groins. When tinea cruris is widespread it is often helpful to give a course of griseofulvin for six weeks, combined with an imidazole ointment.

Tinea corporis *(Plate 9.4)*

Circular lesions on the skin are usually not due to fungi, and ringworm is not necessarily circinate, although it may be.

Primarily zoophilic fungi, such as *Microsporum canis* and *T. verrucosum* attack the skin, causing varying degrees of inflammation. *T. mentagrophytes*, especially the granular variety sometimes called gypseum, is carried by small animals and rodents and may produce inflammatory ringworm. *M. canis*, from dogs and cats, causes single, occasionally multiple lesions which are often ringed with scaly edges. Sometimes it causes multiple concentric rings. *T. verrucosum* from cattle may produce a similar picture, especially in children, but often the lesions are much more inflammatory, with pustulation around hair follicles, sometimes so gross as to resemble a carbuncle, but without much pain or systemic upset (kerion). *T. rubrum* usually produces non-inflammatory lesions, which may be round; alternatively areas of scaling, or a gyrate edge; it can produce bizarre patterning. A high index of suspicion is necessary to detect such lesions. The commonest differential diagnosis is discoid eczema. Clinical differentiation is occasionally difficult. The herald patch of pityriasis rosea is commonly and reasonably mistaken for tinea; the established eruption less justifiably. Psoriasis of the trunk, if it lacks the typical silvery scale, can be mistaken for widespread *T. verrucosum* infection without much inflammation. Annular fixed drug eruptions and rare migratory erythemas can cause difficulty. Malignant reticuloses such as mycosis fungoides (*Plate 17.4*) (which has nothing whatever to do with fungi), Hodgkin's disease and other forms of lymphoma may present as itchy circinate or gyrate lesions.

It is especially important to establish the diagnosis of tinea corporis, or to exclude it, before distorting the picture by fungicides or topical steroids, which can convert *T. rubrum* infections into weird pictures, sometimes called tinea incognita.

Single rings may be treated with a topical agent. In *T. verrucosum*, infections with multiple secondary lesions require griseofulvin, although this drug will not much shorten the course of established pustular ringworm.

All these conditions may occur on the face (*Plate 9.5*). In men, inflammatory ringworm of the beard is frequently thought to be pyococcal and inappropriately treated. The laboratory diagnosis of this type of tinea can be difficult, as scrapings seldom show mycelium. It is necessary to pluck infected hairs from their follicles. The dermatologist can often spot infected hairs on naked eye appearance, and then confirm the diagnosis microscopically by finding characteristic large spores outside the hair shaft. *T. verrucosum* is very slow to appear in culture, and will be missed by the laboratory unfamiliar with fungi.

Tinea unguium *(Plate 9.6)*

Ringworm may affect a single nail, a few nails, or nearly all the finger and toe nails. If one looks carefully enough one can usually, but not always find some evidence in the skin of the feet.

Typically affected nails are yellow, crumbly and distorted, with heaped up debris under the free edges, but they may be atrophic and thin, or they may resemble almost any other described nail disorder, including typical psoriasis. They are usually painless and show little inflammation, except when the big toe nails are grossly thickened and pressed into tight shoes.

Differential diagnosis includes all other nail disorders, especially 'monilial' nails (*see under Candida* infections). Psoriasis without skin lesions can be difficult to distinguish. Leuconychia, eczema of the nails, subungual warts and even melanoma have been diagnosed as tinea. In infancy and childhood tinea is an unlikely diagnosis.

Laboratory diagnosis is made by shavings taken down almost to the nail bed, by clippings, or, in specialist units, by dental drill. The infecting fungus is almost always *T. rubrum*, and its isolation can be difficult unless good material is provided. Various other non-dermatophyte fungi may be isolated from nails if looked for, but will not grow on the usual media which contain inhibitory antibiotics. Some of these may be genuinely pathogenic; they are all resistant to griseofulvin.

The treatment of choice is with griseofulvin. This will need to be given for at least six months in a young adult with finger nails only affected; perhaps for a year or more in an elderly patient with thumb nails as well. It may be helpful to rub in an imidazole fungicide during this course of treatment.

Treatment of infected toenails is unsatisfactory and seldom

indicated. Whatever one does, reinfection from the interdigital skin is likely sooner or later. Some advise removal of all the toenails before starting griseofulvin.

After apparently successful early results, new nails often become infected, sometimes by *C. albicans* or other fungi.

Tinea capitis *(Plate 9.7)*

This is now rare in the UK.

Classic small spored ectothrix ringworm is caused by the anthropophilic *Microsporum audounii*. It is uncommon but can cause epidemics in closed communities. *M. canis*, carried by dogs and cats, causes sporadic cases and small local epidemics in pet owners and breeders. This type of ringworm on the scalp produces circular, partly bald patches, with stumps of hair broken off just above the surface. It can also affect other parts of the body (*Plate 9.8*). Scaling and inflammation are variable. Bright green fluorescence is visible under Wood's light, often in areas of apparently normal scalp, and epilation of hairs from suspect areas is essential for microscopy and culture.

T. verrucosum conveyed by cattle is a cause of scalp ringworm occasionally seen in country districts in Britain. It is often violently inflammatory and its diagnosis is important because it may cause permanent alopecia. Actual contact with infected cattle is not necessary. Children may acquire it from climbing over stiles, coming in contact with fences, cowsheds, or infected clothing. Ringworm is also occasionally acquired from horses and from small rodents.

T. tonsurans and *violaceum*, the latter usually imported, are rare causes of ringworm, of unusual appearance with patchy, minimal alopecia. The hairs break off flush with the scalp, causing an appearance of black dots. The fungal elements are in the hair shaft, so called endothrix involvement.

Favus, caused by *T. schoenleini*, is so rare that it need only be mentioned.

Microsporum ringworm of the scalp occurs only in children and disappears at puberty. *T. rubrum* infections of the neck may creep up beyond the hair line.

When tinea capitis was common, all scalp disorders in children were 'ringworm' until proved otherwise, and the diagnosis must still be considered today. Kerion, a manifestation of cattle ringworm, is often misdiagnosed as carbuncle (*Plate 9.9*), and even accepted as such by surgeons.

Differential diagnosis

(1) Alopecia areata: circumscribed smooth bald patches showing exclamation mark hairs when active.
(2) Seborrhoeic dermatitis: diffuse scaling with no circumscribed hair loss.

(3) Trichotillomania: broken hairs without scaling. The affected areas are usually on the anterior part of the scalp within easy reach of the patient's hands.
(4) Psoriasis: patchy, palpable, discrete scaly areas with no hair loss.

Treatment

The treatment of scalp ringworm in prepubertal children (*M. audouinii, M. canis*) has been revolutionized by the fungistatic drug griseofulvin which avoids the necessity of x-ray epilation. A satisfactory dosage schedule for a child is one tablet (125 mg) of the fine particle griseofulvin twice daily. Cases of *M. audouinii* and *M. canis* should be examined under Wood's light and the antibiotic continued until most of the affected hairs show a normal zone proximal to the infected part. This usually takes three to four weeks and the hair should then be clipped off or shaved close to the scalp. After this the child should be examined daily, or at least twice weekly, and any infected stumps removed manually with epilating forceps. Treatment with griseofulvin should be combined with a topical application of a fungicide and twice weekly washing of the hair. Infected brushes and caps should be destroyed. In endemic areas mass treatment with griseofulvin is justified.

Kerion from cattle ringworm requires griseofulvin in full dosage: in an adult 500–1000 mg daily. Ketoconazole, which is an orally administered imidazole derivative, has recently become available for treating a wide range of dermatophyte, yeast and other fungal infections. Its clinical effectiveness has been demonstrated in short-term studies, but recurrences seem common and its side effects remain to be assessed.

Candida albicans

Candida albicans may be cultured from the bowel, skin, mouth or vagina of healthy people. When behaving as a pathogen *Candida albicans* is mycelial in form, but on culture it appears simply as a budding yeast. When diagnosing *Candida* infection it is necessary to find mycelium in scraping or in vaginal material and not to rely on swabs for culture.

This yeast—and other *Candida* species, which need not concern the non-specialist—are, however, associated with several specific clinical pictures. Tinea pedis, microscopically confirmed, may on culture yield only *Candida*. In many such cases all the toe webs are involved with more maceration than is usual in dermatophyte infections.

All forms of intertrigo may be associated with this yeast, especially in the groins, round the anus and under the breast. When this is so it may be diagnosed by finding mycelial elements on microscopy. Culture is not of diagnostic significance.

Candida albicans may often be found in napkin rashes in babies, usually in association with a variety of bacteria. Getting rid of the plastic pants may be more effective than applying fungicides, especially strong ones, which may worsen the condition.

Angular stomatitis may show *Candida* mycelium and spores on microscopy. This often occurs in the elderly who wear an upper denture overnight. Scrapings from such dentures may show *Candida* in pure culture.

Vaginal candidiasis may often be accompanied by perivulval skin lesions, often tiny superficial ruptured vesicles. A positive vaginal culture does not mean that a woman has an infection needing treatment. *Candida* may cause a frank balanitis, or simply penile itching with little to be seen but vast amounts of mycelium microscopically. It is a common presentation of diabetes.

Monilial paronychia is common (*Plate 9.10*). Typically it is chronic, affecting one or several nail folds, with bolstering of the fold and a creamy discharge, which may be absent. The course of chronic paronychia is often interrupted by episodes of acute or sub-acute bacterial infection. Usually there is some onychia. Chromogenic micro-organisms may give to monilial onychia a wide range of colours, varying from bright green through various shades of brown to black. Distinction from tinea unguium due to *T. rubrum*, which is often improved by griseofulvin, is important. Nail clippings and scrapings should be cultured.

Erosio interdigitalis blastomycetica is rare (*Plate 9.11*). It usually affects the space between the ring and middle fingers and is commonly bilateral. It may be seen in barmaids and those whose hands are constantly wet.

Most *Candida* infections of skin respond to imidazole applications. Nystatin and amphotericin are of great value in mucosal infections, but of limited value on the skin. Onychia and paronychia may defy all efforts. Clotrimazole solution sometimes helps. Repeated applications of a drying antiseptic such as 2 or 4% thymol in chloroform to the nails and folds for many months is useful. Advice to housewives to keep their hands out of water is easy to give but not likely to be followed.

While *Candida albicans* may affect the skin in apparently perfectly healthy people, it must be recognized as a powerfully opportunist organism. Unusual infections and systemic infections may indicate underlying organic disease such as diabetes mellitus or other endocrine disorders. They are also seen in patients undergoing immunosuppressive or cytotoxic therapy. Other less common fungi may invade the skin, blood or central nervous system in such patients. There are rare disorders of humoral or cell mediated immunity in which *Candida* may play a part, including chronic muco-cutaneous candidiasis, of which there are many types. These conditions require specialized immunological investigation.

Nystatin and amphotericin are not absorbed from the gastrointestinal tract. While they may be administered orally to remove *Candida* from the bowel, such treatment is of no value in systemic or widespread cutaneous mycoses. Griseofulvin has no suppressive action against candida.

Tinea (Pityriasis) versicolor *(Plate 9.12)*

Characteristic eruptions of this condition are easily recognized with yellow or brown, slightly scaly plaques scattered over the upper trunk and neck, appearing darker than untanned white skin, or lighter than suntanned or naturally brown or black skin. Unusual presentations or inactive cases can be very difficult. Scanty lesions in patients from endemic areas may raise fears of leprosy.

Lesions which do not look scaly may yield plenty of material for microscopy, which shows the short, fat mycelial forms and the round blastospores of *Pityrosporum orbiculare* (formerly *Malassezia furfur*), resembling 'meatballs and spaghetti'. Cultures are not available as a routine diagnostic measure. Wood's lamp may make the lesions easier to see and demonstrate infections on areas of skin hitherto unsuspected.

In the short term treatment is easy, for it will respond to almost any fungicide, but relapses are common. The whole trunk and proximal limbs should be treated. At present the imidazole fungicides are expensive for such widespread use. Greasy ointments such as Whitfield's are unacceptable.

Selenium sulphide shampoos work well and are cheap. They may be applied to the wetted skin and showered off after five minutes, or left on overnight. Treatment daily for a week, then weekly for a month is satisfactory. Selenium can give rise to contact reactions. Treatment of sexual partners may be advisable, although patient to patient infectivity is low. Recrudescence of an apparently cured infection may follow a tropical holiday or a febrile illness.

Erythrasma

This is uncommon in temperate climates, though habitual users of Wood's lamps may diagnose it more often.

It is of some importance in the differential diagnosis of tinea cruris. It causes a defined, slightly scaly or smooth sheet with a distinctive brown or reddish colour. Under Wood's light there is brilliant red fluorescence. *Corynebacteria* can be isolated on special media. They respond to broad spectrum antibiotics, topically and by mouth, better than to conventional fungicides. Imidazoles are effective topically.

Erythrasma may also affect the toe webs and can be indistinguishable from ordinary tinea unless Wood's light examination is carried out. In tropical countries it can also cause infections of the trunk which may resemble tinea versicolor.

Table 9.1 Differential diagnosis

Foot T. pedis	Groin T. cruris	Body T. corporis	Body T. versicolor	Nails T. unguium	Hands T. manuum	Beard T. faciei	Scalp T. capitis
Contact dermatitis	Flexural seborrhoeic dermatitis	Pityriasis rosea	Seborrhoeic dermatitis	Psoriasis, nail-bed and subungual	Irritant and allergic eczema	Sycosis vulgaris	Alopecia areata
Eczema, various	Flexural psoriasis	Discoid eczema	Pityriasis alba	Candidal onychia and paronychia	Pompholyx, dysidrosis, 'ide'	Seborrhoeic dermatitis	Alopecia, traumatic
Juvenile plantar dermatosis	Candidal intertrigo	Psoriasis	Vitiligo	Eczema of nail-bed	Atopic discoid eczema	Contact eczema	Seborrhoea capitis
Psoriasis, vulgaris and pustular	'Sweat rash'	Seborrhoeic dermatitis	Pityriasis rosea	Nail dystrophy—trauma	Psoriasis, discoid and pustular	Pustular rosacea	Psoriasis
'Id' eruptions	Erythrasma	Erythema multiforme	Pityriasis lichenoides chronica	Nail dystrophy—chemical	Granuloma annulare	Carbuncle	Fausse teigne, sheathing pityriasis
Sweaty feet	Pemphigus, Hailey–Hailey	Erythema annulare	Other pigmentary disorders	Lichen planus	Erythema multiforme	Traumatic folliculitis	Lichen planopilaris
Hyperkeratosis, soft corn etc.	Fixed drug eruption	Drug eruptions	Secondary syphilis	Alopecia areata	Secondary syphilis	Secondary rupial syphilis	Lupus erythematosus

Many of the differential diagnoses mentioned do not really resemble tinea, but are commonly diagnosed as such. In British hospital practice most of these conditions are much commoner than ringworm

10 Viral infections

Rodney Dawber

The commonest viral infections affecting the skin are: (1) warts (verrucae); (2) molluscum contagiosum; (3) herpes simplex; and (4) herpes zoster.

Warts

Warts (verrucae) are classified according to site and morphology. Any part of the body surface or mucous membranes may be affected. Morphological variants include common, plane, filiform and digitate, plantar and acuminate types. All are caused by the wart virus, a papova virus approximately 45 µm in size; it is possible that the acuminate (venereal or condylomata acuminata) type is caused by an antigenically distinct variant. Clinical evidence suggests that the wart virus does not penetrate normal, healthy, intact skin very easily; most warts occur at sites where the skin is subject to friction, hydration or minor damage.

Common warts

Common warts are most frequently seen on the hands, fingers and knees. They may be single or multiple and occasionally coalesce to produce a verrucose plaque. Periungual warts are a particularly ugly and recalcitrant type affecting the finger nail folds of those who over-manicure or traumatize the cuticle and nail folds, e.g. nail biters.

Plane warts

Plane warts are flat, smooth or slightly elevated, and either skin-coloured or grey; on the face they are sometimes pigmented. The face, dorsa of hands and shins are favoured areas and numbers vary from a few to hundreds.

Plane and common warts may form at sites of trauma, e.g. scratches. This is the isomorphic or Koebner phenomenon (*Plate 10.1*) also seen in psoriasis, lichen planus and vitiligo.

Filiform or digitate warts

Filiform or digitate warts (*Plate 10.2*) are more often seen in men. They have a projecting hyperkeratotic tip; they are usually found on the face, scalp, eyelids, nostrils and genitalia.

Plantar warts

Plantar warts (*Plate 10.3*) affect the weight-bearing parts of the soles. They are commonly acquired at swimming pools or sports complexes where bare-foot communal showering or bathing takes place. They are often painful, particularly on walking. If differentiation from corns is difficult, paring of the surface with a scalpel helps: warts show punctate black specks (blood or blood pigments) or bleeding. Corns have a smooth surface with continuity of the dermatoglyphic ridges overlying them. Warts are generally painful on lateral pressure; corns on direct pressure. Plantar warts may be single, multiple or grouped. Large numbers adjacent to each other are called mosaic warts; this is the more persistent type which usually lasts for many years.

Acuminate or genital warts

Acuminate or genital warts (*Plate 10.4*) are now classified as a venereal infection. In studies carried out in major cities, concurrent syphilis or positive serology has commonly been found, particularly in homosexual men with penile or perianal lesions. They form soft, pink, elongated lesions that may coalesce into cauliflower-like growths on the vulva, penis or perianal areas. The condyloma lata of secondary syphilis are not easily confused: warts have a verrucose surface, while the syphilitic type are flat and have an indurated base. When warts affect the perianal skin, the anal canal and rectum are also frequently involved.

Treatment

The multiplicity of treatments for warts reflects the fact that at present there is no certain or ideal method. *Table 10.1* shows the common modes used. In practice the regime adopted is determined more often by the doctor's personal experience, the age of the patient and the number of warts. Many dermatologists are content to use placebos, since most warts remit within six to nine months, though plane, periungual and mosaic warts are notoriously persistent.

Cryotherapy has been traditionally carried out by applying a cotton wool swab dipped in liquid nitrogen to each wart for a few seconds; alternatively solid CO_2 is applied with pressure. More recently, cryosprays and probes have become available, which are quicker to use, cheaper and more effective, particularly for resistant types, e.g. mosaic warts.

Keratolytics act by removing surface keratin, the strength used

Table 10.1 Commonly employed wart treatments

Common warts	(1) Cryotherapy
	(2) Curettage and silver nitrate cautery
	(3) Keratolytics and caustics
Plane warts	(1) Bland topical agents
	(2) Weak keratolytics
	(3) Cryotherapy
	(4) Diathermy or electrocautery
Digitate/filiform warts	(1) Curettage
	(2) Cryotherapy
Plantar warts	(1) Curettage
	(2) Cryotherapy
	(3) Keratolytics
	(4) Formalin soaking or topical glutaraldehyde
Acuminate (genital) warts	(1) Podophyllin paint
	(2) Cryotherapy
	(3) Surgical removal—large lesions

depending on the site and type of wart to be treated, e.g. for plane warts of face: 2% salicylic acid ointment; for mosaic warts 40% salicylic acid plaster.

Podophyllin is a cytotoxic agent and a severe irritant. It is used for genital warts as 15–25% podophyllin in tinct. benz. co. or in spirit. It should never be used in pregnancy and always limited to use by experienced medical or nursing staff. Residual liquid should be washed off not later than three to four hours after treatment to prevent severe irritant dermatitis.

Diathermy and electrocautery may scar and are gradually being replaced by cryotherapy.

Formalin is used for plantar warts as a 5% solution. The affected area is soaked in the liquid for 20 minutes each evening.

Molluscum contagiosum

The virus causing this disease is a member of the pox virus group, which also includes varicella, variola and orf. In the UK the highest incidence is in schoolchildren, particularly those who frequent swimming, sauna and Turkish baths. Boys are more often affected than girls.

Individual lesions are sessile, bulbous and smooth; follicular infection may give prominent inflammatory signs having the appearance of furunculosis (boils). Most typically it takes the form of clusters of umbilicated skin-coloured or pink papules 2–5 mm in diameter (*Plate 10.5*). Patchy eczema often develops around the clusters, even in non-atopic subjects; atopic patients may get hundreds of papular lesions. Any area may be affected but sites of predilection are perianal orificial skin and around the eyes; in adults they are generally confined to genital areas. The condition is not highly contagious.

Treatment

Successful treatments are either irritant, painful, or both. Since most cases remit spontaneously within six to nine months, small, unexposed areas may be left untreated.

Individual lesions may be punctured with a pointed orange stick or scalpel and the contents expressed. A small number can be treated by curettage. Some dermatologists combine the puncturing procedure with the application of cantharidin in flexible collodion, phenol or trichloracetic acid. Cryotherapy, preferably with a liquid nitrogen spray—5–10 seconds to each lesion, depending on size—is also effective.

Herpes simplex

Herpes simplex is caused by the herpes hominis virus, probably the commonest infection in man. There are two antigen types: Type I causes the common labial and non-genital infection, and Type II the genital variety. The latter is transmitted as a venereal disease.

The infection occurs as primary and recurrent forms. It may present at any time from birth onwards, but the primary type usually develops between two and 15 years of age as an acute vulvo-vaginitis or stomatitis. Once infection has occurred the virus persists in the body for life. Neonatal herpes occurs only in infants whose mothers have never been affected, i.e. no passively transferred antibodies are present. In contrast to most viral skin infections, herpes in the first few months of life can be fatal, particularly in babies with atopic eczema.

The commonest clinical manifestation is herpes labialis, seen as groups of vesicles around the lips (*Plate 10.6*). Overt vesiculation may be preceded by paraesthesia or itching felt for several hours. Any part of the body may be involved, commonly the cheeks and genitalia. Periocular involvement may lead to corneal dendritic ulceration. Recurrent herpes tends to affect the same site with each attack, at intervals varying from a few weeks to years. Specific attacks may be precipitated by a variety of factors, e.g. upper respiratory tract infections, menstruation, sun exposure or psychological stress.

Less commonly, primary herpes may present as a group of painful vesicles on a finger (*Plate 10.7*). If it occurs around the fingernail, acute bacterial paronychia is often misdiagnosed, but in herpes incision fails to reveal much pus and pain is not relieved. This type of herpes is mostly seen in dental and medical staff. In the Western world herpes simplex is the commonest cause of erythema multiforme, which may recur ten to 14 days after each episode of herpes.

Kaposi's varicelliform eruption (eczema herpeticum or eczema vaccinatum) (*Plate 10.8*)

This is the most important complication of atopic eczema and is due to infection with the herpes simplex or vaccinia viruses. It appears as groups of umbilicated, varicelliform lesions mainly affecting eczematous sites, but in severe cases the whole body may be involved. Many areas become haemorrhagic and pronounced lymphadenopathy is common. The patient is always ill. Viraemia or serious secondary bacterial infection gave a high mortality in the past, and deaths still occur. A similar eruption may be seen in burns and as a rare complication of Darier's disease and pemphigus foliaceus.

Treatment of herpes simplex

Most clinical types are no more than a temporary, non-scarring inconvenience and treatment can safely be left to the patient, e.g. with proprietary antiseptics to prevent secondary bacterial infection, or astringents such as acetic acid. Most medically-prescribed treatments given for larger lesions with more morbidity are based on the same principles. Severe recurrent herpes in any family member of an atopic eczema sufferer requires more specific treatment. Examples of the latter group are eczematous (atopic) children and immune suppressed patients, i.e. due to disease or drugs. Thymidine analogues (antiviral) are used topically for severe, recurrent disabling herpes. They may be used systemically for severe cases of Kaposi's varicelliform eruption or immunodeficient patients. However, systemic treatment with thymidine analogues is hazardous due to their cytotoxicity, and patients should therefore be admitted to an infectious diseases unit for careful nursing and particularly to monitor bone marrow function. The only specific topical antiviral agent in general use is 5-iodo-2-deoxyuridine (IDU). It is used in a powerful solvent, dimethylsulphoxide (DMSO). In the UK it can be prescribed from retail chemists as 5% IDU in 100% DMSO (Herpid).

Strengths up to 40% IDU can be made in DMSO but such preparations are usually only available from specialist (hospital) pharmacy departments. The spectroscopic brand of DMSO should be used. Most authorities agree that topical IDU is useful for severe recurrent herpes simplex, though not all agree on the correct strength. For routine practice it is recommended that 5% IDU in 100% DMSO be used hourly for the first two days of each attack. Five ml may be enough for several episodes. (It is very expensive.) IDU certainly shortens the infection considerably but only rarely is further recurrence prevented.

Herpes zoster (shingles) (*Plate 10.9* and *Figure 10.1*)

Zoster (shingles) and varicella (chickenpox) are due to the same virus. Invasion of a susceptible host by the zoster–varicella virus results in primary infection: 70 per cent develop overt chickenpox, the other 30 per cent subclinical infection detected by antibodies in the blood. In both groups the virus remains dormant in the host for an indefinite period. Chickenpox usually affects children, while zoster is commonest in the middle-aged and elderly. Zoster is not associated with a high incidence of neoplasia, as popularly believed, but recurrent and generalized zoster is a frequent and often serious complication in patients with grossly disturbed immune mechanisms, e.g. lymphatic leukaemia, Hodgkin's disease, myeloma, other reticuloses, and patients on immunosuppressive drugs.

The eruption may be preceded by generalized malaise and paraesthesia or pain over the affected neural segment. This prodrome may last for several days before the rash appears as a unilateral and segmental eruption with grouped vesicles set on an erythematous base. The vesicles often coalesce and in the severest cases the whole dermatome can be affected; local haemorrhage and necrosis may be seen and secondary bacterial infection is common, particularly in the second week.

Pain during the eruption and post-herpetic neuralgia are unpredictable, though in general the older the patient the more likely is such pain to occur. In elderly subjects intractable pain may persist for years.

The eye is commonly affected in trigeminal zoster and it is wise to solicit the help of an ophthalmic surgeon with this type, since blindness may supervene if care is inadequate.

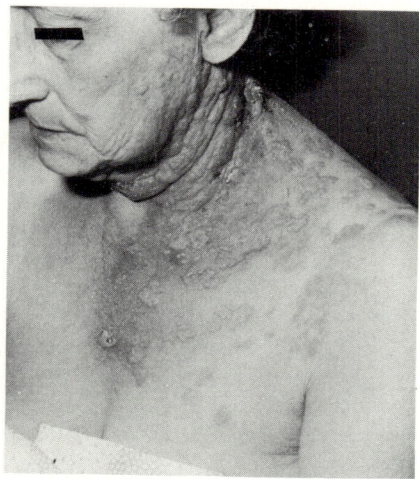

Figure 10.1   *Herpes zoster (shingles)*

Treatment

Therapy may be symptomatic or specifically antiviral. In patients under 50 years of age symptoms are usually mild and treatment should therefore be with analgesia, e.g. oral aspirin as required, together with 'comforting' and antiseptic topical agents such as calamine lotion or cream as necessary, while Vioform cream, twice daily, helps to inhibit secondary bacterial infection and so lessen post-zoster scarring.

Severe cases require more intensive treatment. Idoxuridine (IDU) in 100% dimethylsulphoxide (DMSO) is specifically antiviral. IDU 5% applied intermittently to affected areas for the first week shortens the eruption and decreases pain. Some authorities advocate 35% IDU applied to the whole dermatome as a wet dressing for five to seven days. Known systemic antiviral agents are too toxic for general use, but increased efficacy may be achieved by combining topical IDU with systemic cytarabine in life-threatening cases. This treatment should be restricted to inpatient use only, since bone marrow suppression may occur. The question of using oral prednisolone or amantadine to reduce post-herpetic pain should also be left to specialist judgement.

Hand, foot and mouth disease

This is a vesicular eruption due to A strains of Coxsackie virus. It may occur in epidemic form. Typically, after an incubation period of five to seven days, small vesicles develop on the sides and backs of the fingers and toes, palms and soles, and scattered about the oral cavity. The lesions usually fade within a week of onset.

Orf (contagious pustular dermatitis of sheep)

Orf is caused by a pox virus with a distinctive woven appearance on transmission electron microscopy. It is a vesico-pustular eruption affecting the mouth and udders of sheep, particularly lambs. Human orf is largely an occupational disease of farmers and veterinary surgeons. Normally, one attack gives life-long immunity. In England human orf presents most commonly in Northumbria and the rural south-western counties.

The lesion starts as a small reddish papule, usually on a finger, which enlarges in five to six days to form a vesico-pustule 2–5 cm in diameter; it may be haemorrhagic (*Plate 10.10*). It is generally painless, in contrast to herpetic whitlow, from which it requires differentiation. A generalized maculo-papular eruption is not uncommon during the second week.

Treatment

Treatment is symptomatic. Secondary bacterial lymphangitis and regional lymphadenitis occur so frequently that many authorities recommend prophylactic oral antibiotic treatment. Vioform cream is useful topically.

11 Parasitic infestations

Mark Hewitt

Skin infestations may conveniently be grouped into: (1) those transmitted from man to man (anthropophilic); (2) from animal to man (zoophilic); and (3) mites of foods, dusts or vegetation which will attack man (geophilic).

(1) Anthropophilic—primarily parasitic on humans:
    (i) Scabies—human.
    (ii) Pediculosis—capitis, corporis, pubis.
    (iii) Fleas—human.
    (iv) Bed bugs (cimex lectularius).
(2) Zoophilic—transmitted from animals to man:
    (i) Fleas—cats, dogs, rodents, hedgehogs.
    (ii) Scabies—dogs, horses, camels, foxes.
    (iii) Cheyletiella—dogs, cats, rabbits.
    (iv) *Dermanyssus gallinae*—fowls, starlings, cage birds.
    (v) *Ophyonissus natricis*—pet snakes.
(3) Geophilic—mites of foods, dusts or vegetation which will attack man:
    (i) *Acarus siro*—grain or cheese.
    (ii) Tyrophagus species—grain or cheese.
    (iii) Glycyphagus species—house dust.
    (iv) *D. pteronyssinus*—house dust.
    (v) *Trombicula autumnalis*—vegetation.
    (vi) Pyemotes species—vegetation, grain, wood and insect larvae.

The nature and type of noxae and reactions

Individuals vary greatly in their reactions. Atopic subjects are the most severely affected and the reactions vary according to anatomical site, secondary infection, age of the patient and medication. Host reactions may be caused by mechanical trauma from puncture wounds; injection of injurious substances, e.g. venom; injection of antigen into a sensitized host, e.g. flea bites, causing an allergic response; secondary infections from scratching with scabies or

122

pediculosis. Contact hypersensitivity is also caused by sensitization from living or dead mites, and reactions may be initiated by retained mouth parts or excreta, e.g. harvest mites. Lice can cause disease, e.g. relapsing fever. The nit and scabetic burrow are diagnostic. Other common manifestations of ectoparasites are general pruritus, papular rashes, papular urticaria, pleomorphic papular urticaria, generalized papular prurigo, eczema, bullous eruptions, especially on the lower legs, dermatitis herpetiformis-like eruptions and impetiginous skin lesions.

Types of infestation

Human scabies is pandemic and prevalent. The diagnosis must always be considered when a patient complains of itching which is worse at night. Other members of the family may be affected. Burrows are visible on the hands and forearms and male genitalia; the head and neck are unaffected. There can be a widespread papular rash. The acarus can be demonstrated (*Plate 11.1*) and the disease responds to appropriate treatment.

The female mite is 200–400 μm long and the male 100–200 μm. Both are non-segmented, with four pairs of legs—the two anterior with suction pads and the two posterior ending in bristles. The fertilized female travels up to 2.5 cm/minute on the skin surface, burrows into the selected site of horny layer within an hour, lays two to three eggs a day for 60 days and in doing so produces a burrow. The eggs hatch in three to four days, mature through larval and nymphal stages in four to six days, copulate and the cycle is repeated. Males and mites in various stages spend much time on the skin surface. Only pregnant females burrow and the number of burrows is called the parasite rate. The average parasite rate is 11, but this varies. In clean, hygienic persons burrows may be difficult to identify. Burrows are seen as grey-white tortuous lines 5–15 mm long (*Plate 11.5*). The mite may be visible at the anterior end as a tiny white dot, 'grain of wheat' or vesicle. She may be seen on the surface and can be extracted with the point of a needle to which she clings. She can be placed on a glass slide, is frequently mobile and can be identified with low microscopic power. Ninety per cent of patients have burrows on their hands and forearms, notably the interdigital spaces, accompanied by scaliness, the ulnar border, flexures of wrists, and in infants and children along the palmar creases and soles. The genitalia are almost always affected, female breasts frequently, and also the feet (*Plates 11.3, 11.4, 11.5* and *11.6*).

Infection occurs through close bodily contact and may be venereal. Irritation only develops three to four weeks after a primary infestation due to a general allergic reaction, although during this initial phase the patient is infected and infective. There may be minimal cutaneous signs. The secondary allergic manifestations are a generalized fine papular erythematous rash with increased skin sensitivity and frequently secondary eczematization, infection and excoriation. The rash is maximal on the abdominal wall, inner thighs, axillary folds and buttocks. The patient must be stripped to search for burrows and to confirm the pattern of the secondary eruption.

Norwegian crusted scabies

This is a massive infestation, usually by millions of mites, is highly contagious and leads to epidemics in contacts. It occurs in geriatric and mental institutions and is encouraged by long-term steroids or immunosuppressive drugs. Thick crusted lesions resembling psoriasis are found on limbs and trunk, and the nails may be brown and teem with parasites.

Differential diagnosis

(1) Canine scabies and cheyletiella from dogs, cats and occasionally rabbits.
(2) Papular rashes from fleas, including papular urticaria.
(3) Atopic eczema—peripheral lesions in children and of disseminated neurodermatitis pattern.
(4) Pityriasis lichenoides chronica et varioliformis acuta.
(5) General pruritus.
(6) Delusional parasitosis.
(7) Lichen planus.
(8) Dermatitis herpetiformis.
(9) Onchocerciasis.

Many patients are seen with rashes resembling infestation but in whom no ectoparasite is identifiable. There is much scope for further study.

Treatment

(1) Benzyl benzoate emulsion 25% BPC (this tends to sting; gamma benzene hexachloride is preferred in infants and children).
(2) Gamma benzene hexachloride 1% lotion (Quellada).
(3) Gamma benzene hexachloride 1% cream (Lorexane).
(4) Sulphur ointment 5% for children and 10% for adults can still be used.

Treatment should preferably be supervised by trained staff and must include all patients, even if lesions are secondarily eczematized or infected; all members of the household should be treated and all intimate contacts. The routine to be followed is:

Day 1: Hot bath—scrub thoroughly with soap and flannel, especially sites of burrows; dry; apply preparation with paint brush from chin to soles and allow to dry; leave on for 24 hours. The skin applications will kill mites in clothes and bedding.

Day 2: Repeat application as before.

Day 3: Bath; clean clothes, night attire and sheets.

Residual irritation may persist for weeks; for this 10% crotamiton cream (Eurax) is helpful. There may also be persistent vesicles and papules on the trunk; this is not an indication for further treatment, which could provoke a contact dermatitis. Enquiries will reveal if treatment has been adequate.

Sarcoptes scabiei var canis

One per cent of dogs are believed to be infested. The parasite is morphologically indistinguishable from the human variety but does not burrow into human skin. Usually the onset of symptoms dates back to acquisition of the dog, and all the litter will be affected. All contacts should be traced. Clinically there is an immediate papular rash at the site of contact, in most cases the lower legs, thighs, lower abdominal wall, wrists and flexures of the forearms. There is generalized erythema, increased skin sensitivity, eczematization and pigmentation from scratching similar to human scabies but without burrows.

Signs on animals

Puppies may be scaly, frantic with irritation and even paralytic with diarrhoea. Low grade chronic infestation in older animals may go unrecognized. Veterinary assistance should be sought.

Cheyletiella species

These are free-living parasites, in the fur of domestic and pet rabbits 46–83 per cent, dogs (mostly long-haired) 18 per cent, while up to 3 per cent of cats (mostly long-haired) are infested. There is a seasonal incidence which is highest in the spring; the distribution is worldwide. The mites are host-specific but the morphological differences are minute. There may be no visible skin changes, or there may be scaliness over the dorsal aspects of the trunk and neck, with pruritus causing constant scratching. Cheyletiella spp. (*Plate 11.7*) are small grey-white oval-shaped mites, barely visible to the naked eye. They live on the skin surface of the host, do not burrow, but move about among the skin debris at the base of the hairs. The eggs, resembling but much smaller than nits, are loosely attached to the base of the hair shaft by means of a cocoon-like structure of finely woven thread. They are acari, like scabies, and pass through the same stages of development. The adults have characteristic claw-like palpal hooks by which they attach themselves to the hair, and prominent stylet-like chelicerae which are used to puncture the skin and can penetrate clothing. They have characteristic tarsal brushes. They are present in large numbers in the spring, are believed to exist for only short periods away from their host but, contrary to popular belief, can be hard to eradicate.

Cheyletiella produce a variety of skin reactions in humans which are influenced by the degree of sensitivity of the subject and the extent of the animal infestation. In about one-third of patients the lesions occur in crops at the site of contact, starting as small erythematous macules which may develop a central papule, become vesicular, then pustular, and finely rupture to produce a yellow crusted lesion, sometimes with intense inflammation but well demarcated from normal skin. There is sometimes a central area of necrosis. This well-defined clinical picture will justify the label of cheyletosis. Individual lesions subside in about three weeks but grouped pigmented relics may be visible for three to six months (*Plate 11.8*).

About two-thirds of patients present with widespread and bizarre cutaneous changes, the commonest being an extensive papular eruption. Some patients complain of general pruritus but have no visible cutaneous change, while others exhibit dermographia. Cheyletiella may produce papular urticaria, bullous eruptions on the feet and lower legs, increased skin sensitivity and migratory eczematous eruptions on the chest and upper arms.

Treatment is of the infested animal. Simple measures may be adopted against the environment similar to those recommended for fleas (*see Table 11.1*).

Diagnosis of animal infestation

The animal should be placed on a sheet of newspaper and brushed down vigorously. Alternatively the bedding may be shaken into a plastic bag. The detritus should be examined directly by stereomicroscope or, after clearing in 10% KOH by flotation technique. Unfortunately, with the exception of scabies, acari are not easy to identify.

Fleas

Human parasitic skin reactions due to fleas are common. They range from the human type (pulex irritans) to cat, dog, rodent, hedgehog and rabbit, and fowl varieties. They are host-specific for breeding but not for feeding. The numbers of fleas and rate of maturation of all developmental stages are affected by warmth, humidity and darkness of their environment. Fleas lay eggs in the sleeping quarters of the host; the eggs hatch in two to 12 days; larvae live in floor crevices and under carpets and take nine to 200 days to pupate. The pupae take seven to 300 days to hatch out. The breeding cycle may be as short as two weeks or extend to 21 months. Minor disturbances, especially vibration, seem to stimulate emergence of mature fleas.

Fleas can survive for long periods in all stages of development with little or no food.

Flea bites

Groups of erythematous macules with a central punctum are commonly associated with weals and excoriation, but papules are most frequently seen. They may vary in number with differing degrees of erythema, from a few scattered lesions in linear pattern to a confluent papular eruption with much erythema and swelling of tissues.

Papular urticaria is a common sign of flea infestation in children, and is characterized by crops of weals (so-called hives) surrounded by inflammation and intensely itchy lesions, which may be excoriated and occasionally infected and pustular. New crops erupt as old ones fade. Perhaps the commonest picture is of isolated classic papules with lesions in all stages of development. In adults the papule is the common reaction; it may be extensive and present as papular prurigo. Lengthy exposure to infestation at all ages can lead to pigmentation, eczematization and secondary infection. Management is primarily of the host animal and its environment and is summarized in *Table 11.1*.

Lice

Lice are wingless, host-specific insects. Man can be infested by lice on the head (*Pediculosis humanus capitis*), on the body (*P. humanus corporis*), and in the pubic area (*Phthirus pubis*) (*Plate 11.9*).

Lice live on blood and pierce the skin with stylets. Their salivary secretion prevents blood coagulation. The female lives for a month and lays 12 eggs per day. The egg is attached to the base of a hair by a cement collar and its grain-like quality can be palpated between thumb and index finger. This differentiates the eggs of lice from scale. The eggs hatch and achieve maturity in approximately 21 days, and the life-cycle recommences.

P. capitis remains a major problem in spite of improved public health measures and better insecticides. No less than 10 per cent of children in urban areas are still said to be infested, and rural areas are little better. It is a golden rule to search the scalp hair for nits in any itchy dermatosis of the head, neck and chest, especially in females. Besides itching, there may be sores on the scalp, impetigo, secondary eczematization, and enlarged neck and occipital lymph nodes, together with a feeling of being dirty and lousy.

Treatment of *P. capitis*

Gamma benzene hexachloride BPC 1% cream (Lorexane) or 1% lotion (Quellada) should be massaged into the scalp and left for 24 hours, then washed off with a detergent cleansing shampoo. Nits

Table 11.1 Control—joint veterinary/medical/public health exercise

Fleas—life-cycle up to 21 months	**(A)** *Environment*
NB Adult can live for long periods away from host.	(1) Vacuum and burn debris
	(2) Change, wash or destroy bedding frequently
	(3) Use insecticide sprays and strips, e.g. flea collar, e.g. pyrethrum, malathion, dichlorphos
	(4) Use of flaked naphthalene or paradichlorbenzene (old insecticides—the latter is an active ingredient of moth balls)
	(5) Fumigation can be used, but is best avoided.
Dependent on host:	**(B)** *Host*
Impractical to shampoo cats or vacuum animals. Flea collars can cause contact reactions and are not very effective. Medical practitioners may not treat animals (*Vet. Act 1946*).	(1) Comb and brush animal and destroy combings
	(2) Shampoo dogs weekly for many weeks—1% Gamma BHC (Quellada) or 1% Bromocyclen (Alugan)
	(3) Powders, e.g. 12.5% Pyrethrum, usually combined with piperonyl butoxide. Pybuthrin (Wellcome), 3.5% Malathion powder (Taskil, Tasman Lab, Bury St Edmunds), organic phosphorus compound. 0.1% Gamma BHC
	(4) Use aerosol insecticides, e.g. organic phosphorus (Nuvan Top, Ciba-Geigy) Dichlorphos 0.2% ⎱ organic Fenitrothion 0.8% ⎰ phosphorus
	(5) Flea collars
	(C) *Patient*
	Crotamiton 10% cream or lotion. Calamine lotion with 1% phenol Antihistamines by mouth.

should be cleaned out with a special comb. Alternatively a malathion 0.5% lotion (Prioderm) or carbaryl 0.5% (Derbac) incorporated in a shampoo can be applied to the scalp, left on for 30 minutes and then cleansed out of the scalp with a detergent shampoo. In all cases the treatment should be repeated in seven days.

Effective management and control of pediculosis depends on the cooperation of the infested person, all members of the family, and other contacts, notably schoolmates. If at all possible supervised measures are desirable. It seems probable that ineffective management, apathy and lack of cooperation rather than resistant strains are responsible for the perpetuation of head lice.

P. pubis is a separate genus. The lice are broad and are visible as brown dots. They occur especially on pubic hair but may be present on eyebrows, eyelashes or axillae. Itching is invariable and there may be small red papules with a tiny central clot and intense local irritation, residual pigmentation, local or general urticaria, eczema and impetigo.

The same application as for *P. capitis* is used.

P. corporis is now rarely seen. The lice and eggs occur in the seams of clothing. The same application as for *P. capitis* is used but the clothing must be disinfested. A simple machine washing in detergent is adequate.

Other bites

There are great variations in individual susceptibility to the bites of gnats, mosquitoes or sandflies, and they are an especial problem to foreign travellers. To be effective, insect repellents must be applied widely and frequently; they tend to lose their potency in about four hours. A good application available in the form of 'wipes' (Smith & Nephew) contains 20% diethyl toluamide and 10% dimethyl phthallate.

When the subject has been bitten topical steroid creams are probably the most effective counter-inflammatory agent. Antihistamine creams are potent skin sensitizers, particularly with light exposure, and are not recommended. Antihistamine can be given orally, e.g. chlorpheniramine maleate (Piriton), promethazine hydrochlor (Phenergan), and brompheniramine maleate (Dimotane LA).

Bee and wasp sting reactions

Pain and minor reactions are commonplace. The more rapid the onset of symptoms the more severe the reaction is likely to be. The same seems to apply to the proximity of stings to the head and neck. The major problem is severe anaphylactic reaction after bee and wasp stings, and a patient with a record of increasingly severe reactions to successive stings should be advised to give up bee keeping.

Ampoules of adrenalin 1:1000/1 ml are no longer available for self-injection when anaphylaxis seems probable. Potential subjects might carry hydrocortisone for injection and tablets of prednisolone. Dermatologists are divided on the efficacy of desensitization. Skin tests can be done to confirm sensitivity. The vaccine should be administered commencing with a very weak dose. Some patients appear to be helped and desensitization can reassure the apprehensive patient.

12 Imported skin diseases

R. R. M. Harman
R. J. Cairns

Imported diseases which affect the skin come chiefly from the tropics and subtropics, are infective, treatable and above all important. They provide interest and challenge against a background of European skin complaints which are often of dubious aetiology, poorly responsive to treatment and may be relatively trivial.

Among the imported diseases largely confined to the skin are larva migrans, a number of mycoses including deep mycoses (mycetoma), as well as infestation with diptera larvae (myiasis) such as the Tumbu fly (cordylobiasis) and the burrowing flea *Tunga penetrans* (tungiasis or jiggers).

More serious and important to recognize are leprosy, mycobacterial ulceration (Buruli ulcer), African histoplasmosis, yaws, leishmaniasis, cutaneous amoebiasis, onchocerciasis, dracontiasis (guinea worm infestation) and both Bancroftian and Malayan filariasis.

The most frequently met and important conditions are described in this chapter, whilst a reference textbook on tropical dermatology may be consulted for information on the others.

Leprosy (Hansen's disease)

Leprosy is a chronic infective disease due to *Mycobacterium leprae*. Although it is difficult to diagnose in its earliest stages, the disease produces characteristic and sometimes mutilating effects in the later stages. The clinical manifestations are determined by the antigenic load and the individual pattern of immunological response to the infected person. In addition to the delicately balanced host-parasite relationship the course of the disease is influenced by race, and local factors, especially a low skin temperature, influence the distribution of the eruption. The protean manifestations of leprosy may first present in any department of a general hospital in any part of the world.

Mycobacterium leprae has fastidious micro-environmental requirements and is cultured only with difficulty in the armadillo or in thymectomized and irradiated mice.

Aetiology

The mode of transmission of the organism from person to person is unknown, but there is now strong evidence that it is acquired by nasal droplets from inhalation or ingestion rather than by prolonged bodily contact with a contagious case as used to be assumed. The incubation period is uncertain—probably ranging from six months to 20 years, with a usual range of four to seven years. The disease is sometimes acquired after only a brief stay in an endemic area. The incidence is related to poor socio-economic conditions and overcrowding rather than climate, and in these conditions familial cases are common. The disease is now most prevalent in tropical and subtropical regions and the physician should be alerted to the possibility of leprosy in any patient from an endemic area regardless of race. Once infection has occurred the organism invades Schwann cells ensheathing cutaneous nerves and in the absence of an effective defence mechanism the organisms proliferate and spread throughout the body. With high innate resistance a localized skin lesion (preleproma) may occur and then resolve with spontaneous cure of the disease.

Three main clinical types of leprosy are recognized: (1) tuberculoid, (2) borderline and (3) lepromatous. These are designated TT, BB and LL respectively (*see Table 12.1*). Intermediate types between tuberculoid and borderline are designated BT, and between borderline and lepromatous BL. The three major types represent three groups on the immunological spectrum of host-parasite resistance. In fact, BT and BL are commoner than the pure polar forms.

Tuberculoid leprosy

Because the tissue resistance to the invading organism is high—although not high enough to eliminate the organism—localized and self-limiting skin patches with a well marked cellular response appear. The lepromin test is positive. Areas 'out in the cold' such as the face, buttocks, extensor surfaces of the arms, are particularly affected. Tuberculoid lesions are usually scanty and asymmetrical. They appear as discrete, erythematous macules or plaques (*Plate 12.1*). The surface is dry, scaly, anhidrotic and anaesthetic. The centre is often depressed and hypopigmentation is a characteristic feature. In spreading lesions the hypopigmentation spreads in amoeboid pattern beyond the boundaries of the initial macule or plaque. Nerve involvement with neurological signs *within* the patches is another characteristic of tuberculoid leprosy. Thermal analgesia, anaesthesia and autonomic denervation are coterminous with the lesions and sometimes a tell-tale 'feeder nerve' can be detected by running the examining finger around the periphery of the lesion. Another feature is thickening of the 'cool nerves', the great auricular, ulnar and peroneal. These are best demonstrated by examination under oblique lighting and by careful palpation.

Table 12.1   Major types of leprosy

	Tuberculoid (TT)	*Borderline (BB)*	*Lepromatous (LL)*
Race	Indian	African	European, Eurasian and Chinese
Infectivity	None	Slight	Marked
Host resistance	High	Variable	Low
Course	Often self-limiting	Variable	Often progressive
Extent	Peripheral nerves, skin	Peripheral nerves, skin	Peripheral nerves, skin and RE system
Skin lesions	Often scanty Asymmetrical	Scanty to profuse Non-characteristic	Profuse Symmetrical
	Round, annular, oval, amoeboid Bright red	Arciform, annular or bizarre shaped Bright and dusky red	Diffuse infiltrate, nodules, plaques Dusky red
	Hypopigmented Dry scaly surface Well-defined margin	Hypopigmented Variable Ill-defined margin Well-defined 'notches'	Erythematous Shiny surface Ill-defined margin
	Anaesthesia confined to lesions	Variable sensory loss	Normal or anaesthesia not confined to lesions
Peripheral nerves	Early involvement Moderate Filaments	Early involvement Severe Filaments and trunks	Late involvement Moderate Trunks
	Unilateral Anaesthesia confined to lesions	Asymmetrical Non-diagnostic	Symmetrical Glove and stocking distribution
General examination	Normal findings	Normal findings	Hepatospleno-megaly γ globulin increase
Lepromin test	Positive	Weak positive or negative	Negative
Skin smear	Negative	Occasional bacilli	Many bacilli

Increased redness, tumidity and tenderness to percussion of the skin lesions indicate a so-called reversal reaction with increasing cell-mediated immunity and may herald spontaneous clearing of the skin. Neuropathy with cutaneous sensory denervation is the basis of the absent axon flare following stroking of the skin or histamine injection. Autonomic denervation causes absence of sweating and of pilo-erection after injection with pilocarpine or mecholyl.

Histological examination shows a non-caseating tuberculoid granuloma with foci of epithelioid cells, scanty giant cells and numerous lymphocytes. Bacilli are rarely found. The granuloma is situated in the upper dermis and the definitive perineural, perivascular and perisweat gland localization of the tuberculoid granuloma of leprosy helps to distinguish it from other dermal granulomas.

The diagnosis of tuberculoid leprosy is sometimes difficult: for example, a neurological presentation with peripheral neuropathy and ulceration of the digits, or a painless burn, may be the initial findings. Moreover, the patient with paraesthesia with normally brisk reflexes may be mistakenly diagnosed as an hysteric; in such an individual careful examination of the skin and the discovery of anaesthetic hypopigmented areas is a valuable aid to the diagnosis.

The differential diagnosis of scattered papules and plaques includes sarcoidosis, lupus vulgaris, tertiary syphilis, granuloma annulare and tinea circinata. Pityriasis alba, seborrhoeic eczema and tinea versicolor can sometimes cause diagnostic difficulties in patients from an endemic area. Plaques of follicular mucinosis can closely mimic tuberculoid leprosy because the infiltrated plaques may show some sensory loss, absent histamine flare and a negative mecholyl test. The *depigmentation*—i.e. total pigment loss—of vitiligo differs from the *hypopigmentation* of the anaesthetic patches of leprosy.

Borderline leprosy

Both in distribution and appearance the eruption of borderline leprosy is intermediate between tuberculoid and lepromatous leprosy. Nevertheless lesions with features of both tuberculoid and the lepromatous type sometimes coexist in the borderline disease which was formerly called dimorphous leprosy. Borderline leprosy is immunologically unstable and usually 'drifts' particularly to the lepromatous end of the spectrum. The lepromin test may be positive or negative; a change from positive to negative is particularly significant, heralding transformation towards the lepromatous disease (downgrading). An increase in cellular immunity towards the tuberculoid disease is termed a reversal reaction (*see Table 12.2*). Annular, arciform and gyrate plaques are characteristic; they are violaceous and the outer margin is ill-defined whereas the inner margin is usually clear-cut. This sharply defined central area of normal skin gives the plaques a 'punched out' appearance. Some loss of melanin is common and some slight loss of thermal and tactile sensation is usual. Neurological signs are often present, with nerve palsies based on leprous neuritis showing muscle wasting, foot-drop, etc.

The histology shows epithelioid cells and a few lymphocytes, admixed with small areas of foam cells.

Lepromatous leprosy

This is a widespread and progressive form of the disease, often with bacillaemia. The host response is minimal and the invading organisms proliferate unhindered throughout the body; hence large numbers of bacilli are found in the RE system of the bone marrow, liver, spleen and lymph nodes, as well as the skin. Ill-defined macules (sometimes scarcely visible), plaques and nodules (lepromas) are widely scattered symmetrically over the skin (*Plate 12.2*). The warm intertriginous zones are spared. The lesions are dull-red, shiny and commonly affect the face, where multiple oedematous plaques and nodules produce the characteristic leonine facies. Early infiltration of the eyebrows gives rise to alopecia, and ear lobe infiltration is also a feature. Hand involvement, with neurotrophic changes, is seen late in the disease. Sometimes nodules ulcerate and exude serum containing many leprosy bacilli. Similarly a highly infective nasal discharge from intranasal mucosal lesions contains many viable organisms.

The disease often follows a stormy course with febrile exacerbations (lepra fever) and the appearance of new lesions. Although the lepromin test is negative, vasculitic lesions characteristic of immune complex disease and autoimmune phenomena are sometimes encountered (erythema nodosum leprosum). Neurological manifestations appear late in lepromatous disease and the histological changes show little or no lymphocytic reaction, but groups of leprae cells (foam cells) containing large numbers of bacilli are found.

The diagnosis of lepromatous leprosy is confirmed by demonstrating acid fast bacilli using the slit skin smear technique (Wade test). Similarly nasal scrapings may reveal many acid fast organisms.

The differential diagnosis of lepromatous leprosy includes the following: lymphomas—mycosis fungoides, lymphatic leukaemia, lymphosarcoma; metabolic disease with cutaneous infiltrates—myxoedema, lichen myxoedematosus, lipoid proteinosis; granulomatous vascular disease—Wegener's granulomatosis and lymphomatoid granulomatosis.

Leprosy reactions

Two major types of reactions are seen in leprosy and each has an immunological basis. Ridley and Jopling denote these as Type I and II, and the characteristics of each type are shown in *Table 12.2*.

Lepromin test

The lepromin test is *not* used in diagnosis but only to aid the classification of the disease and to monitor the immunological status of the host.

Treatment

Tuberculoid leprosy is non-infectious and isolation is not required. Dapsone, 50–100 mg daily, is given for an initial period of two years.

Table 12.2 Types of leprosy reaction

Common usage	Reversal reaction	Downgrading reaction	Erythema nodosum reaction
Ridley–Jopling type	I	I	II
seen with	BB, BL, LL	BB, BL	BB, BL, LL
precipitated by	ALD*	Spontaneous infections, etc.	ALD*, pregnancy, infections, etc.
Clinical features			
existing lesions	red, oedematous	red, oedematous	no change
new lesions	none	rare	always
systemic upset	rare	rare	common
nerves	tender, swollen	tender, swollen	no change
Investigations			
blood	normal	normal	ESR ↑, γ globulin, leucocytosis antinuclear factor positive
	bacteraemia absent	bacteraemia absent	bacteraemia present
Histology			
organisms	rapid decrease	rapid increase	slow decrease
infiltrate	increased lymphocytes	decreased lymphocytes	LCA* and macrophage granuloma
Immunological mechanism	CMI*	CMI*	CMI* unchanged, immune complex disease
Treatment	reduce dapsone to 50 mg daily prednisone 30 mg daily for a few days	reduce dapsone to 50 mg daily prednisone 30 mg daily for a few days	dapsone 50 mg daily prednisone 20–60 mg daily clofazimine 300 mg daily
	nerve decompression	nerve decompression	?thalidomide, ?colchicine

* ALD—antileprosy drug, including dapsone, rifampicin
* CMI—cell mediated immunity, type IV, of Gell and Coombs' classification
* LCA—leucocytoclastic angiitis with neutrophil infiltration

Lepromatous leprosy requires isolation until the patient is non-infective. Due to the emergence of dapsone resistant strains on *M. leprae* monotherapy should be avoided. Rifampicin 600 mg daily for three to six weeks together with dapsone 100 mg is recommended. Dapsone 100 mg should be continued for life. Clofazimine 100 mg may be given on alternate days in addition. Attention is paid to the prevention of trophic ulcers; splints are required for nerve palsies and physiotherapy is important.

Prophylactic BCG inoculation may modify the host response in childhood by producing cross immunity, but its value in practice is not proven.

For the management of reaction states *see Table 12.2.*

Leishmaniasis

Three clinical forms of the disease due to morphologically identical protozoa are described:

(1) Cutaneous leishmaniasis—*Leishmania tropica.*
(2) American cutaneous and mucocutaneous leishmaniasis—*Leishmania braziliensis.*
(3) Visceral leishmaniasis (kala-azar)—*Leishmania donovani.*

A small proportion of patients with kala-azar develop the hypopigmented and erythematous macules and nodules of post-kala-azar dermal leishmaniasis.

The American forms are rarely met in Europe.

Cutaneous leishmaniasis (Oriental sore, Baghdad boil) *(Plate 12.3)*

This important disease is endemic in parts of the tropics and subtropics, especially in North Africa and the Middle East, causing much misery in children and scarring in adults. It is transmitted by sand fly bites (commonly *Phlebotomus papatasii*) which inoculate the easily bitten face, arms and hands. A variable time later ulcerating nodules 1–4 cm in diameter form with discharge and crusting. These are particularly distressing on the face; they progress for a few months and then tend to heal with unsightly cribriform scarring over the course of a year with the development of immunity.

Chronic cutaneous leishmaniasis (recidivans or lupoid) *(Plate 12.4)*

In about 10 per cent of cases of oriental sore a chronic lupoid stage develops. This often resembles lupus vulgaris clinically and histologically and is highly resistant to treatment. As in lupus vulgaris, no infecting organism can be found in the chronic granuloma.

Diagnosis

In the acute form smears are taken from the edge of a lesion and stained to demonstrate *Leishmania tropica.*

Cultures are also made on NNN medium. There will be a positive leishmanin intradermal test.

Treatment

Pentavalent antimonials still form the basis of treatment for all forms of leishmaniasis; but the effect of treatment in oriental sore is hard to discern and there is no agreement as to the best remedy in the lupoid form.

Claims for newer drugs such as metronidazole and rifampicin have not been substantiated.

Larva migrans (creeping or sandworm eruption) *(Plate 12.5)*

Larva migrans describes a distinctive eruption which has many causes. The essential features are that the lesions creep or migrate and that they are due to parasites moving in the skin. Visceral larva migrans also occurs due to human infestation with the common roundworms of dogs and cats *(Toxocara)*.

Parasitic migrating cutaneous eruptions are classified as follows:

(1) Larva migrans: *Ankylostoma braziliense, Ankylostoma caninum* and other roundworm species.
(2) Larva currens: *Strongyloides stercoralis*.
(3) Migratory myiasis: *Gasterophilus spp.* (horse bot fly), *Hypoderma spp.* (cattle warble fly).

Ankylostoma braziliense is the commonest cause of larva migrans in the Americas and the tropics. Dogs infested by these hookworms deposit ova in their faeces and the larvae which develop can penetrate human skin where there is direct contact. Favourable conditions for development are in sandy, moist ground and those who develop the eruption are usually holiday-makers who have been lying or walking on otherwise attractive tropical beaches, or builders and farm workers doing awkward jobs under out-buildings.

An irritant dermatitis may occur at the site of penetration of the larvae (ground itch) which, after a few days or months, begin to wander, causing intensely itchy moving pink serpentine patterns beneath an intact epidermis. Lesions may be single or wild tortuous patterns may develop. The larvae move erratically, 1–5 cm daily; secondary vesicular and crusting dermatitis with bacterial invasion due to scratching is common.

The disease is self-limiting and confined to the skin, for the larvae have entered a 'dead end' host and eventually die. Estimates of spontaneous cure times vary considerably.

Treatment

The traditional treatment is by freezing, using CO_2 snow, ethyl chloride spray or liquid nitrogen just ahead of the advancing burrows, but the effect of this is very doubtful.

Recently the topical application of thiabendazole suspension under occlusion has been found highly effective. Two per cent Gammexane cream and 25% piperazine ointment have also been used successfully.

Systemic thiabendazole though effective can have unpleasant side effects.

Larva currens

The rapidly moving tracks of larva currens due to the larvae of *Strongyloides stercoralis* are similar to those of larva migrans but move as far in half an hour as larva migrans does in a day. They tend to fan out from the anus onto the buttocks and back and are always accompanied by intestinal *Strongyloides* infection.

The giving of prednisone or immunosuppressives in strongyloidiasis can give rise to a fatal ulcerative enteritis.

Treatment is with systemic thiabendazole.

Migratory myiasis

Cutaneous myiasis is the infestation of the skin by fly larvae of the order *Diptera*. Many of these form painful furunculoid lesions or invade wounds but do not migrate and travel in the skin like the larvae of the horse bot fly or cattle warble fly.

Onchocerciasis (Blinding filariasis; river blindness)

Onchocerciasis is a filarial disease caused by the roundworm *Onchocerca volvulus*. In the New World it is known as *Onchocerca caecutiens*. The majority of the victims are in tropical Africa and Central America where the infestation causes endemic blindness in young adults as well as severe skin changes.

The disease is transmitted by *Simuliidae* (buffalo gnats) which inject infective larvae into the skin as they bite. The larvae mature into adult worms which reside in subcutaneous nodules (onchercomata) and form microfilarii. These migrate into the dermis in huge numbers. More seriously they also invade the eye causing keratitis, iritis, choroiditis and eventually blindness. They may also be found in lymphatics in small number but *not* in blood.

Endemic areas are close to streams where the *Simuliidae* breed and the earliest symptom is of widespread itching. Skin changes (onchodermatitis) progress to an extensive papular rash, sometimes with slight oedema. The worst affected areas are the shoulders, buttocks, thighs and upper arms (*Figure 12.1*). Lichenification, hyperpigmentation, drying, crusting, loss of elasticity due to dermal destruction and white scarring due to deep scratching slowly develop. In severe Negro cases 'hanging groins' (*Figure 12.2*) due to

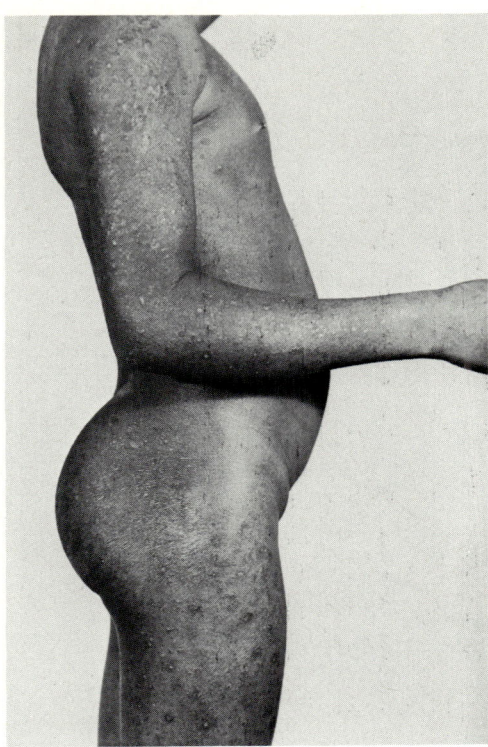

Figure 12.1 *Onchodermatitis (by courtesy of Professor Anezi Okoro, Enugu, Nigeria)*

this elastic loss, and gross spotty loss of pigment on shins and thighs are seen (onchocercal depigmentation, 'leopard skin').

Onchocercomata are mainly around the pelvic girdle and rib cage in Africa but on the skull in Central America.

Diagnosis

The diagnosis can be proved by demonstrating microfilaria under the microscope in skin snips taken from affected areas. The tip of a straight cutting needle is lightly inserted into thickened skin; this tip is then elevated while the body of the needle is held parallel with the skin so as to raise a little 'tent'. This is shaved off with a sharp blade without going so deep as to cause bleeding and the 'snip' is examined in a drop of saline under a coverslip. It may help to tease this out a little and the microfilariae can be seen swimming about close to it. There will also be positive filarial complement fixation and fluorescent antibody tests, leucocytosis and relative eosinophilia.

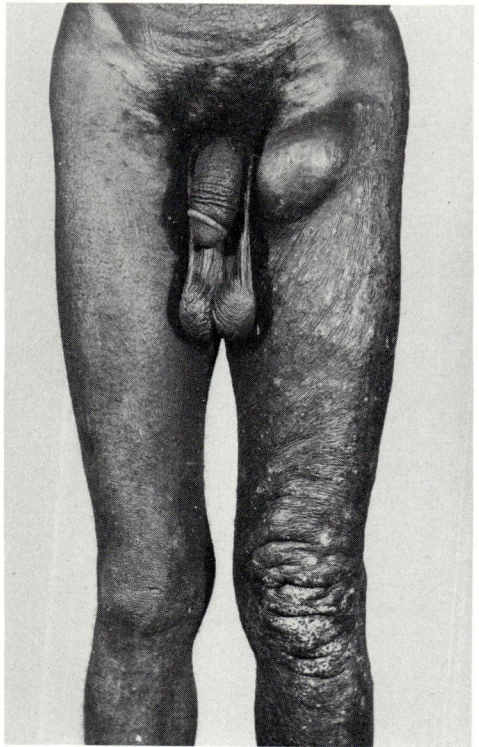

Figure 12.2   *Onchocerciasis—hanging groins and spotty depigmentation (by courtesy of Professor Anezi Okoro, Enugu, Nigeria)*

Treatment

Treatment is with repeated courses of Banocide (diethylcarbamazine). Suramin (BP) is a toxic intravenous drug which may be used with great caution to kill adult worms. Surgical removal of onchocercomata (nodulectomy) is also practised.

13 Bullous diseases

Martin Black
Martin James

The bullous diseases comprise a heterogeneous group of disorders with blistering at some stage of the disease process. The important bullous disorders are listed in *Table 13.1*. Only those diseases most frequently seen will be considered in this chapter.

Table 13.1 Classification of the bullous diseases

Relatively common	*Rare*
Bullous impetigo	Bullous ichthyosiform erythroderma
Bullous cellulitis	Epidermolysis bullosa
Bullous papular urticaria (insect bites)	Incontinentia pigmenti
Erythema multiforme	Mastocytosis
Bullous drug eruptions	Toxic epidermal necrolysis
Bullous eczematous eruptions (contact dermatitis)	Cicatricial pemphigoid
Bullous pemphigoid	Herpes gestationis
Dermatitis herpetiformis	Bullae associated with diabetes, lichen
The pemphigus group	planus, morphoea, lichen sclerosus et
Porphyria cutanea tarda	atrophicus, carcinoma, leukaemia and
	barbiturate overdose

The age of the patient, the history, the clinical examination, the histology of the early vesicles or bullae and the immunofluorescence findings in peribullous skin and serum will enable the correct diagnosis to be made in most cases. In recent years immunofluorescence (IF) techniques have greatly facilitated the diagnosis and classification of the major bullous diseases. Direct IF enables tissue fixed antibodies in the patient's skin biopsy to be detected. Indirect IF detects circulating antibodies in the patient's serum.

Epidermolysis bullosa (EB)

This rare group of inherited disorders is characterized by the early
onset of blistering of the skin following trauma (*see* Chapter 21).
Blistering is subepidermal in the dystrophic forms but more
superficial in the non-scarring types. The pathogenesis is unknown
but the absence of anchoring fibrils at the dermo-epidermal junction
may be important in the dystrophic types.

Clinical features

EB simplex (autosomal dominant) (*Figure 13.1*)

Trauma produces blisters on the palms and soles. Other sites of
friction may be affected particularly during the first year of life.
Lesions heal without scarring even in severe cases. Warm weather
exacerbates the disorder.

EB of hands and feet (Weber Cockayne) (autosomal dominant)

Trauma produces blisters on the feet in childhood or early adult life.
The hands may be involved. Scarring does not occur. Warm weather
exacerbates the disorder.

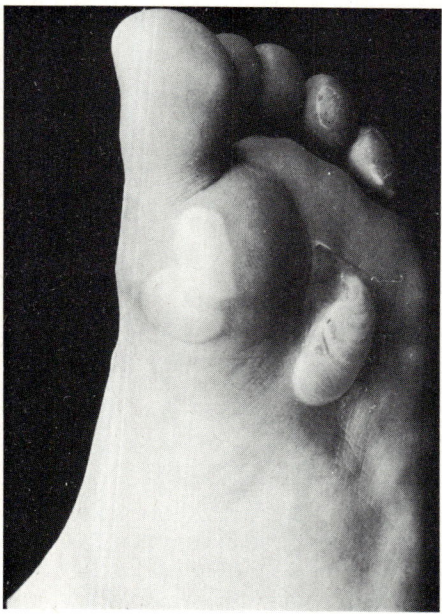

Figure 13.1 *Typical blistering of autosomal dominant epidermolysis bullosa
(Photograph by Dr F. M. Pope)*

EB dystrophica (autosomal dominant)

Patients usually present in the first year of life with bullae on the extensor surfaces of the limbs following trauma. These heal to leave scars which may contain numerous milial cysts. The nails are usually abnormal but involvement of the mucous membranes is uncommon. Improvement occurs with ageing.

EB dystrophica (autosomal recessive) (*Figure 13.2*)

Extensive, large, flaccid and haemorrhagic bullae appear on the skin or mucous membranes at birth or soon after. Scarring leads to pseudo-webbing of digits, loss of nails, a constricted mouth, oesophageal stricture and blindness. Eventually, squamous cell carcinoma and systemic amyloidosis may complicate the disease. Improvement with age may occur.

EB letalis (autosomal recessive)

Severe blistering of the skin with loss of nails occurs and is usually present at birth. Paradoxically, palms and soles are spared. The mucous membranes including the upper and lower gastrointestinal and respiratory tracts may be extensively involved. Early death is frequent though long-term survivors do occur.

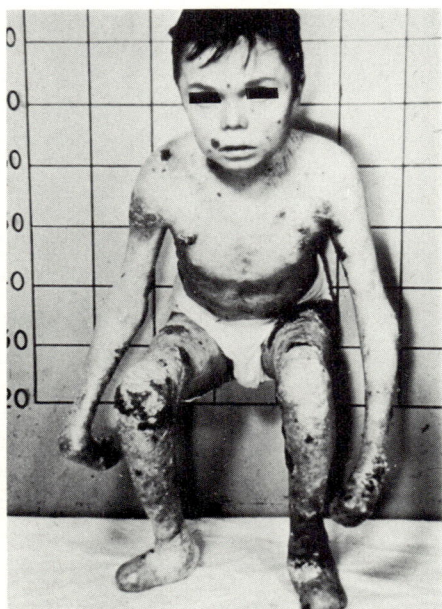

Figure 13.2 *Extensive mutilating fibrosis and contracture in patient with severe autosomal recessive dystrophic epidermolysis bullosa (Photograph by Dr F. M. Pope)*

Acquired EB

Patients present in adult life with the clinical picture of EB dystrophica. Investigations should be undertaken to exclude any underlying disease. The diseases which may be associated with acquired EB include Crohn's disease, ulcerative colitis, primary systemic cutaneous amyloidosis, myeloma, diabetes and drug reactions, notably to frusemide and penicillamine.

Treatment

Avoidance of trauma and control of secondary infection are important. High dose systemic steroids may limit scarring in the dystrophic types. Plastic surgery may be required. Genetic counselling is essential.

Benign familial pemphigus (Hailey–Hailey disease)

This is an autosomal dominantly inherited disease and despite its name is really quite unrelated to pemphigus. Immunofluorescence investigations are negative. In the second or third decade vesicles and bullae appear on the sides of the neck, axillae, groins and scalp. These rupture to form peripherally spreading erosions which heal to form flexural vegetations. Secondary infection, heat and sweating exacerbate the condition. Long remissions may occur and the prognosis is good.

Dermatitis herpetiformis (DH) (*Figure 13.3*)

Dermatitis herpetiformis is a pruritic vesiculo-bullous eruption which can affect any age group. Males are affected twice as often as females.

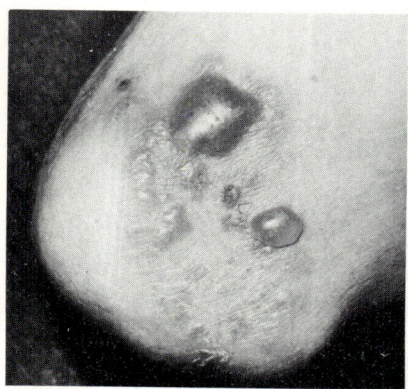

Figure 13.3 *Dermatitis herpetiformis—vesicles arising on the elbow*

Aetiology

The cause of DH is unknown. Genetic factors are now known to be important as between 80 and 90 per cent of patients are HLA-B8 and DW3 positive. Gluten sensitive enteropathy and DH are closely associated diseases. Relatives of patients with DH have a higher incidence of jejunal mucosal abnormalities than the normal population. An association with circulating autoantibodies, other autoimmune disease and the presence of immunoglobulin (IgA) in the skin raises the possibility of an autoimmune basis for this disease.

Histopathology *(Figure 3.6,* p. 31)

The earliest changes are of oedema, fibrin deposition and neutrophil invasion into the subepidermal papillary tips. Later, progressive oedema leads to subepidermal vesicle formation.

Immunofluorescence

Direct IF of uninvolved skin demonstrates granular deposits of IgA in papillary tips. In a few cases a linear deposition of IgA is seen along the basement membrane zone (BMZ).

Clinical features

Pruritic erythematous macules evolving into vesicles within 36 hours are the hallmark of this disease. Scratching removes the blister roof and relieves the itching. Thus, excoriations and scarring may be the principal physical signs. Clinical differentiation from eczema or scabies may at times be difficult. Inexplicably, ingestion of inorganic iodine salts may make the disease worse and it may be useful as a diagnostic pointer. The main sites of involvement are the elbows, buttocks and sacral area, shoulders and interscapular area, scalp, face, knees and thighs. Oral involvement is not uncommon. The eruption is usually symmetrical except in juveniles. DH in children usually starts after the age of five in contrast to juvenile pemphigoid which can start at an earlier age. The lesions often take on gyrate forms and are less symmetrical. The course of the disease does not differ from that of adult DH. Pruritic vesicles appear continuously though the disease does tend to wax and wane in severity. Natural remissions are unusual but may occur in a few patients after many years. DH is associated with an increased incidence of circulating antithyroid antibodies, antinuclear antibodies, splenic atrophy and diabetes.

Enteropathy

About 80 per cent of patients with DH have a gluten sensitive enteropathy similar to, though less severe than, that of coeliac disease. Jejunal biopsy will show partial or subtotal villous atrophy in a significant proportion of cases. The mucosal abnormality may be patchy and diminishes in severity towards the distal small bowel. Severe malabsorption is unusual, though increased faecal fat excretion and abnormal xylose excretion may be demonstrated. Decreased serum levels of calcium, folate and iron may occur but tend not to be associated with significant osteoporosis or anaemia. General malaise, tiredness, diarrhoea and weight loss may be the presenting features. A significant proportion of patients with DH have achlorhydria, atrophic gastritis and circulating gastric parietal cell antibodies, though intrinsic factor secretion is normal and overt pernicious anaemia seldom seen. Intestinal lymphomas may develop after many years. A gluten-free diet reverses the morphological and biochemical abnormalities in the small bowel. It is, however, a rather unpalatable diet and it seems justifiable to reserve it for those patients who are found to have clinical or biochemical evidence of malabsorption or those needing a large maintenance dose of dapsone.

Treatment

Dapsone in a dose of 100–150 mg/day stops the itching and blistering dramatically in 12–48 hours in most cases. A maintenance dose of between 50 and 200 mg/day is then required. Dapsone inhibits hyaluronidase activity, inhibits alternate complement pathway activation and stabilizes lysosomal membranes. It is not known if any of these properties are important in the control of DH.

Some authorities claim that a strict gluten-free diet may eventually enable the maintenance dose of dapsone required to control the disease to be lowered or occasionally discontinued. Side effects of dapsone are not uncommon. Sulph- and methaemoglobinaemia may occur soon after treatment is started, causing cyanosis and shortness of breath. Haemolytic anaemia is also an early side effect. Almost all patients have a reticulocytosis. Haemoglobin and reticulocyte count should be estimated at each visit. Rashes, including exfoliative dermatitits may occur. Rare but important side effects include agranulocytosis and peripheral motor polyneuropathy which are not always reversed by stopping dapsone.

Sulphapyridine, 1-3 g/day, is a useful alternative drug, especially in children who do not tolerate dapsone as well as adults. Methaemoglobinaemia, haemolytic anaemia, neutropenia and rashes are the principal side effects. Potent topical steroids suppress the disease locally and may be useful if serious side effects prevent the use of dapsone or sulphapyridine.

The pemphigoid group

This group of diseases has certain histological and immunopathological features in common. Their aetiology is unknown but an autoimmune pathogenesis is most likely.

Bullous pemphigoid (BP) (*Plate 13.1* and *Figure 13.4*)

This is a bullous dermatosis, often pruritic, most commonly affecting the elderly.

Histopathology (*Figure 3.5,* p. 31)

The characteristic lesion is a subepidermal bulla containing fibrin, eosinophils and neutrophils.

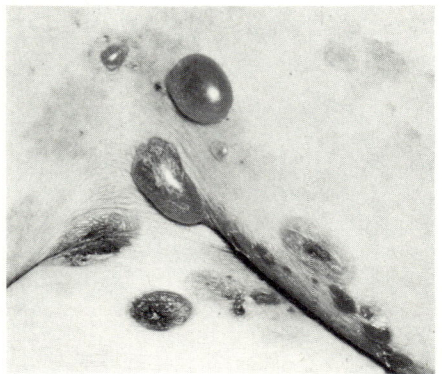

Figure 13.4 Bullous pemphigoid— tense bullae arising on erythematous skin

Immunofluorescence

Nearly all patients show linear BMZ fluorescence to IgG and C3 on direct IF of peribullous skin. About 70 per cent of patients have a circulating antibasement membrane antibody detectable by indirect IF. The titre does not usually parallel disease activity.

Clinical features

The disease may start as a pruritic erythematous or urticarial rash. Tense bullae eventually appear either on a figurate erythematous background or on normal appearing skin. Oral lesions are uncommon and not usually painful. The flexural aspects of the limbs and abdomen are the sites predominantly affected. The bullae heal without scarring. The disease is self limiting and lasts about two years on average. A possible association of bullous pemphigoid with internal malignancy has been postulated but recent evidence indicates that this is not so. Despite widespread blistering the patient's general condition is usually good.

Treatment

Systemic prednisone in a dose of 60–80 mg /day will control the disease in most cases and it can then be lowered to a maintenance dose of 10–20 mg/day. Topical steroids may control mild or localized disease. The use of immunosuppressive drugs such as azathioprine may enable the dose of steroid to be reduced. Occasionally pemphigoid will respond to dapsone. Periodically, steroid reduction should be attempted to establish whether a remission has occurred.

Cicatricial pemphigoid

This disease is largely confined to the elderly and affects the mucous membranes predominantly. Recurrent bullae occur in the mouth, eyes, pharynx, larynx and genital area. Bullae may occur on the skin in a peri-orificial situation and on the scalp. The latter lesions give rise to a scarring alopecia. Oesophageal, urethral and anal strictures, fusion of oral mucosal surfaces, conjunctival scarring (*Plate 13.2*) and blindness may result. The disease has little tendency for natural remission and may not respond completely to systemic steroids. Intraconjunctival steroid injections may be helpful.

Herpes gestationis (HG)

This is a rare pruritic bullous disease of pregnancy and the puerperium which histologically resembles pemphigoid. Direct IF demonstrates C3 and sometimes IgG along the BMZ. Indirect IF may demonstrate a circulating HG factor capable of fixing C3 at the BMZ. This factor can cross the placenta and cause an identical but self-limiting disease in the newborn. HG does not usually occur in the first pregnancy.

Itchy urticated papules, vesicles and bullae appear on the hands, feet, flexures and around the umbilicus in the second or third trimester. Skin lesions may become widespread and oral lesions may occur. The disease settles spontaneously within a few weeks post partum, only to reappear at an earlier stage in each succeeding pregnancy, with a tendency to become increasingly severe. Exacerbations may occur with each menstrual cycle or if the contraceptive pill is used. Systemic steroids and antipruritic drugs will control the disease.

The pemphigus group

This group of diseases has histological and immunopathological features which clearly distinguish it from the pemphigoid group. Evidence suggests that this group also has an autoimmune pathogenesis.

Pemphigus vulgaris *(Plate 13.3)*

This disease occurs equally in males and females in the 40 to 60 age group and is more commonly seen in Jews.

Aetiology

In almost all cases an antibody directed against a component of the intercellular space in the epidermis can be detected in the patient's serum. The pathogenic role of this antibody has been confirmed in animal and *in vitro* tissue culture experiments. The association of pemphigus with SLE, circulating antithyroid antibodies, myasthenia gravis and thymoma and an increased incidence of HLA–A10 and B13 provide further evidence for an autoimmune pathogenesis.

Histopathology *(Figure 3.3, p. 27)*

The early bullae are intraepidermal in situation. Suprabasal epithelial cells separate from one another, round off and lie singly or in clumps in the blister cavity (acantholysis). Exfoliative cytology of the base of an early blister (Tzanck smear) demonstrates clumps of acantholytic cells.

Immunofluorescence

Almost all cases show the presence of IgG and sometimes C3 in the epidermal intercellular space on direct IF of peribullous skin. Indirect IF usually demonstrates circulating intercellular antibody. Changes in antibody titre parallel disease activity and can be used to monitor response to treatment.

Clinical features

Over 50 per cent of cases present with painful oral ulceration several months before the generalized skin eruption occurs. At this stage it may be difficult to exclude aphthosis, lichen planus or cicatricial pemphigoid. Flaccid blisters appear on the skin and may remain localized for several months but eventually other areas become involved, especially the scalp, face, flexures and pressure areas. The thin roof of the blisters is rapidly broken. The lesions crust, bleed and spread peripherally whilst healing occurs centrally without scarring but leaving post-inflammatory hyperpigmentation. Laterally applied pressure at the site of an erosion or downward pressure on an intact blister produces lateral extension of the lesion (a positive Nikolsky sign). Without treatment the mucous membrane and skin involvement extend and death occurs in about two years.

Pemphigus vegetans

This rare disease is essentially a modified form of pemphigus vulgaris but it may start at an earlier age. Flexural lesions form large hypertrophic vegetative masses which become secondarily infected. Axillae, groins and perineum are the principal sites involved. Typical pemphigus vulgaris lesions can be found in the mouth and on other parts of the skin.

Pemphigus foliaceus (*Plate 13.4*)

Blistering is less often seen in this type of pemphigus as the split occurs higher in the epidermis and the roof of the blister is quickly broken. The patients usually present with scaly erosions of the scalp, face, chest and back simulating seborrhoeic dermatitis. Oral involvement is unusual. The prognosis is better than for pemphigus vulgaris.

Pemphigus erythematosus

Lupus erythematosus-like lesions occur on the face with features of pemphigus foliaceus elsewhere. The ANF may be positive. Direct IF of facial skin may show linear BMZ fluorescence to IgG typical of LE, as well as intercellular fluorescence.

Endemic pemphigus (Fego selvagem)

This type of pemphigus is found among children and young women in Brazil. It resembles pemphigus foliaceous and may be due to an infective agent.

Eosinophilic spongiosis

Although this is not a specific bullous disease, the term eosinophilic spongiosis is used because of the histological appearance of intra-epidermal abscesses containing eosinophils. Clinically it may resemble DH or pemphigoid but usually evolves into pemphigus. Most cases have IF findings typical of pemphigus even at a relatively early age.

Drug induced pemphigus

D-Penicillamine may cause a vesiculo-bullous process which clinically, histologically and immunologically cannot be distinguished from pemphigus, usually of the foliaceus type. Pemphigus has also been caused by rifampicin and phenylbutazone. The disease sometimes remits when the drug is stopped.

Treatment

Before the corticosteroid era mortality of patients with pemphigus vulgaris was almost invariable. The mortality now in all form of pemphigus is about 24 per cent (1960–1970), most of these deaths being due to side effects of steroids and/or cytotoxic drugs, especially infections and gastrointestinal bleeding. The initial dose of prednisone needed to control the disease is usually 100 mg/day or more and maintenance treatment may necessitate a dosage in excess of 20–30 mg/day. After several years the disease may remit spontaneously in some patients.

The use of azathioprine or methotrexate may allow the maintenance steroid dose to be reduced and these drugs are now being used with increasing frequency in conjunction with early steroid treatment.

Topical steroids may be useful for localized pemphigus foliaceus or benign familial pemphigus. Control of secondary infection is important in all types of pemphigus. Gold has also been used with some success. Excision and grafting of flexural lesions in pemphigus vegetans and benign familial pemphigus has sometimes led to prolonged remissions.

Erythema multiforme (EM) *(Figure 13.5)*

Erythema multiforme presents as a polymorphous erythematous vesiculobullous eruption which occurs at any age and is provoked by a number of agents.

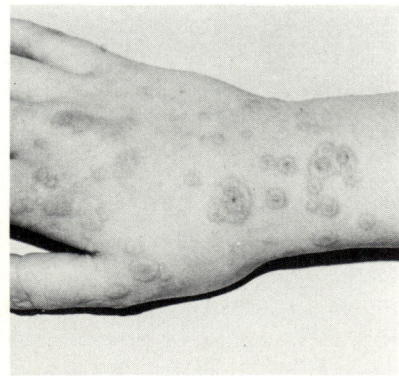

Figure 13.5 Erythema multiforme —target lesions on dorsum of hand and wrist

Aetiology

The cause of EM is unknown but it is thought to be a hypersensitivity reaction. In only about 50 per cent of cases can a likely provoking factor be found. The commonest prediposing causes are herpes simplex infections, mycoplasma infections and drug reactions, notably to co-trimoxazole, sulphonamides, phenylbutazone and barbiturates. Many other bacterial, viral and fungal infections can cause EM. Autoimmune diseases such as SLE, carcinomas and lymphomas, especially following radiotherapy, may also cause EM.

Histopathology

Histological changes vary from mild perivascular lymphocytic infiltration and dermal oedema to gross oedema and subepidermal bulla formation. Epidermal cell necrosis is an early feature and when severe, complete epidermal necrosis and ulceration occurs. IF investigations are negative.

Clinical features

The mildest form commonly occurs one to three weeks after a herpes simplex infection. Crops of erythematous macules erupt symmetrically on the dorsa of the hands, wrists, feet and around the knees and elbows. The lesions are 1–2 cm in diameter with an annular configuration (*Figure 13.3*, target or iris lesions). New lesions may continue to erupt for a few days but spontaneous recovery occurs in one to two weeks. Recurrent herpes simplex infections often provoke further attacks. In the more severe form the symmetrical acral lesions may be larger and become bullous. Oral involvement is common.

In the most severe form (Stevens–Johnson syndrome) (*Plate 13.5*) there may be preceding malaise, headache or sore throat before the rapid onset of fever, painful oral ulceration and a widespread maculopapular bullous EM eruption. Haemorrhagic crusts form on the vermilion of the lips, palate and buccal mucosa. The genital mucosa is often involved. Exudative conjunctivitis may eventually lead to corneal scarring and blindness. Lung, renal and joint involvement can occur. Death may result from this type of EM. Recovery usually takes several weeks.

Treatment

In the mildest form only symptomatic treatment is required. Mouth washes may help those with oral involvement. In the severe forms corticosteroids are thought to be beneficial but there is no evidence to suggest that these shorten the recovery time.

Toxic epidermal necrolysis (TEN) (Lyell's syndrome)

This disease is characterized by widespread desquamation of the epidermis and may occur at any age (*see Plate 8.6*).

Aetiology

Two types of TEN are recognized:

(1) The staphylococcal 'scalded skin' syndrome is caused by an epidermolytic toxin produced by the staphylococcus group 2, phage type 71. The pathogenic role of this toxin has been confirmed in human and animal experiments.

(2) Drug induced TEN is probably a hypersensitivity reaction caused by certain drugs, principally those which also cause erythema multiforme. This type of TEN is probably related to the severe form of EM, as are bullous drug eruptions (*Plates 23.2 and 23.3*).

In many cases no cause can be found and it must be classified as idiopathic.

Histopathology

In the staphylococcal scalded skin syndrome separation occurs at the level of the granular layer and acantholytic epithelial cells lie in the cleft. In drug induced TEN the basal epidermal cells are destroyed and inflammatory cells lie in the resultant cleft. Tzanck smear and frozen section histology of a blister roof may allow rapid differentiation between the two types.

Clinical features

Staphylococcal scalded skin syndrome

Infants and neonates are most commonly affected. Conjunctivitis, rhinorrhoea or impetigo with associated fever and malaise may precede the eruption by a few days. The skin of the face, flexures and trunk becomes erythematous and tender. Flaccid bullae appear and the Nikolsky sign may be positive. After a few days widespread sheeted desquamation of the epidermis occurs (resembling scalded skin) which rapidly heals in one to two weeks. Staphylococci may be isolated from the nasopharynx, skin, eyes or perineum. The mortality is low except in neonates. Treatment with antibiotics is essential. Corticosteroids do not help.

Drug induced TEN

Adults are more often affected. Conjunctival, oral or genital mucosal inflammation may precede the generalized rash. Flaccid bullae appear on erythematous skin, especially of the axillae and groins. The rash may remain localized but involvement of the whole body may lead to widespread desquamation of the epidermis, fluid and electrolyte imbalance and has a high mortality. Healing occurs in two to four weeks. Withdrawal of any provoking drug is essential. High dose corticosteroids should be given. Control of secondary infection and correction of fluid and electrolyte imbalance may be required.

Porphyria cutanea tarda (PCT)

This disease is due to an abnormality of porphyrin metabolism. Excess uroporphyrins and coproporphyrins derived from the liver are found in the urine. PCT may be precipitated by ethyl alcohol, oestrogen or chloroquine. Blisters appear on the sun exposed skin of the forehead and backs of hands following trauma and heal to leave scars and milial cysts. Periorbital hypertrichosis may be prominent. Many of the patients have cirrhosis and elevated total body iron stores. Phlebotomy is the treatment of choice and abstention from further alcohol ingestion is essential.

Bullous impetigo (*see* Chapter 8)

Bullae lasting a few days may appear during the course of impetigo. They are clear at first but rapidly become filled with pus and hypopyon formation may be apparent. This is the only type of impetigo found during the neonatal period. Antibiotics are curative.

Bullous papular urticaria (*see* Chapter 11)

Severe insect bite reactions may become bullous especially on the legs. They are often grouped and more typical papular urticarial lesions may also be present.

Bullous cellulitis (*see* Chapter 8)

Large, often haemorrhagic blisters may be seen with acute streptococcal cellulitis, particularly when the lower limbs are involved.

14 Hair and nails

Rodney Dawber

Hair and nails are synthesized by specialized groups of cells in the hair root and nail matrix respectively. Both are composed essentially of the same substance, the protein alpha-keratin, as in the stratum corneum. In fact, the cells producing hair and nail have a common origin embryologically being derived from the primitive epidermis that also forms the stratum corneum. Hair and nail keratin is hard and, unlike that of the stratum corneum, is produced without an intervening granular layer (stratum granulosum).

Hair

The characteristic covering of mammalian skin probably evolved as modified epidermal scales from reptiles. Though man no longer needs hair for survival, in health hair is an important organ of touch and the pattern of hair is important in the sexual and psychological sense.

Anatomy and physiology

Hair follicles with the capability to produce hair are found early in the human embryo. Follicles develop in a cephalocaudal direction; by the fifth month of development all areas have formed follicles except the palms and soles, which remain the only parts of the body without hair throughout life. Each primordial follicle forms a bud-like down-growth from the epidermis, the primary epithelial germ, which elongates and then canalizes, whilst a mesodermal condensation below the epithelial bud provides blood vessels for the future hair root.

Three types of hair are recognized. Primary or lanugo hair which first appears in fetal life is replaced *in utero* at about 32–36 weeks by secondary or vellus hair that characterizes post-natal life in all areas bar the scalp, eyebrows and eyelashes, where tertiary or terminal pigmented hair is found. At puberty, further terminal hair develops— the secondary sexual hair. This change is under the influence of androgens in both sexes. The final pattern of body hair is the result of interplay between racial, genetic and hormonal factors.

The hair follicle is in effect an invagination of the surface epithelium with the specialized inner root sheath and a germinal zone providing the cellular basis of the hair shaft by intense metabolic activity. The growing hair consists of six concentric cylinders of cells growing longitudinally towards the skin surface (*Figure 14.1*). The root sheaths probably exist to control the rate of movement of cells within them, i.e. the cuticle, cortex and medullary cells. The internal root sheath hardens before the layers inside it and it therefore defines the overall shape of the hair, i.e. normally a cylindrical tube of uniform bore.

All human hair undergoes cyclical periods of growth throughout life. Three stages are recognized: anagen, catagen and telogen (*Figure 14.2*). Anagen is the growing phase during which hair is synthesized. The duration of this stage determines the final length of the hair. Catagen is characterized by cessation of growth and involution of the follicle. Telogen is the resting phase which continues until the commencement of the next anagen; in this phase the root is club-shaped—easily seen by plucking hair, and it normally remains in the follicle until being displaced by a new anagen hair. However, scalp hair may be lost in telogen due to washing, combing, etc.

The growth phase on the scalp lasts from two to five years, whereas hair on the trunk, limbs and other areas grows for only four to six months. Unlike lower animals, in man the cycles of adjacent hairs are not synchronous. If this random or mosaic pattern of follicle activity is disturbed and local synchronization develops, then alopecia inevitably occurs when the hairs enter telogen.

The normal scalp has approximately 100 000 follicles with a normal daily loss of up to 100 hairs. Alopecia is clinically visible only when more than 25 per cent of terminal hairs are lost. In health, hair root analysis reveals approximately 85–95 per cent in anagen, 1 per cent in catagen and 4–14 per cent in the telogen phase. Anagen may last up to five years, catagen up to three weeks and telogen a maximum of four months.

The hair matrix or germinal epithelium is particularly susceptible to toxic influences during the growth phase. Thus x-irradiation, thalium salts and cytotoxic drugs induce sudden cessation of hair growth with loss of hair sometimes within days (anagen effluvium). If the injurious stimulus is less severe, e.g. malnutrition, fever, diabetic coma and anticoagulants, then hair diameter may decrease temporarily or more follicles are precipitated into telogen, i.e. greater hair loss will occur (telogen effluvium); this transformation to telogen is slower than anagen loss, the period between noxious stimulus and increased hair fall being approximately six to eight weeks.

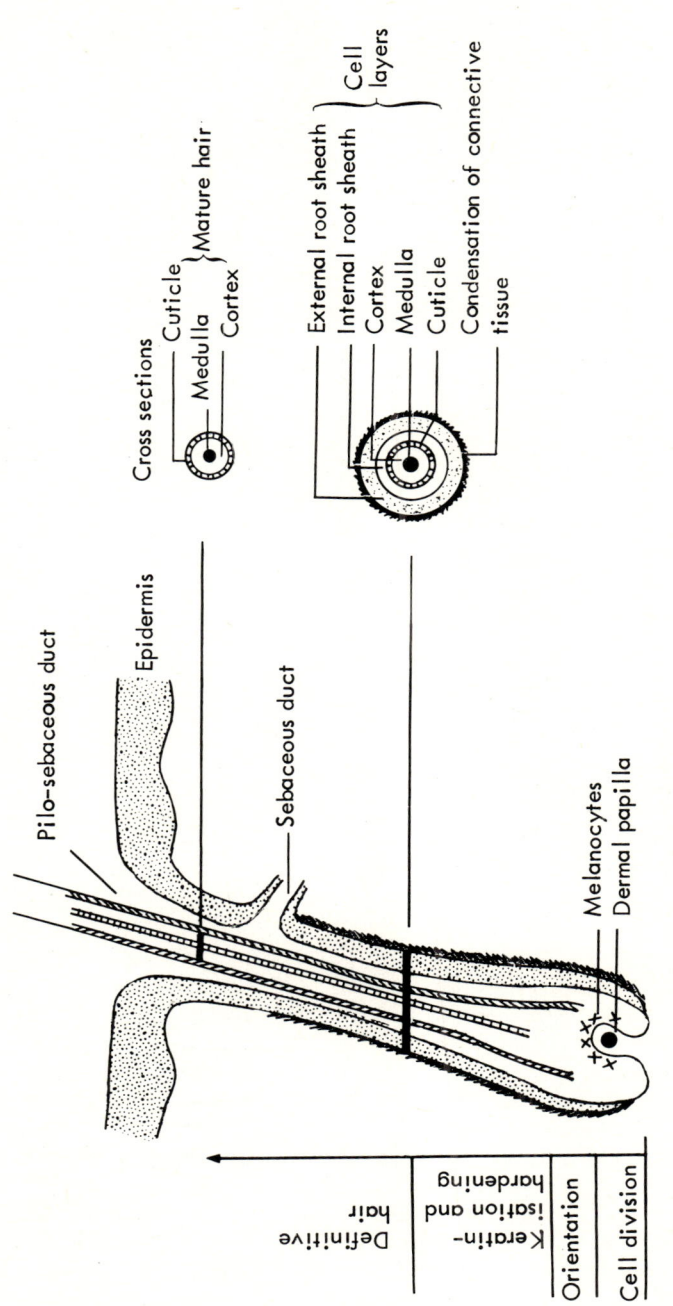

Cross sections

Cuticle
Medulla — } Mature hair
Cortex

External root sheath — } Cell
Internal root sheath — } layers
Cortex
Medulla
Cuticle
Condensation of connective tissue

Epidermis

Pilo-sebaceous duct

Sebaceous duct

Melanocytes
Dermal papilla

Definitive hair

Keratin-isation and hardening

Orientation

Cell division

Hair bulb

Figure 14.1   Structure of hair follicle in growing phase

157

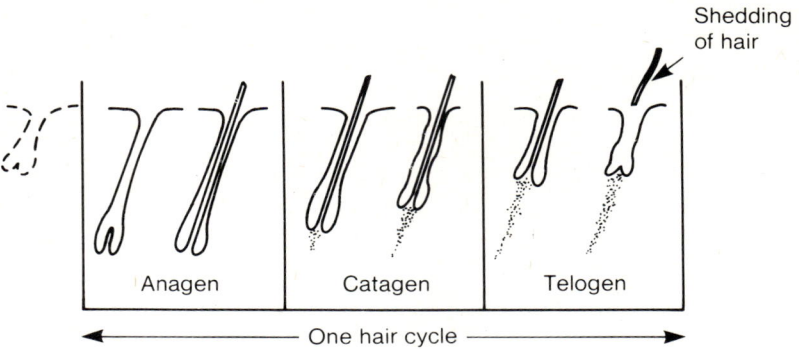

Figure 14.2 *Hair follicles during the hair cycle*

Alopecia

The term alopecia signifies loss of hair, though the complaint by the patient may be of increased shedding of hair, particularly after combing or washing, decreased density of hair or finer hair.

Congenital alopecia

Congenital alopecia is rare and may be part of a congenital ectodermal defect involving associated abnormalities of skin, nails and teeth. The hair is commonly short and sparse with no microscopic abnormalities; rarely specific shaft defects are found, such as monilethrix (beaded hair), pili torti (twisting), trichorrhexis nodosa (nodal fracture and fragility of hair) and pili annulati (banded hair). They are usually inherited as autosomal dominant traits (*see* Chapter 21).

Traumatic alopecia

The commonest form is seen in infancy affecting the occipital region from rubbing the head on the bed. Older children may twist, tug or rub localized areas of scalp hair causing it to break short. The abnormality is misnamed trichotillomania. In childhood and early adolescence it is no more than a habit and ceases spontaneously. In adult women this condition has a poor prognosis and often affects the whole of the vertex—'tonsure' trichotillomania (*Figure 14.3*); obvious psychological or psychiatric symptoms are the rule in this group.

Hair is a dead structure and consequently begins to degenerate ('weather') as soon as it leaves the scalp. The breakdown is normally so minimal that hair is able to attain its full anagen length. However, various procedures can exaggerate this weathering, causing the hair to fracture, break or be lost, e.g. over-zealous massage, bleaching, 'perming', or traction from a variety of styles, e.g. 'pony tails' and plaits, and cosmetic implements such as curlers; 'hot or cold' combing

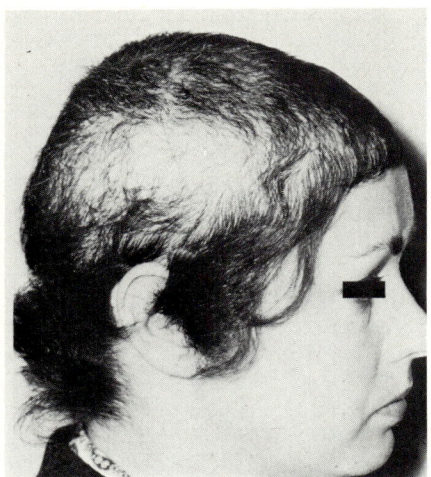

Figure 14.3   *Trichotillomania*

used to straighten negroid hair can damage both the hair and follicles with scarring of the treated areas.

Alopecia areata

Alopecia areata is the commonest form of alopecia seen in medical practice. Areas of patchy baldness occur on an otherwise normal scalp; other body hair is affected less often. Complete scalp loss is called alopecia totalis and loss of terminal hair from the whole body alopecia universalis.

The cause is unknown but a family history is elicited in 20–30 per cent of cases. Autoimmunity has been proposed because of the histological appearance of follicular infiltration with lymphocytes and the known association with autoimmune Addison's disease, thyrotoxicosis, hypothyroidism and pernicious anaemia. Vitiligo is also commonly associated. Emotional stress is frequently a precipitating factor.

Onset is usually sudden, hairs being shed over a circumscribed area; in the active areas diagnostic 'exclamation mark' hairs are seen. These are broken off hairs 2–8 mm long with a pigmented, wider distal part and a club root proximally. The bald areas are not hairless because close inspection reveals downy vellus hair over the whole surface. Because of the absence of symptoms, hairdressers often notice the hair loss before the patient. Characteristically only a single patch is seen initially but within a few weeks several patches appear on the scalp or also on sites such as eyebrows, eyelashes and beard area (*Plate 14.1*). Alopecia totalis and universalis are fortunately rare. Regrowth is usually evident within a few months but initially the new hair often lacks pigment.

It is impossible to give an accurate prognosis in the early stages. Adverse factors include prepubertal onset, universal hair loss, concurrent atopic eczema, a positive family history of alopecia areata and the presence of nail dystrophy, i.e. pitting or shedding of nails.

Differential diagnosis is from secondary syphilis which produces diffuse patchy scalp alopecia without exclamation mark hairs; other syphilitic stigmata are usually present and serology is positive. All other causes of patchy alopecia either have retained broken off hair over the affected areas or abnormal scalp, e.g. scaling in tinea capitis and loss of follicles in scarring alopecia.

No consistently successful curative treatment is known, though many agents can induce regrowth to a limited extent. Most cases with only a few inconspicuous bald patches have a good prognosis and reassurance alone is satisfactory. Of the treatments that give some regrowth, few can hope to maintain the improvement when they are stopped, i.e. the effects are only suppressive and temporary. It is therefore logical to limit treatment to the milder cases, i.e. those with the best prognosis, but few doctors adhere to this principle. Topical irritants, e.g. Trafuril, cantharidin and ultraviolet radiation therapy, and chemical induced contact dermatitis, e.g. dinitrochlorobenzene (DNCB) may help regrowth. Sedatives and hypnotics are frequently necessary since severe hair loss leads to considerable psychological problems which can precipitate further exacerbations. Topical, intralesional and oral steroids are advocated by many authorities and can often induce some regrowth; however the effect is usually only temporary.

Scarring alopecia

Discoid lupus erythematosus

Discoid lupus erythematosus is the main cause. Individual lesions are red, scaly and telangiectatic and later show atrophic changes as the patch enlarges. Plugs of keratin are typically seen protruding from follicular openings. The scales often show 'carpet tacking' and the presence of discoid lupus erythematosus on other sites, particularly the face, helps to confirm the diagnosis. Immunofluorescence techniques on biopsied tissue are useful in difficult cases, demonstrating under ultraviolet microscopy C3 complement and IgG deposited at the dermo-epidermal junction.

Lichen planus

Lichen planus, a follicular variant lichen planopilaris may present with scarred patches on the scalp and no lesions elsewhere. New lesions resemble 'old' lesions of discoid lupus erythematosus, i.e. central scarring with peripheral follicular keratotic plugs. Signs of lichen planus elsewhere aid diagnosis; histology is quite characteristic and immunofluorescence often shows IgM deposited at the dermo-epidermal junction. An appearance similar to scarring lichen planus can be seen as a side effect from treatment with gold salts.

Pseudopelade

Pseudopelade, a name coined by the French to differentiate it from alopecia areata, is a rare type of progressive scarring alopecia affecting the vertex of the scalp in adults, in men more than women. Multiple atrophic patches like 'white footprints' along the top of the head with no inflammatory signs present no diagnostic difficulty. Small areas of scarring eventually coalesce to produce disfiguring large cicatricial areas. No effective treatment is known.

Other diseases less commonly cause irreversible scarring of the scalp, including *localized scleroderma (Plate 14.2)*, *inflammatory fungal infections* and a chronic follicular staphylococcal disease termed *folliculitis decalvans*.

Hair in systemic disease

A variety of general diseases cause diffuse hair fall, mostly by precipitating many follicles into telogen. Systemic lupus erythematosus, syphilis, malignant disease, any fever and iron deficiency may induce this, as can various drugs such as anticoagulants, antithyroid drugs, high doses of vitamin A, selenium and amphetamines. Stopping such therapy, or treating the cause, is curative.

Hair in endocrine disease

The pattern of hair in each individual is governed by genetic, racial, familial and hormonal factors. Changes in the hair pattern, i.e. male type loss in women, and hirsutism, may be the earliest signs of adrenal, ovarian or pituitary disease.

Development of secondary sexual hair in both men and women depends on the presence of androgens. The female type, i.e. axillary and lower abdominal and genital pubic hair, is produced by adrenal androgens in both sexes, with a contribution by ovarian androgens in women. Men acquire greater hair development from the influence of testicular androgens. It is important to note that skin can manufacture more virilizing androgens, i.e. dihydrotestosterone from testosterone, mediated by the enzyme 5-alpha-reductase perhaps enhanced by prolactin. Interrelated endocrine factors are thus important determinants of the pattern of hair seen in adults.

The characteristic male pattern (common) baldness shows recession of the fronto-temporal region and thinning of the vertex. In severe examples loss may continue until only lateral temporal, parietal and lower occipital hair remains. The degree of loss is probably inherited as an autosomal dominant trait with decreased and variable penetrance. It never occurs in the absence of androgens, i.e. in eunuchs, or prepubertally, even with a strong family history. Females are probably protected from fully developing common baldness by oestrogens. However, women with a genetic predisposition, plus relative androgen excess, e.g. low androgen binding globulin or slightly raised circulating androgens may get a mild form. Most women presenting with diffuse alopecia are examples of the female type of common (androgenic) baldness. After the menopause the full male pattern of common baldness may occur due mainly to a progressive fall in oestrogen production (*Plate 14.3*).

In Addison's disease both pubic and axillary hair is scanty and the scalp hair normal. Myxoedema causes dry, brittle, lustreless often thin hair on the scalp with associated thinning of the eyebrows.

Hirsutism

This is defined as excessive growth of hair of male type and distribution in a woman. Excess hair is found on the face, arms, legs and trunk, often resulting in severe psychological disturbance. Most patients have no definable endocrine disease but minor hormonal changes may be detectable with recent refined investigations. Common baldness of the scalp may be associated with hirsutism.

The following types of hirsutism are recognized:

(1) Racial and constitutional cases with no overt clinical or laboratory abnormality. It is suggested that endorgan hypersensitivity causes this type.

(2) Defeminization. After the menopause or oophorectomy, loss of oestrogen leads to amenorrhoea and breast atrophy and frequently hirsutism with or without associated common baldness. The hair changes are probably due to a relative increase in androgen function with the falling oestrogen levels. No marked virilization is seen.

(3) Cortisol excess, due to pituitary or adrenal hyperfunction (tumour or hypertrophy) or glucocorticosteroid therapy causes hirsutism, obesity and a tendency to bruise. Urinary hydroxy-corticosteroids are raised.

(4) Adrenal virilization. In the adrenogenital syndrome, androgen/cortisol imbalance can occur due to a metabolic block in the synthetic pathway of adrenal corticosteroids. Androgenic influence causes seborrhoea, acne, male type alopecia, enlargement of the clitoris and hirsutism.

(5) Hirsutism is seen with drugs such as androgenic (anabolic) steroids, ACTH and testosterone.

(6) Ovarian virilization. In this group 17-oxogenic (ketosteroid) excretion is often normal. The commonest type is the polycystic ovary (Stein–Leventhal) syndrome of hirsutism, infertility, amenorrhoea and obesity; the ovaries may be palpable or only detectably enlarged at laparoscopy or laparotomy. This syndrome has been described without polycystic ovaries but still with increased ovarian androgen production detected by ovarian vein catheterization. Rare ovarian tumours including the arrhenoblastoma and hilar cell and lipid cell tumours may underlie ovarian virilization, as may the adrenal rest tumour.

(7) A cryptogenic group with no genetic, racial, familial or hormonal abnormality.

Clinical features in mild cases consist only of coarse, dark hairs on the upper lip and the nasolabial folds and less often the chin, the sides of the face, the breasts and chest presternally. The complete masculine pattern of secondary sexual hair may occur even in the absence of overt endocrine disease, i.e. as well as the above sites, terminal hair develops in the infraumbilical area, thighs, shins and forearms.

All patients presenting with hirsutism require careful endocrine investigation, in particular to assess adrenal, ovarian and pituitary function. The initial screen will depend on the clinical findings; serum cortisol and testosterone (and 5-alpha dihydrotestosterone, if possible), urinary 17-oxosteroid (ketosteroid) and 17-oxogenic steroid corticotrophin stimulation, dexamethasone suppression and meta-pyrone tests, androgen binding globulin and tissue 5-alpha-reductase may all be relevant, as well as air insufflation radiography to assess adrenal morphology. In selected cases laparoscopy or laparotomy will be indicated.

The majority of hirsute patients have no detectable specific endocrine disease. In general, women are revolted by the presence of 'excess' body hair and treatment of some sort is necessary. Most will be satisfied with the effect of some combination of bleaching, shaving, wax removal, hair remover, e.g. thioglycollates or electrolysis. Only a small minority need more specific medical treatment. Prednisolone 5 mg daily for six to nine months to inhibit adrenal function, combined with an oestrogen/antiandrogen regime, e.g. oestradiol valerate 1 mg/day plus cyproterone acetate 75 mg daily for 21 days of each menstrual cycle, always decreases the degree of pigmentation and amount of coarse hair on objective testing; however not many women are satisfied by the decrease in hair, and such hormones are potentially toxic, i.e. glucocorticosteroid (Cushingoid) side effects and cardiovascular occlusive disease may occur. Consequently only patients with severe hirsutism and its psychological consequences should receive treatment.

Hypertrichosis

Excessive growth of long, often apigmented hair can occur rarely in a wide variety of systemic disorders. It may occur in either sex and the hair distribution is not of the male type, though the face is often affected. Causes include disseminated neoplasia, visceral carcinoid syndrome, anorexia nervosa and drugs, e.g. hydantoinates, diazoxide, minoxidil and topical corticosteroids.

Hair colour and discoloration

Normal hair colour is due to melanin pigment: eumelanin in brown or black hair and phaeomelanin in red and blonde-haired individuals.

Cosmetically this may be bleached with hydrogen peroxide or dyed shades of brown to black using the dyes paraphenylenediamine (PPD) or paratoluenediamine (PTD); the greater the strength of PPD or PTD and the longer it is applied without neutralization, the blacker the hair becomes. Temporary rinses can now produce virtually any desired colour if the hair is light coloured or grey.

Greying hair (canities) is a physiological, senescent failure of melanocyte function. Premature greying, defined as significant colour loss before 20 years of age, is significantly associated with a tendency to pernicious anaemia, malabsorption syndrome and vitiligo. Focal congenital white hair (leucotrichia) may be inherited as a dominant trait, e.g. familial white forelock. It is a consistent physical sign in oculo-cutaneous albinism. Acquired patchy white locks can be caused by vitiligo and alopecia areata. Chloroquine, an antimalarial, may cause complete loss of hair colour.

The nail

The nail plate is a relative of the more grandiose claw of primitive mammals. The flattened nail plate of man probably represents only the dorsal elements of the claw, and the occasional contribution to the nail plate by the distal area of the nail bed, forming the so-called ventral nail, is interpreted as an atavistic relic.

The structure and terminology of the nail and surrounding tissues is seen in *Figure 14.4*. The germinative area, the nail matrix, is in

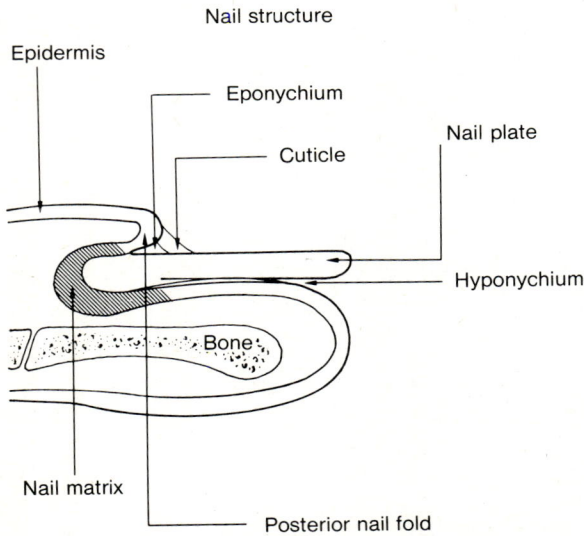

Nail structure

Figure 14.4 *Nail structure*

continuity with the epidermis of the dorsal skin, the nail bed and fingertip. The whole nail structure differentiates from the primitive epidermis *in utero* beginning in the ninth week; by the twentieth week nail growth (hard keratin) is well established. Complete nails are usually present at birth. During the first few months of life the nail plate is relatively thin, soft and flat, or even showing inverted curvature—spooning or koilonychia.

In health, fingernails grow at about 100 μm (0.1 mm)/day, i.e. approximately 1 cm/three months. Thus a distorted or avulsed nail may take up to a year to return completely to normal, particularly in old age, since nail growth decreases with age—from 200 μm/day in childhood to 40–50 μm/day at 80 years of age. Clinical observations suggest that the nail matrix has not functionally differentiated from the epidermis as completely as the hair follicle since the nail is frequently involved in diseases affecting the epidermis, e.g. psoriasis or hereditary ectodermal disease.

Congenital abnormalities

In cases of widespread ectodermal defect a variety of nail abnormalities may be seen, e.g. hidrotic ectodermal dysplasia causes either shortened atrophic or thickened nails; in anhidrotic ectodermal dysplasia excessive transverse curvature may be seen. Complete absence of nails (anonychia) rarely associated with absent patellae may be a dominant condition, as may congenital thickening (pachyonychia). Typically all ten digits will be affected in these disorders. Hereditary koilonychia often affects the 'working' nails most obviously, i.e. thumbs and index fingernails. In tuberose sclerosus (synonym: epiloia or adenoma sebaceum) fibromatous protrusions of the nail fold are common.

Traumatic disorders

Nail biting results in the loss of the free margin of the nail; in extreme cases over 70 per cent of each fingernail may be lost. Often one nail is bitten more than the others, while less often one will remain unbitten. Contrary to popular belief, nail biting is not related to psychological or psychiatric instability. Three to five per cent of adults are chronic nail biters, while more than 50 per cent of children are affected temporarily, usually for no more than one or two years. The habit should be ignored, since childhood nail biting rarely persists into adult life. The only factor that consistently 'cures' adults is the loss of natural teeth, since dentures are rarely 'subtle' enough to allow nail biting. Manual workers, e.g. bricklayers, suffer continual minor trauma to the nails which leads to an increased rate of nail growth (as with nail biting) and occasionally splinter haemorrhages.

Brittle nails usually occur in women and are due to frequent hydration and dehydration from immersion in water; the nails may break off terminally or split into layers. Similar changes sometimes occur due to exposure to chemicals such as alkalis, formalin, and degreasing agents. Terminal oncholysis, separation of the nail from the nail bed, may occur from the same insults.

Laddering, or multiple transverse ridges of one nail, usually a thumb (*Plate 14.4*), is caused by rubbing or pressing on the posterior nail fold of the affected thumb with the adjacent index fingernail. Affected individuals may not admit to inflicting the damage. Minor degrees of transverse ridging are very common and are due to over-zealous manicuring of the cuticle and posterior nail fold.

Nail infections

Acute paronychia

Acute paronychia is due to focal bacterial infection of the lateral or posterior nail fold. The commonest organism is *Staphylococcus aureus* and rarely streptococcus. Infection can only gain entry when the protective cuticle and eponychium is lost; nail biters are the commonest group affected. The nail fold becomes swollen, tender and painful; increasing amounts of pus accumulate in the paronychial space and lymphangitis may occur with regional lymphadenopathy. Very early cases respond to systemic antibiotic therapy alone but the majority require surgical incision and drainage.

Chronic paronychia

Chronic paronychia is common in those whose hands are frequently immersed in water, e.g. housewives, domestic and kitchen workers and nurses. The protective cuticle is always absent at the site of the inflammatory process due to hydration and minor trauma. The wet environment enables a variety of organisms to be carried into the paronychial space, particularly *Candida albicans*. The hydrated nail fold provides a magnificent substrate for the growth of organisms. The nail fold becomes progressively more swollen and the nail plate develops non-specific irregularities due to inflammation of the nail matrix. Intermittently focal symptoms and signs occur similar to acute paronychia and represent entry into the nail fold of virulent organisms: staphylococci, streptococci or *Candida albicans*; rarely *Pseudomonas pyocyanea* invasion occurs, causing the nail to become dark green, brown or even black. Specific antibacterial and antifungal agents only succeed if the affected fingers are kept scrupulously dry. In view of its broad spectrum, topical miconazole nitrate cream twice daily is the treatment of choice. Treatment should be continued until the nail fold thickening has remitted and the eponychium and cuticle have reformed. The latter structures prevent further infection.

Fungal infection

Fungal infection of the nails is discussed elsewhere (p. 108), as are *herpetic paronychia or whitlow* (p. 117) and *periungual virus warts* (p. 114).

Primary syphilis

Primary syphilis rarely occurs as a primary chancre of the nail fold; doctors and nurses are especially at risk. Atypical cases of acute (non-purulent) paronychia, particularly if induration and regional lymphadenopathy are present, should be investigated for syphilis (*see* p. 94).

The nail in skin disease

Eczema

Both exogenous and endogenous eczema may be accompanied by nail changes. In general exogenous eczema only causes nail signs when it is severe and affecting the terminal phalanges, whereas even mild endogenous eczema can be associated with severe nail disruption. The nail develops pits, typically few in number and larger than those in psoriasis, and varying degrees of irregular transverse troughs and ridges (*Plate 14.5*).

Psoriasis

Over 90 per cent of adult psoriatics develop nail signs at some stage of the disease. Such signs may rarely be the first or only evidence of psoriasis. Children are much less likely to have a nail dystrophy even when the psoriasis is severe. Pitting, onycholysis—patchy separation of the nail from the nail bed—and subungual thickening are seen frequently affecting all ten nails. Thickening is usually distal and more evident on the toe nails, while the pitting and separation are more obvious on the hands (*Plate 14.6*). No other disease exhibits this triad of signs though pitting may occur in eczema, alopecia areata and vitiligo; psoriatic pits are small ('thimble' pits), numerous and may be regimented into lines. Psoriatic onycholysis characteristically has a brown/pink margin to the white or yellow onycholytic areas. Fungal disease does not cause pitting and commonly only affects one or two toe nails. Psoriatic nail dystrophy fluctuates like psoriasis elsewhere. Routine psoriatic treatments are not successful when applied to nails because of failure to penetrate to the nail matrix or nail bed in adequate concentration. Temporary improvement may occur following the application of potent topical steroids for several months, e.g. Dermovate cream. Injecting steroids into the nail matrix using the dermajet or Porton pressure jet produces good early results in many patients, but relapse is general and atrophy is common at the site of injection. PUVA treatment is currently under evaluation in several centres and some good results have been reported.

Lichen planus

At least 10 per cent of patients with the common type of skin and oral lichen planus show nail changes, including longitudinal ridging, loss of lustre and brittle nails; typically all nails are affected. These changes eventually remit completely. Rarely nails may atrophy and become permanently scarred in atrophic lichen planus. As in psoriasis, the nail changes can be the sole presenting sign in lichen planus; nail biopsy shows specific and diagnostic microscopic findings as with lichen planus of the skin (p. 77).

Alopecia areata

Alopecia areata may be associated with diffuse pitting or shedding of nails. Similar findings can occur in vitiligo, with which alopecia areata is linked four times more frequently than expected by chance alone.

Other dermatoses

In systemic lupus erythematosus (SLE) and dermatomyositis (DM) nail fold capillaries at the cuticular base are abnormal, probably reflecting similar circulatory changes in other organs. In SLE the capillaries are classically tortuous like 'candelabra', while in DM they are longitudinally rigid like 'soldiers standing to attention' and associated with ragged cuticles. Subungal splinter haemorrhages are sometimes seen in SLE, bacterial endocarditis and trichinosis. Darier's disease and epidermolysis bullosa consistently show nail dystrophy. The nails become thickened, simulating fungal infection in Norwegian scabies; subungual debris is teeming with mites and ova.

The nail in systemic disease

Beau's lines appear as a transverse furrow on every nail associated with some episode of ill-health, e.g. fever or severe psychiatric shock. Similar factors may concurrently cause epidermal desquamation and hair changes, i.e. either telogen effluvium or a narrowing of hair fibres (Sims' nodes). Since nails grow approximately 1 cm/three months and hair 1 cm/month, it is possible to date an illness retrospectively by the position of Beau's lines or Sims' nodes.

Mee's lines are transverse white lines seen on the nail in arsenic poisoning. Broad white bands frequently occur across the nails in hypoalbuminaemia of whatever cause (*Figure 14.5*); the condition is immediately reversed on correcting the protein deficiency. The 'ground glass' white nails of cirrhosis are permanent.

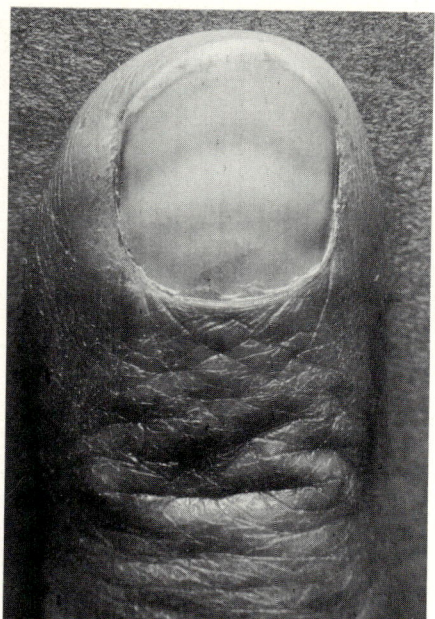

Figure 14.5 *Showing broad white horizontal nail bands as a result of hypoalbuminaemia*

Koilonychia (spoon nails) is seen in chronic iron deficiency anaemia, probably due to a failure to incorporate cystine-containing sulphur into the keratin molecule allowing natural pressures to reverse the convex curvature. Any factor which softens the nail plate may produce koilonychia, e.g. constant contact with industrial oils, Down's syndrome and chronic peripheral arterial disease.

Hyperthyroidism, and rarely hypothyroidism may cause patchy onycholysis (Plummer's nails), while hypoparathyroidism is frequently associated with candidal nail dystrophy. In the mucocutaneous candidosis syndromes a similar nail dystrophy is seen, often with concomitant iron deficiency.

Vascular disease

Chronic progressive arterial disease alters nail structure in relation to the severity of the circulatory occlusion. The mildest changes are an exaggeration of those of old age, i.e. thinning of the nails, longitudinal ridging and rarely koilonychia. In more severe arterial disease, e.g. Raynaud's disease and systemic sclerosis, the nails become increasingly atrophic (pterygium). Loss of the terminal phalanx and finger pulp in systemic sclerosis leads to curvature of the nail plate over the end of affected digits.

In the yellow nail syndrome (Samman's disease) slowed nail growth is associated with increasingly obvious greenish-yellow nail discol-

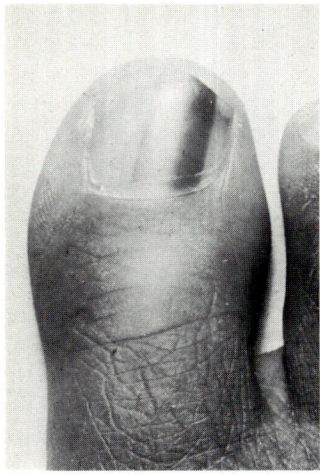

Figure 14.6   Showing longitudinal linear pigmentation as seen in Addison's disease

oration; individual nails may be shed. This disorder is accompanied by hypoplastic lymphatics which sometimes manifest as chronic lymphoedema. Chronic cryptogenic serous effusions, e.g. pleural or pericardial effusion, purulent chest disease and rarely hypothyroidism can occur, therefore the syndrome must be taken as a sign of internal disease.

   Addison's disease leads to widespread pigmentary signs which also affect the nails, causing diffuse nail pigmentation and rarely longitudinal linear pigmentation (*Figure 14.6*). The latter more often occurs as a naevoid change in dark-skinned races.

15 Skin colour and pigmentation

J. A. A. Hunter

Normal skin colour

Haemoglobin, oxyhaemoglobin, melanin and carotene are the pigments which give skin its colour. The pink appearance of the untanned Caucasoid is due to the reddish pigment oxyhaemoglobin in the blood within the capillary plexus of the superficial dermis. This colour can be partly obscured by the production of melanin in the overlying epidermis as occurs in suntanning. Melanin is, of course responsible for the various shades of brown seen in Negroids. Other hues are produced by the combination of these pigments with the fourth one, carotene, a yellow substance found in the subcutaneous fat and epidermis. There is no blue pigment and when this colour is seen it is due to either an optical effect involving normal pigments or the presence of an abnormal pigment.

Abnormal skin colour

An abnormal skin colour may be produced by either an imbalance in the proportion of these normal pigments as seen, for example, in cyanosis, naevus anaemicus, melanosis and carotenaemia, or an abnormal pigment (*Table 15.1*).

Sometimes it is not easy to distinguish the colours produced by different pigments. For example, the gingery brown colour produced by haemosiderin is often confused with the colour of melanin.

In practice most patients seek advice for a disorder of melanin pigmentation.

The melanocyte and melanogenesis

Melanin is produced in the skin by melanocytes seen mainly in the basal layer of the epidermis (*Figure 1.1*, p. 2). These specialized dendritic cells contain the enzyme tyrosinase (dopa oxidase) which initiates a complex sequence of reactions converting the substrate tyrosine, derived from the essential amino acid phenylalanine, to the

Table 15.1   Some pigments responsible for abnormal skin colour

Haemoglobin products		
Methaemoglobin	}	'Enterogenous cyanosis'
Sulphaemoglobin		
Carboxyhaemoglobin	Pink	
Bilirubin	}	Yellow to green
Biliverdin		
Haemosiderin	Brown	
Metals		
Gold	Chrysiasis	Blue-grey
Silver	Argyria	Blue-grey
Bismuth	Grey	
Drugs		
Mepacrine	Yellow	
Clofazimine	Red	
Phenothiazines	Blue-grey	
Tattoo pigments		
Carbon	Blue-black	
Cobalt	Blue	
Chrome	Green	
Cadmium	Yellow	
Mercury	Red	
Iron	Brown	

extremely stable and insoluble polymer melanin. Dihydroxyphenylalanine (dopa) is formed by the oxidation of tyrosine, and further enzyme action results in the formation of dopaquinone. Eumelanin, a brown or black pigment is then formed by random polymerization of dopaquinone with other intermediaries in the pathway.

As melanocytes are the only cells in the epidermis which contain tyrosinase they can be specifically demonstrated by the histochemical dopa reaction. Here skin is incubated in dopa and enzymic conversion of dopa to melanin occurs only in melanocytes, which appear as dark brown dendritic cells.

The colour of red hair is due to the pigment phaeomelanin. Its synthesis in the melanocyte is similar to that of eumelanin until the formation of dopaquinone. Cysteine then reacts with this intermediate and polymerization of cysteinyldopa with its derivatives forms phaeomelanin. It is probable that oxidation products of both dopa and cysteinyldopa intermesh in the formation of many melanins including human melanin.

Biochemical, ultrastructural and autoradiographic research has indicated that melanogenesis occurs in the melanocyte within discrete organelles called melanosomes. These tiny particles measure about $0.1\,\mu m \times 0.7\,\mu m$ and are shaped like rugby footballs. The melanin is laid down on a helical protein skeleton limited by a unit membrane. Eventually the fully melanized organelles pass into the dendritic process of the melanocyte and are then injected into, or ingested by, neighbouring keratinocytes where they are seen distributed in packets, or singly, throughout the cytoplasm. The melanocyte together with the group of keratinocytes which surround it and acquire its synthetic product have been called the 'epidermal melanin unit'.

There is no difference in the number of melanocytes between Negroids and Caucasoids. However, those in the Negroid produce more melanosomes and melanosomes which contain more melanin. The Negroid melanosomes tend to be slightly larger than those of the Caucasoid and fewer are packaged into melanosomal complexes when they are transferred to the keratinocyte. Melanosomal packaging appears to be a size dependent phenomenon. As these melanosomal complexes contain lysosomal enzymes Negroid melanosomes are broken down less quickly than those of the Caucasoid.

The control of melanogenesis

There is no doubt of the fundamental genetic basis of skin colour differences between and within races. The Negro who lives in Britain and the Caucasoid who settles in Africa remain respectively black and white. There is however some phenotypic variation in skin colour, for example to sun tanning. In fact genetic factors may influence numerous points in the process of melanin production by the melanocyte and melanosomal transfer to the keratinocytes. They could regulate events in melanoblast migration from the neural crest, melanocyte morphology, melanosomal structure, tyrosinase activity, types of melanin synthesized, melanin transfer to keratinocytes and melanosomal degradation within keratinocytes.

Ultraviolet irradiation affects primarily the melanocyte and surrounding keratinocytes of the epidermal melanin unit. Within five minutes of exposure to ultraviolet light there is some darkening of the skin probably due to the migration and redistribution of already existing melanosomes from basal to more superficial keratinocytes, and to an oxidization reaction occurring in the melanosomes which may convert them temporarily to more dense structures. This immediate pigment-darkening reaction, which lasts only for about 15 minutes after cessation of exposure, is mediated by long-wave ultraviolet light (UVA, 360 nm) and is responsible for the well known 'false tan'.

The more delayed process of *new* pigment formation begins some 24 hours after ultraviolet exposure. It depends on an increase in number of melanocytes, an increase in tyrosinase activity and melanosome production and an increase in transfer of new melanosomes to the surrounding keratinocytes in the epidermal melanin unit. It is mediated by medium wave ultraviolet light (UVB, 290–320 nm).

A neat intraepidermal control mechanism involving glutathione has been postulated. Reduced glutathione in the epidermis, produced by the action of glutathione reductase on glutathione, inhibits tyrosinase by combining with the copper present in the enzyme and by forming complexes with intermediates in the tyrosine to melanin pathway. Ultraviolet and some inflammatory skin conditions may cause pigmentation by oxidizing glutathione and blocking its inhibitory effect on melanogenesis.

Melanocytes produce more melanin under the influence of certain *pituitary melanotrophic hormones*. In man there appear to be only three such melanotrophic peptides, adrenocorticotrophin (ACTH), β-lipotrophin (β-LPH) and γ-lipotrophin (γ-LPH). All are produced in the same cells of the anterior pituitary. Their melanocyte stimulating activity is due to a common heptapeptide sequence at positions 4 to 10 in the amino acid chain. ACTH is the most biologically potent being about twice as strong as γ-LPH and five times more powerful than β-LPH. Recently it has been shown that β-melanocyte stimulating hormone (β-MSH) like immunoreactivity is an extraction artefact of the radioimmunoassay procedure (probably a cleavage product of both β- and γ-LPH) and is not a distinctive melanotrophic hormone. It appears that the melanotrophic hormones are not involved in the physiological control of pigmentation. Hypophysectomy does not cause Negroid skin to lighten and only large doses of ACTH, such as occur in pathological states, increase skin pigmentation. Melatonin has been isolated from human pineal glands but it has not been shown to produce skin lightening.

It seems likely that both oestrogens and progestogens have a melanocyte stimulating effect.

Disorders of melanin pigmentation

All forms of nosology have their drawbacks and the traditional classification which has been chosen here can be criticized on the grounds that it provides little information on the pathogenetic mechanism of the disorders. Nevertheless, it is suitable for clinical application. The conditions are conveniently grouped into those with decreased and those with increased pigmentation.

Decreased pigmentation (hypomelanosis)

Most conditions associated with a lack or loss of pigmentation are listed in *Table 15.2*.

Albinism

Melanocytes are present in this disorder but there is an inherited abnormality in their tyrosinase, resulting in depigmentation. Two forms exist; total (oculo-cutaneous albinism) inherited as an autosomal recessive, and partial (piebaldism) inherited as an autosomal dominant.

The whole skin is white in *oculo-cutaneous albinism* and there is

Table 15.2 Hypopigmentation (Leukoderma)

Genetic	Albinism (*see* Chapter 21)
	Piebaldism
	Phenylketonuria
	Vitiligo
	Tuberous sclerosis (Chapter 21)
	Chediak–Higashi syndrome (Chapter 21)
	Waardenburg syndrome (Chapter 21)
Endocrine	Hypopituitarism
Chemical	Pityriasis versicolor
	Substituted phenols
	Chloroquine
Post-inflammatory	Pityriasis alba
	Eczema
	Psoriasis
	Tuberculoid leprosy
Tumours	Halo naevus
	Malignant melanoma
Miscellaneous	Idiopathic guttate hypomelanosis

also a lack of pigment in the hair, iris and retinal epithelium. Affected individuals frequently have poor visual acuity, photophobia and a rotatory nystagmus. The hair bulb test, in which plucked hairs are incubated in dopa, distinguishes two types. Those in which the hair bulb turns black (tyrosinase positive) are less severely affected than tyrosinase negative individuals. The occurrence of lentigines, pigmented naevi and malignant melanomas provide clinical evidence for the presence of melanocytes. In the tropics these unfortunate individuals develop numerous skin tumours even when they are young, demonstrating the photoprotective effect of melanin.

Patients with *piebaldism* often have a white forelock of hair and patches of depigmentation distributed symmetrically on the limbs, trunk and central part of the face especially the chin. The depigmentation may improve with ageing.

Phenylketonuria

Phenylketonuria is a rare metabolic cause of depigmentation. Affected individuals often have a lighter complexion than non-affected family members. Blonde hair and blue eyes are characteristically, though not invariably, seen in this condition. The liver enzyme catalysing the hydroxylation of phenylalanine to tyrosine is absent. This amino acid and alternative metabolites accumulate causing damage to the brain during a phase of its rapid development just before and after birth. The skin signs are of minor importance in the diagnosis of the condition; if blood and urinary screening tests of the newborn are routinely performed they can alert suspicion. It is essential that treatment, with a low phenylalanine diet, is instituted as soon as possible to prevent further neurological damage.

Vitiligo

Vitiligo is a common form of depigmentation (*Plate 15.1*). The cause is unknown but occasionally there is familial clustering of the condition. There is also an association with other organ specific autoimmune diseases such as pernicious anaemia, diabetes, thyroid disorders and alopecia areata. Vitiligo may develop at any time in life but usually in the first three decades. Sometimes the onset follows emotional stress or physical trauma. Sharply marginated white patches, often with a hyperpigmented rim appear and enlarge. The patches are frequently symmetrical and sites of predilection include the flexures, around the body orifices, the backs of the hands and the skin overlying bony prominences.

Histologically a complete absence of melanocytes is seen within the depigmented patches.

Spontaneous repigmentation may occur but it is rare. When seen it usually stems from the hair follicles. Treatment is disappointing, but beneficial results have been reported with photochemotherapy. Psoralens are either applied locally or taken as a tablet. Shortly afterwards the involved patches are exposed to natural sunlight (if there is enough) or long wave ultraviolet irradiation (UVA) provided by an artificial source. Careful monitoring of the psoralen dose and the amount of ultraviolet is essential to avoid burning of the skin. If long-term treatment is initiated then the precautions taken should be similar to those suggested under the PUVA treatment of psoriasis (*see* Chapter 6). Local steroids have also been used in the treatment of vitiligo but the results are disappointing. Unfortunately less than 25 per cent of patients show an encouraging response to any form of treatment and the most important part of the management may be to warn the patient about excessive sun exposure. The use of a standard local sun barrier preparation may prevent unpleasant sunburn reactions. Preparations containing dihydroxyacetone ('artificial tans') and masking makeups may also disguise the disfigurement.

The skin signs of *hypopituitarism*, although of minor importance to the patient, may be typical enough to alert the astute physician of the diagnosis. There is thinning, or loss, of the sexual hair and the skin appears pale and atrophic. Characteristically the complexion acquires a pasty yellowish tinge. The hypopigmentation is due to decreased or absent pituitary melanotrophic hormones.

Pityriasis versicolor

Pityriasis versicolor (*Plate 9.12*) is remarkable in that it appears as discrete scaly light brown patches on the upper trunk of untanned subjects, but as depigmented areas compared with the surrounding sun-tanned skin after sun exposure. The yeast-like fungus, *Malassezia furfur*, apparently produces carboxylic acids which are toxic to melanocytes.

Some chemicals, especially the substituted phenols, cause depigmentation by a direct toxic effect on the melanocyte. For example depigmentation of the finger-tips has occurred in individuals contacting hydroquinone and related compounds used in the manufacture of rubber. This property may be put to advantage in the formulation of depigmenting preparations for the treatment of hyperpigmented disorders (p. 180).

Post-inflammatory depigmentation

Post-inflammatory depigmentation may be seen in the wake of some skin conditions. This is, of course, more of a problem in the skin of Negroids and Asians. Psoriasis (*see* Chapter 6) can cause quite dramatic depigmentation after resolution. The distinction between vitiligo and the depigmentation caused by leprosy (*see* Chapter 12) is an important one. Sensation is normal within a patch of vitiligo and the distribution of the lesions, follicular repigmentation and hyperpigmentation of the surrounding non-inflamed rim of the lesion may all help in confirming this diagnosis. Frequently there is an inflammatory element at the periphery of a hypopigmented patch of tuberculoid leprosy and the peripheral nerves may be enlarged and palpable.

Pityriasis alba

Pityriasis alba, a low grade eczematous process, seen often on the cheeks of infants, also causes some degree of depigmentation. There is fine scaling of the affected patch.

White hair (poliosis)

The activity of melanocytes in hair bulbs decreases with age with the result that grey and white hair is an almost universal sign of ageing in man. Localized patches of poliosis may be due to partial albinism, vitiligo, a halo naevus, alopecia areata (during regrowth phase) and irradiation with x-rays.

Hyperpigmented conditions

The most common disorders associated with hypermelanosis are listed in *Table 15.3*. Lentigines, pigmented naevi and tumours are considered in Chapter 18.

Freckles (ephelides)

Freckles (ephelides) are so common that description of these gingery brown mini-macules is hardly necessary. They are seen often in redheads, but also on the exposed skin of fair-haired individuals. They become more numerous and darken after sun exposure. Histologically there appear to be fewer melanocytes than in the surrounding skin, but the dopa reaction reveals that they are more active.

Table 15.3 Hyperpigmentation due to hypermelanosis

Genetic	Freckles
	Lentigines
	Café au lait macules
	Peutz–Jeghers syndrome
	Xeroderma pigmentosum
	Albright's syndrome
	Leopard syndrome
Endocrine	Pregnancy
	Addison's disease
	Cushing's syndrome
	Nelson's syndrome
	Ectopic ACTH syndrome
Metabolic	Liver disease
	Biliary cirrhosis
	Haemochromatosis
	Porphyria
	Hepatic cutaneous porphyria
	Erythropoietic porphyria
Nutritional	Kwashiorkor
	Pellagra
Drugs	ACTH and synthetic analogues
	Oestrogens and progesterones
	Psoralens
	Arsenic
	Fixed drug eruptions
Post-inflammatory	Lichen planus
	Eczema
	Herpes zoster
	Secondary syphilis
	Poikiloderma
	Systemic sclerosis
	Lichen and macular amyloidosis
Tumours	Pigmented naevi
	Malignant melanoma
	Mastocytosis

Café au lait macules

Café au lait macules (*Plate 15.2*) are distinctive brown areas measuring from 1 to 5 cm. Their presence, especially if there are more than five in an individual, may be an early sign of neurofibromatosis. These pigmented patches may also be seen in tuberous sclerosis though solitary lesions are frequently found in normal people.

The Peutz–Jegher's syndrome

The Peutz–Jegher's syndrome (*see Figure 21.6*, p. 309) is of interest only because the characteristic peri- and intra-oral macular pigmentation is associated with gastrointestinal polyposis. The macules are brown to black and even dark blue. Until recently malignant degeneration of the intestinal polypi was thought to be common but it is now appreciated that this is rare. Recurrent incomplete intussusception may occur.

Chloasma (melasma)

Chloasma (melasma) is a term used originally to describe any type of facial pigmentation, but now most often restricted to a type of patterned hyperpigmentation of the face occurring in pregnancy and when taking the oral contraceptive. It seems likely that oestrogens and progestogens are responsible and the circulating melanotrophic peptides are not raised. The pigmentation is more pronounced in summer but ultraviolet light is not essential as pigmentation also occurs on covered areas such as the nipples, abdominal midline and genitalia.

Hyperpigmentation may be most striking in Addison's disease. It may be generalized or limited to areas such as the body folds, skin creases of the palms, scars and buccal mucosa. The increased secretion of ACTH, with the melanocyte stimulating properties of the heptapeptide core, is the most likely cause. Other conditions (*see Table 15.3*) with increased endogenous ACTH production and the administration of ACTH and its synthetic analogues may also be associated with similar hyperpigmentation.

Formed *porphyrins*, uroporphyrins, are produced in excess in cutaneous hepatic porphyria and erythropoietic porphyria. These endogenous photosensitizers may cause hyperpigmentation on exposed areas but other features of photosensitivity such as blistering may be more obvious. Porphyrin precursors such as as porphobilinogen and delta aminolaevulinic acid (raised in acute intermittent porphyria) do not photosensitize.

Photosensitizing drugs

Photosensitizing drugs include the phenothiazines, sulphonamides, chloroquine, hydantoin, thiazides (*Plate 23.5*) and demethylchlortetracycline. Pigmentation on exposed areas may occur, but once again it is usually another sign of photosensitivity that brings the patient to the doctor. Psoralens are used in the photochemotherapy of psoriasis (*see* Chapter 6) and vitiligo. Dramatic pigmentation may be seen on the exposed areas.

Nowadays preparations containing arsenic are seldom used therapeutically but the pigmentation produced by them was most characteristic. Generalized bronze pigmentation occurred from one to 20 years after exposure to the drug, and scattered throughout the pigmented areas were small 'raindrop' spots of depigmentation.

Some cosmetics contain 5-methoxypsoralen in the form of oil of bergamot. This is a potent photosensitizer and may cause reticulate pigmentation, often on the side of the neck, at the site of application.

It is wise to remember that the male cosmetic industry (pre- and after-shaves etc.) is a thriving one.

Poikiloderma (*see* Chapter 22)

Poikiloderma is characterized by the triad of pigmentation, atrophy and telangiectasia. It is not a disease but a reaction pattern of multiple aetiology. Causes include x-irradiation, photocontact reactions, connective tissue and lymphoreticular disorders. Congenital variants also occur.

Hyperpigmentation may also be seen in the malabsorption syndrome and in *grave systemic illness* such as terminal cancer. The mechanism is not known.

Treatment of hyperpigmentation

The cause should be established and, if possible, eliminated. Occasionally patients request treatment for unsightly facial pigmentation for which a cause may not be evident. Similarly the hyperpigmented margins of a vitiliginous patch may cause cosmetic embarrassment. There have been good reports of the use of a depigmenting solution containing:

Hydroxyquinone	5%
Hydrocortisone BP	1%
Retinoic acid	0.1%
Butylated hydroxytoluene	0.5%
Polyethylene glycol	47%
Methylated spirit 74 op to	100%

The lotion is applied at night once to twice weekly and washed off in the morning. It is stable for only one month after constitution and should be kept in the dark at a low temperature.

16 The skin in systemic disease

R. J. Cairns
F. M. Pope

The importance of an accurate medical history and direct observation of the patient's skin combined with a full clinical examination cannot be over-emphasized. The history and examination remain of paramount importance despite the many complex and valuable diagnostic procedures that have become available in recent years. The history of course reveals the evolution of the disease and, combined with observation of the 'whole patient', provides an invaluable pointer to possible underlying disease manifested as a cutaneous disorder. The dermatologist is often in a better position than most clinicians to decide whether the cutaneous changes are diagnostic or only suggestive of internal disease, or merely coincidental. The diverse lesions and changes that may be encountered in the skin are shown in *Table 16.1*.

The skin in internal malignancy

The late features of visceral malignancy that include cachexia, pallor, melanotic pigmentation and cutaneous metastases (*see* p. 253) are well known. Other signs such as finger clubbing are well recognized and provide valuable guideposts and early warning, demanding a thorough examination for an occult neoplasm. However, not all physicians are acquainted with the non-metastatic manifestations of malignancy that may appear in the skin. For convenience of presentation many of these diverse cutaneous manifestations are discussed alphabetically.

Acanthosis nigricans

In this rare but distinctive disorder the skin becomes both pigmented and thickened in the flexures, notably the axillae, umbilicus and groins. Sometimes the skin darkening is generalized and the flexural thickening sufficient to cause rugosity. The palms become thickened with prominent dermal ridges, the so-called 'tripe palms' or 'velvet palms'. Warty lesions appear on the lips and tongue and eruptive skin tags are prominent on the neck, while florid seborrhoeic warts

Table 16.1   Major skin changes seen with systemic disease

Colour:
> Erythema, pallor, cyanosis, sallowness, jaundice, melanosis, hypopigmentation, depigmentation, haemosiderosis, blushing, flushing.

Texture and thickness:
> Dry, moist, coarse, smooth, thinning, thickening.

Exanthems:
> Morbilliform, rubelliform, scarlatiniform, pustular, eczematous.

Widespread and generalized dermatoses:
> Eczematous, erythroderma, toxic epidermal necrolysis, impetigo herpetiformis, migratory necrolytic erythema, acrodermatitis enteropathica.

Lesions resulting from scratching, rubbing, picking, pressure:
> Excoriations, prurigo, weals, lichenification, 'pick' ulcers, neurotrophic ulcers.

Vascular lesions:
> Urticaria, inflammatory purpura, haemorrhagic necrosis, anaemic infarcts, non-inflammatory purpura, bruising, ecchymoses, telangiectasis, livedo reticularis, ulcers, pyoderma gangrenosum, gangrene, oedema, lymphoedema, dilated veins.

Sweating:
> Hyperhidrosis, anhidrosis.

Hyperkeratosis and acanthoses:
> Xerosis, eczema craquelé, ichthyosis, acanthosis nigricans.

Nodules, plaques, cysts:
> Metabolic infiltrates, metastatic deposits, xanthomata, granulomas.

Scars, striae distensae, skin tags.

Changes in hair growth and distribution:
> Hypertrichosis, hirsutes, hypotrichosis, alopecia.

Nails:
> Onycholysis, discoloration, banding, subungual haemorrhage.

particularly on the arms and legs (Leser–Trélat sign) complete the clinical picture. When acanthosis nigricans first appears in a patient over the age of 40 a meticulous search must be made for internal cancer, particularly of the gastrointestinal tract. Acanthosis nigricans sometimes precedes the appearance of the neoplasm by several years.

Bullous eruptions

Certain bullous dermatoses may appear with visceral malignancy, but this could be an age association. The morphology of these dermatoses may resemble pemphigoid, or erythema multiforme. Thymoma is sometimes associated with the pemphigus type of eruption.

Cushing's syndrome

The clinical features are based on an excess of circulating corticotrophin of nonpituitary origin. Ectopic hormone production arises from adrenal or lung carcinoma.

Dermatomyositis (*see* Chapter 19)

Both dermatomyositis and its systemic counterpart polymyositis have an autoimmune basis. In an adult the antigenic stimulus responsible for the dermatomyositis is frequently an occult neoplasm. The common sites of such tumours include the gastrointestinal tract, ovary and uterus. Removal of the tumour often causes amelioration of the skin and muscle disorder and recrudescence of the tumour may be accompanied by the reappearance of dermatomyositis.

Erythroderma

This widespread dermatosis shows erythema and exfoliation (exfoliative dermatitis) and it is sometimes a presenting feature of a lymphoma such as Hodgkin's disease or mycosis fungoides and, less commonly, of visceral carcinoma.

Flushing attacks

These constitute a noticeable feature of a functioning carcinoid tumour of the intestine, bronchus or ovary. Attacks can be provoked by alcohol, over-breathing or injection of noradrenaline. They sometimes appear spontaneously and are probably prostaglandin mediated. By contrast the catecholamine producing tumours—the adrenal phaeochromocytoma and neuroblastoma—produce attacks of blanching, sweating and paroxysmal hypertension. The rarer adrenaline producing tumour produces vasodilatation, hypotension and even shock. Pancreatic insulinomas which may become malignant cause sweating by virtue of hypoglycaemia.

Gyrate eruptions

Gyrate erythemas particularly on the trunk sometimes appear with carcinoma of the lung (Gammel syndrome). A recently recognized characteristic eruption is seen with benign or malignant glucagonoma of the pancreas. The eruption is a migratory necrolytic erythema with superficial pustulation. Other features of the glucagonoma syndrome include anaemia, a red glazed tongue, diabetes and weight loss.

Hypertrichosis

What is sometimes termed 'malignant down' or hypertrichosis lanuginosa is a rare initial finding with an internal malignancy. Removal of the tumour is usually followed by clearing of the skin.

Intraepidermal epithelioma

Patches of Bowen's disease (Chapter 18) should always alert the clinician to the possibility of internal carcinoma. Lung cancer, hepatic, gastrointestinal and urinary tract malignancy should particularly be excluded. Many cases with combined skin and visceral carcinomas have an arsenical basis. Paget's disease (*see* Chapter 18) is another form of intraepithelial neoplasia which when affecting the nipple indicates underlying ductal carcinoma. The rare extramammary Paget's disease should lead to a careful search for an aprocrine or eccrine carcinoma in the underlying skin or for a distant visceral neoplasm.

Jaundice

A well-known initial finding in visceral malignancy, particularly with carcinoma of the pancreas, ampullary carcinoma and with carcinoma of the stomach with secondary deposits in the porta hepatis. Early jaundice may only be noticeable in the conjunctivae and early jaundice of the skin is easily missed in an artificial light.

Keratoses

Multiple wart-like lesions appear on the hands and feet in patients exposed to inorganic arsenic (*Figure 23.1,* p. 333). Such arsenical warts are premalignant and may coexist with hepatic or lung cancer of arsenical origin. A rare type of palmar keratosis is familial and associated with carcinoma of the oesophagus (Howel–Evans syndrome). Pearly palmar-plantar keratoses are a feature of Cowden's disease (*see Table 16.2*).

Lichen myxoedematosus

This rare scleroderma-like infiltration of the skin with mucin sometimes appears in patients with internal malignancy. A feature of this disorder is monoclonal gammopathy.

Another disorder associated with internal malignancy and mucinous infiltration of the skin is pachydermoperiostosis which shows extreme corrugation of the skin particularly on the forehead and clubbing of the fingers.

Melanosis

Melanotic darkening of the skin appears in severe cachetic states from adrenal insufficiency and with adrenal destruction from metastatic deposits. Individuals with widespread melanomatosis and circulating melanin pigment sometime show extreme darkening of the skin.

Nodules and plaques

Amyloid deposits may be the first finding in individuals with multiple myeloma. However, skin nodules are more often cutaneous metastases which are sometimes the first sign of a visceral tumour especially from gastrointestinal tract and kidney. Nodules appear as painless, discrete, freely movable lesions which may be solitary or multiple (*see* p. 252). Histological examination provides the diagnosis. A special type of secondary deposit in the scalp causes diagnostic difficulties; it appears as a pseudosclerotic patch with associated alopecia (alopecia neoplastica). The usual site of the primary is the breast. A secondary deposit in the umbilicus (Sister Joseph's module) usually arises from a primary gastric carcinoma. Nodules of the leg— lipolytic panniculitis—are sometimes a feature of carcinoma of the pancreas.

'Orange peel' skin

Permeation of the dermal lymphatics with carcinoma cells is the basis of this skin change. It is usually caused by carcinoma of the breast and the changes are seen in the affected breast and surrounding skin. Sometimes the skin becomes red and infiltrated resembling erysipelas (carcinoma erysipelatodes).

Pruritus

Although pruritus has many causes (*see* p. 188) itching is a common first symptom in patients with internal malignancy. Sometimes the basis is skin dryness or sideropenia; occasionally it is due to urticaria. Rubbing and scratching may lead to excoriations and prurigo papules. The label 'senile pruritus' should always be suspect and an intensive search should be made in such patients to exclude visceral malignancy.

Raynaud's syndrome

The sudden appearance of blanching attacks in an adult without any previous history should lead to a search for the presence of circulating cryoglobulins which may be a manifestation of myelopathy or lymphoma.

Seborrhoeic warts

These wart-like lesions are common in the general population. However, the sudden appearance of otherwise typical seborrhoeic warts, particularly on the limbs and when associated with pruritus, should lead to a careful search for internal malignancy (Leser–Trélat sign). The presence of skin tags and acanthosis nigricans completes the clinical picture. Sutton's naevi (halo naevi) appearing for the first time in an adult may be associated with pernicious anaemia which in turn may predate carcinoma of the stomach, and rarely halo naevi may first appear in association with malignant melanoma elsewhere.

Secondary sex changes

In the female the development of hirsutes, seborrhoea with acne and breast atrophy should lead to screening tests to determine the cause of virilization. Ovarian or adrenal tumours may be responsible for abnormal androgen production. It has been recognized recently that a pituitary prolactinoma may be associated with hirsutes and acne. The menses are normal, although these patients are often infertile.

Thrombophlebitis migrans

The association of this disorder with internal malignancy, particularly carcinoma of the pancreas, is now well recognized.

Urticaria

The appearance of urticaria presumably of autoimmune basis is sometimes associated with an internal tumour. Therefore the sudden appearance of urticaria in an elderly patient should alert the clinician, and a careful history and examination, with appropriate screening tests, are mandatory.

Vasculitis

Nodules resembling erythema nodosum sometimes appear with leukaemia or Hodgkin's disease. Histological examination is sometimes non-specific, showing only subacute vasculitis.

Waldenstrom's purpura

Purpura associated with macroglobulinaemia can be an initial finding in multiple myeloma.

X-ray burns

The higher incidence of leukaemia in patients with ankylosing spondylitis is well known. The mutagenic effect of radiation is responsible for the lymphoma. A patch of radiation atrophy (radiodermatitis) over the spinal region may draw attention to earlier radiotherapy.

Zoster (*Plate 10.9* and *Figure 10.1*, p. 119)

This is sometimes a presenting feature of Hodgkin's disease or leukaemia. It is also encountered with spinal tumours involving the dorsal root ganglia. With lymphomas immunological depression is usual and presumably results in reactivation of the zoster varicella virus. The skin lesions may be necrotic, haemorrhagic and sometimes widespread (zoster disseminata).

In addition to these numerous markers and early warnings of internal malignancy there are certain genetic and acquired diseases showing skin changes that should alert the clinician to the possibility of present or future malignancy. The genetic diseases causing non-lymphomatous malignancy are shown in *Table 16.2.* For the genetic diseases predisposing to lymphoma *see* p. 318.

Table 16.2   Developmental syndromes with internal malignancy

Disease	Skin and mucosal lesions*	Site of primary neoplasm
Cowden syndrome	Facial tricholemmomas, papules corners of lips, scrotal tongue, palmar keratoses	Breast, thyroid
Dyskeratosis congenita	Poikiloderma, buccal leucokeratoses	Oesophagus, rectum
Epiloia	Facial angiofibromas Lumbar 'shagreen' patches	Brain, lung, kidney
Fuerstein syndrome	Facial linear naevus	Brain
Gardner syndrome	Epidermal cysts, fibromas, osteomas, lipomas	Small gut especially ampullary region
Gorlin–Goltz syndrome	Multiple basal cell epitheliomas, cysts	Brain, meninges, jaw bones
Howel–Evans syndrome	Palmar-plantar diffuse hyperkeratosis	Buccal mucosa, oesophagus
Leiomyomatosis	Skin leiomyomata	Uterus, kidney (hypernephroma)
Mafucci syndrome	Haemangiomas	Bone
Neurocutaneous melanosis	Giant pigmented naevus	Meninges
Neurofibromatosis (Von Recklinghausen's disease)	Neurofibromatous nodules Cafe au lait patches	Brain, soft tissue (sarcoma) adrenal (phaeochromocytoma)
Oldfield syndrome	Sebaceous cysts of scalp	Colon
Peutz–Jegher syndrome	Multiple lentigines	Small gut, colon, ovary
Sipple syndrome	Mucosal neuromas, lingual labial and peri-anal	Thyroid, adrenal (phaeochromocytoma)
Torre syndrome	Sebaceous adenomas	Head, neck, visceral

* Skin lesions frequently antedate the internal malignancy

The skin and neurological disease

The developmental diseases with combined skin and central nervous system disorder are discussed elsewhere. Some primary neurological disorders exhibit certain characteristic cutaneous changes. The seborrhoeic facies of chronic Parkinsonism is easily recognized and the bullae on the legs and feet seen in patients with cerebral disease and barbiturate overdosage are well known. *Syringomyelia* produces a characteristic dissociated loss of skin sensation, sometimes with autonomic neuropathy and dry hands with nail dystrophy are common. Other rare acrodystrophic syndromes with combined sensory and autonomic loss affects the lower limbs. Burns, minor injuries and neurotrophic ulcers are frequently found.

Neurotrophic ulcers

Neurotrophic ulcers are seen only in anaesthetic skin. They appear as painless, persistent, non-inflammatory ulcers on sites of trauma and pressure. The ulcer first appears as a hyperkeratotic fissured area which soon becomes infected. A small sinus appears forming a cone-shaped ulcer with a narrow neck. Both the appearance of the ulcer and its location provide a clue to the diagnosis. Neurotrophic ulcers on the sole of the foot are seen with tabes dorsalis, diabetic neuropathy, leprosy and spinal tumours. Treatment is unsatisfactory and every effort must be made to relieve pressure and control secondary infection. The causative disease must receive appropriate treatment. In some instances surgical excision of the metatarsal head is helpful for recalcitrant plantar ulcers.

The presence of serious malformation of the vertebral column and lower spinal cord in children should be suspected with anomalies of the skin over the sacral region. These include coarse dark hair (faun tail), a small dimple or capillary haemangioma. If untreated the deformity may cause neurological damage to appear with growth of the child. Evidence of neurological complication includes lower limb weakness or incontinence. Surgical exploration following myelography may be necessary to prevent irreversible neurological damage.

Pruritus

Pruritus is a major symptom of many skin disease and its presence is of diagnostic value in distinguishing certain morphologically similar dermatoses. As a diagnostic label pruritus signifies that the symptom of itching is the primary complaint of the patient in the absence of any visible causative cutaneous disease. However, the skin often shows secondary changes, the result of rubbing and scratching, which lead to frictional and lacerative damage, excoriations, weals, papules or prurigo nodules. Once an itch-scratch-more-itch cycle becomes established it is usually self-perpetuating and difficult to break.

Whilst the severity of the noxious stimulus in the skin may be the same, the perception and the action differ widely in different subjects or in individuals at different times; some patients have a low itch threshold. It should also be remembered that recurrent pruritus may produce secondary psychological effects determined by the basic personality of the individual.

Aetiology

Many instances of pruritus are the result of environmental causes. Simple dehydration of the stratum corneum occurs in winter months from dry cold winds or central heating and in the summer from a dry desert-type environment. Such dry skin is pruritic. On the other hand, certain individuals suffer pruritus in high humidity because of an inefficient sweating mechanism. It is well known that many forms of particulate matter on the skin surface evoke a tickling or itching sensation. This is especially noticeable with foreign bodies such as glass fibre and certain ectoparasites such as *Acarus scabei*.

Certain pruritic dermatoses are associated with particular skin changes; thus lichenification tends to occur with atopic eczema, neurodermatitis and lichen planus. Weals are seen with urticaria and dermatitis herpetiformis. Linear excoriations and excoriated papules are common with scabies, dermatitis herpetiformis, the toxic eruption of pregnancy and cutaneous lymphomas. Linear purpura suggests a contact reaction from clothing although these lesions are also seen in drug-induced purpura and with lymphomata. The Koebner phenomenon is seen with lichen planus and psoriasis.

Many systemic diseases sometimes present as widespread pruritus. These include thyroid disease (both hyper- and hypothyroidism, and hypoparathyroidism) liver and renal disease, diabetes, internal malignancy and lymphomata. The infectious diseases, apart from rubella, varicella and hepatitis B infection, are not usually accompanied by pruritic eruptions. However, secondary syphilis in the Negro is often pruritic and pustular secondary lues is usually accompanied by itching.

Psychogenic pruritus

Psychogenic pruritus is not uncommon although usually confined to one or several small areas such as the anogenital region. Exacerbations occur at times of emotional stress and secondary lichenification is common. Deep excoriations and self-induced artefacts anywhere on the skin suggest the diagnosis of psychosis rather than psychoneurosis, and the prognosis must be guarded in these individuals.

Senile pruritus

Elderly patients sometime complain of intolerable itching for which no cause can be found. It should be remembered that in some instances pruritus is a symptom of early visceral malignancy, and careful examination and evaluation to rule out internal malignancy is important.

Diagnosis

A detailed history is important in evaluating the cause of pruritus. Attention should be paid to occupational exposure, the presence of other members of the household with similar symptoms and the geographical history of the patient is important because certain tropical diseases may present as pruritus many years after residence in the tropical zone has ceased. Again, questioning concerning the periodicity of the pruritus and any relationship to woollens, cold, emotion, etc. is valuable. Scabies is characteristically pruritic when the patient is warm in bed. The pruritus of polycythaemia and sarcoidosis is intensified by hot bathing. Similarly the pruritus of Hodgkin's disease and sarcoidosis may be exacerbated by alcohol. Pruritus evoked by heat, exertion or emotion may have a cholinergic basis.

Complete physical examination is directed to excluding any other systemic disease. The skin is examined minutely for evidence of skin disease with minimal physical signs; thus scabies may show very few papules or burrows. A tell-tale burrow under a ring or penile papules may give the clue to the diagnosis.

Investigations

Initial screening tests in patients with pruritus include full blood count, examination for abnormal cells, ESR, urine and stool examination and chest x-ray. Special investigations are directed to the study of liver, renal and thyroid function. Marrow examination and screening tests for autoimmune disease may be necessary. If malabsorption is suspected serum folate and fat balance studies may be necessary. Serum calcium, serum iron and examination directed towards revealing occult malignancy or lymphoma may be required.

Localized pruritus

Localized pruritus is commonly based on a local cause and the patient complains of a rash rather than itching. However, localized pruritus is sometimes the presenting feature and the physical signs may be minimal. *Pruritus of the scalp* is common with seborrhoeic eczema and psoriasis. Pediculosis capitis is sometimes overlooked. On other sites the important causes of itching are:

Auditory meati: eczema, neurodermatitis, psoriasis.
Eyelids: airborne irritants, allergens (dust or vapour), contact eczema from cosmetics, etc.
Nose: hay fever, intestinal worms, cerebral tumour.
Presternal: seborrhoeic eczema.
Nipples: scabies, atopic eczema.
Forearms: irritant and allergic contact eczema, actinic urticaria.
Fingers: contact eczema, scabies, glass fibre.
Legs: varicose veins, asteatosis, ectoparasitosis.

Treatment

Anogenital pruritus is discussed elsewhere.

When pruritus is due to environmental, cutaneous or systemic disease the treatment should be directed towards the primary cause.

Desiccation and asteatosis due to low humidity is often effectively treated by daily bathing followed by the application of an emollient cream or a urea-containing cream or lotion, such as Calmurid or Aquadrate. Palliative treatment of pruritus may pose a difficult therapeutic problem. In general, cool light clothing should be worn and evaporating lotions such as lin. calamine are helpful. Some patients benefit from 0.25% menthol in lin. calamine. Topical antihistamines and anaesthetic creams should be avoided because of the high risk of cutaneous sensitization. With skin dryness emollient baths are helpful—the patient baths once or twice daily using an oil such as Oilatum bath oil with Oilatum bar for skin cleansing. Promethazine (Phenergan) 25 mg at night or hydroxyzine (Atarax) 25 mg at night is useful in allaying irritation at night. Sometimes when the diagnosis is uncertain a therapeutic trial is valuable; thus if scabies is suspected but not confirmed appropriate treatment may relieve itching within a few days.

Endocrine disease

Abnormalities of endocrine function produce a wide range of changes in the skin. Alterations in cutaneous pigmentation and hair distribution are discussed elsewhere and the reader is referred to larger textbooks of general medicine or endocrinology for details of non-cutaneous features which are deliberately omitted here.

Cushing's disease

The face is round (moon face), the complexion ruddy (resembling rosacea) and the skin greasy with acne papules and pustules although, in contrast with adolescent acne, comedones are absent. Downy hypertrichosis on the trunk is found whilst an increased growth of coarse hairs is seen on the face and limbs. The skin is atrophic and purple striae, purpura and ecchymoses are common findings. Dermatomycosis from *Trichophyton rubrum* and tinea versicolor is commoner in these patients than in the normal population.

Acromegaly

The skin is coarse, thickened and greasy with dark terminal hairs notably on the face and limbs. Hyperhidrosis is usual and corrugation of the scalp (cutis verticis gyrata) is a rare but striking finding. Skin tags are usually present in excess on the neck and trunk, and veins are plainly visible on the hands.

Sheehan's syndrome

A rare disorder from a decrease of all pituitary function. The skin is pale, thin, soft and wrinkled. The facies appear wizened and the skin tans poorly. General thinning of the scalp, axillae and pubic hair is found and erythema ab igne (*Plate 19.1*) is commonly seen on the shins.

Hyperprolactinaemia

A recently recognized syndrome which may be due to excessive production of prolactin by the pituitary or from a prolactin secreting pituitary tumour. The cutaneous manifestations include hirsutes and mild acne. Although gynaecomastia and galactorrhoea are absent Montgomery's tubercles are usually present on the areaolae.

Hyperthyroidism

General hyperhidrosis, flushing of the face and warm, moist, tremulous hands are the usual findings. Widespread pruritus can occur and sometimes excoriations and prurigo may be the presenting features. Rarely pretibial myxoedema (*Plate 16.1*), thyroid acropachy and 'malignant exophthalmos' are encountered. Nail changes including distal onycholysis (Plummer's nails) are common. The hair is often velvety and sparse and sometimes widespread melanosis or melasma is found.

Hypothyroidism

The characteristic facies of myxoedema is general pallor with redness of the cheeks, the so-called 'strawberries and cream' complexion. The facial skin is thickened, dry and sometimes eczematous with 'bagginess' of the eyelids; the scalp hair is sparse and dry and there is general skin dryness with hypohidrosis. The skin is pruritic and may be excoriated. Some individuals show marked palmar and plantar hyperkeratosis; sometimes hyperkeratosis of the heels is a feature. The skin on the front of the shins can be dry simulating eczema craquelé and erythema ab igne is often present.

Pituitary hypothyroidism

In this disorder the skin is pale and thin, in marked contrast to myxoedema. Hair loss on the scalp is severe and thinning of the axillary and pubic hair is commonly encountered.

Hypothyroidism in children

This diagnosis in children is easily overlooked. The skin is pale, dry and covered with downy hairs (lanugo hypertrichosis) while the scalp hair is dull and coarse. Follicular hyperkeratosis may be marked on the limbs and thus any child with xeroderma or keratosis pilaris should be checked for thyroid deficiency.

Hypoparathyroidism

The skin changes resemble those seen in hypothyroidism: the skin is dry, rough and scaly, whilst the scalp hair is sparse and dry; early cataract and epilepsy are encountered; oral candidiasis, paronchia and nail infection are often present; nail dystrophy is common. Hyperkeratotic candidal infection on the palms and soles closely resembles *Trichophyton rubrum* infection. A widespread pustular dermatosis, impetigo herpetiformis, is sometimes the presenting feature of the acute disease; it may proceed to an exfoliative dermatitis.

Diabetes mellitus

Skin changes sometime herald the onset of the disease. Genital pruritus is a frequent initial symptom. Bacterial infections, notably staphylococcal folliculitis, boils and carbuncles, recurrent erysipelas and erythrasma are common in diabetics. Likewise, fungal infections are commoner in diabetics than in the non-diabetic population. The presence of candidiasis should always lead the clinician to exclude diabetes because vulvitis, vaginitis, balanitis, intertrigo and paronychia are well-known first findings of the disease. Vascular disorders which include lipoid necrobiosis, arteriosclerosis of the coronary and limb vessels, are common in diabetics. *Lipoid necrobiosis* appears as a yellow shiny waxy infiltrated plaque on the shin; the appearance resembles glazed porcelain (*Plate 16.2*). The edge of the plaque often shows marked infiltration and telangiectatic vessels. With peripheral extension the central area of the patch becomes atrophic and sometimes ulcerates. Other findings in diabetics include diabetic dermopathy, neurotrophic ulcers (from peripheral neuropathy), bullae and eruptive xanthomata from hypertriglyceridaemia.

Addison's disease

The melanosis on light exposed area, in the flexural regions and buccal mucosae is well known. The axillary and pubic hair is sparse and vitiligo is common. In some patients a presenting feature is darkening of the hair and darkening of pigmented naevi and scars (*see Table 16.3*).

Table 16.3   Skin changes in Addison's disease

Widespread melanosis	Traumatic melanosis, e.g. friction from clothing, belts, straps, etc.
Darkening of scalp hair	Thinning of axillary, pubic hair
Darkening of palmar creases and knuckles	Dirty hands (excessive hand washing)
Darkening of scars	Longitudinal bands on nails
Darkening of naevi	Darkening of nipples
Persistent suntan	Unmasking of vitiligo
Xerosis	Salty sweat

Virilizing adrenal and ovarian tumours

In the female both types of tumour may produce androgens with marked hirsutes affecting the chin, chest and limbs. Seborrhoea, acne vulgaris and the male pattern of alopecia is common with severe virilization. Atrophy of the breasts, clitoromegaly and deepening of the voice is also noted. Similar features are present with the androgenital syndrome when androgenic excess results from a metabolic defect in steroid synthesis.

Hypogonadism

In the male the skin is fine, pale and suntans poorly; the growth of beard hair is greatly diminished; the axillary and pubic hair is thin or absent. The male type of baldness is unknown in eunuchs.

Phaeochromocytoma

This tumour secretes an excess of noradrenalin or adrenalin. When noradrenalin production is predominant hypertension, intermittent sweating and pilo-erection ('goose pimples') are sometimes present. Livedo reticularis is often marked. With an adrenalin-producing tumour flushing and hypotension may present as paroxysmal attacks. In extreme cases the patients may pass into shock.

Nutritional disorders

Tissue malnutrition results from poor food intake, malabsorption, malretention or hypermetabolism.

Malabsorption syndrome

The diverse skin manifestations seen with malabsorption depend on varying degrees of malabsorption of fat, fat-soluble vitamins, carbohydrates, proteins and minerals. The usual features found with gluten sensitive enteropathy include pallor, diffuse melanosis, follicular hyperkeratosis, petechiae and ecchymoses. A widespread seborrhoeic-like eczema may be present. Other skin changes includes xeroderma, pellagra, prurigo and candidal intertrigo. Protein deficiency causes oedema and a kwashiorkor-like dermatosis. Other special syndromes are dependent upon malabsorption of particular minerals. Extreme calcium deficiency may provoke impetigo herpetiformis whilst iron deficiency produces anaemia, alopecia and pruritus. Various vitamin deficiencies will not be detailed here and the reader is referred to a larger textbook.

In malabsorption the scalp hair is usually fine and sparse, and shows early greying. The nails may be clubbed or show koilonychia; transverse banding or longtitudinal pigmentation may be present. Mucosal changes may first draw attention to the possibility of malabsorption with angular cheilitis, oral candidiasis, aphthous ulceration or stomatitis. It should be remembered that any patient with a recalcitrant endogenous eczema, particularly if it is pruritic and heals with post-inflammatory melanosis, may have malabsorption.

Pellagra

Pellagra is exceptionally encountered in individuals taking a normal diet, when it is likely to be due to malabsorption. However, certain drugs such as isonicotinic acid hydrazide cause pellagra. It is also seen from the metabolic deviation of nicotinic acid synthesis from tryptophan as in Hartnup disease and with carcinoid tumours. The classic clinical features include the three Ds: dermatitis, diarrhoea and dementia. To these may be added three further Ds characterizing the dermatosis: the dermatosis appears on light exposed areas and patches of pellagra show a *d*usky melanotic centre with a *d*usky magenta rim surrounded by a *d*esquamating margin. The tongue is glazed and magenta coloured. The light exposed areas of the face and dorsa of the hands are particularly affected. On the face the eruption takes on a butterfly distribution and on the neck the characteristic 'Casals necklace'.

Scurvy

The clinical features of chronic scurvy are less well-known; they include ankle oedema, ecchymoses and dryness of the skin. On the legs follicular petechiae simulate bites, whilst corkscrew hairs clinch the diagnosis. Other features include general apathy, even dementia, and haemorrhagic oedematous gingivitis.

Iron deficiency

The Paterson–Kelly syndrome is due to chronic iron deficiency. The skin is pale and the face wizened, the lips thin and the hair thin and brittle. Sideropenia also causes koilonychia and atrophy of the mucous membranes of the tongue, buccal mucosa and vulva. Like the pharyngeal atrophy associated with webbing the mucosal changes are precancerous.

Metabolic disease

The metabolic diseases are here only briefly described. Certain amino acid disorders may affect the skin. In phenylketonuria the hair is blonde and the skin pale. In Hartnup disease a pellagrous eruption is sometimes present. Another rare metabolic disorder is angiokeratoma corporis diffusum (Anderson–Fabry disease) (*see* Chapter 21). Certain metabolic diseases are characterized by papules and plaques due to the deposition of metabolic infiltrates in the skin; the mucopolysaccharidoses show such skin changes. Some metabolic disorders produce characteristic and diagnostic cutaneous changes. The commonest is *xanthomatosis*, a disorder showing yellow papules, nodules or plaques scattered widely over the trunk and limbs. The sudden appearance of small papular xanthomata sometimes indicates a lipoprotein disorder or diabetes mellitus. The different groups of lipoproteinaemia have been delineated by Fredrickson and designated Types I to V.

Porphyrias (*see also* Chapter 24)

The porphyrias are a group of inherited abnormalities of porphyrin metabolism which produce a systemic disease and light-mediated porphyrin-triggered skin damage from accumulation of abnormal products. Normally the condensation of porphyrin precursors with iron produces haem which then combines with globin to form haemoglobin. Haem formation from glycine, via succinyl coenzyme A and delta amino laevulinic acid (ALA) is complex and a number of defects have been identified (as separate diseases) along the metabolic pathway. This a typical example of an inborn error of metabolism of the type first conceived by Garrod. Enzymatic defects of the biosynthetic pathway at various points then produce a series of related, but clinically and biochemically distinct abnormalities. The pathway is as follows:

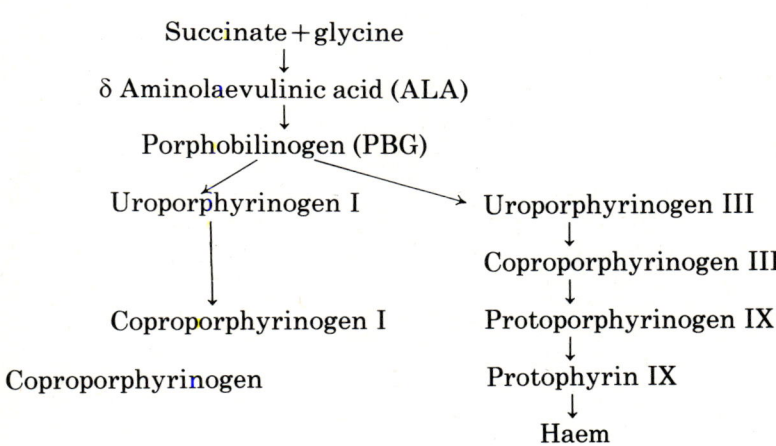

The porphyrias are clinically separated into two groups: erythropoietic and hepatic depending upon the main organs affected. There are two types of erythropoietic and three types of hepatic porphyria.

Erythropoietic:

(1) Congenital erythropoietic porphyria (autosomal recessive)
(2) Erythropoietic protoporphyria (autosomal dominant)

Hepatic:

(1) Acute intermittent porphyria (autosomal dominant)
(2) Porphyria variegata (autosomal dominant)
(3) Porphyria cutanea tarda
    (i) Drugs
    (ii) Liver disease
    (iii) Systemic disease

Congenital erythropoietic porphyria (Werewolf syndrome) Gunther's disease (CEP)

This is an extremely rare form of porphyria characterized by mutilating photosensitivity and large amounts of uroporphyrin I in the urine which varies from pink to wine coloured. Coproporphyrin I is increased in the faeces but serum ALA and PBG leves are normal. Uroporphyrin III synthetase is deficient with inefficient haem formation.

Pink stained napkins allow early diagnosis in childhood and this is later followed by disabling mutilating photosensitivity with cutaneous mutilation. The teeth typically fluoresce red in ultraviolet light and chronic haemolytic anaemia with splenomegaly is common. Raised urinary porphyrin I levels and the severity of clinical changes distinguish the disease from erythropoietic protoporphyria (EPP). Both diseases have excess red cell porphyrins—but uroporphyria is recurrent in CEP and protoporphyria in EPP. Red blood cells fluoresce in both disorders, but permanently in CEP and transiently in EPP. Because of the photosensitivity, scarring and hypertrichosis and the red fluorescence of the teeth, it has been postulated that such affected patients originally gave rise to the werewolf legend.

Treatment

Avoidance of sunlight, treatment of the haemolytic anaemia and infections.

Erythropoietic protoporphyria (EPP)

This is a relatively common autosomal dominant form of porphyria which presents in childhood with eczematous photosensitivity. Protoporphyrin levels are increased in skin, red cells and sometimes the plasma and faeces. Protoporphyrin conversion into haem is impaired (due to ferro-ketolase deficiency). Occasionally the red cell levels are normal. Coproporphyrin can be increased in the faeces but the urine is normal. (In contrast CEP has raised urinary porphyrins.)

Clinical features

The skin is often sensitive to 400 nm radiation and also the 500–600 nm range. Photosensitivity may be unaccompanied by cutaneous changes, but more usually the skin is erythematous and swollen with occasional urticaria but without blistering. Children can present with chronic eczema of the face, mouth and knuckles but without blistering, hypertrichosis and hyperpigmentation. There is usually a PAS positive glycoprotein deposition in the skin. Gall-stones and portal cirrhosis can also occur. Red cells show a transient fluorescence when diluted in saline and exposed to ultraviolet light.

The differential diagnosis includes other porphyrias, polymorphic light eruptions, lipid proteinosis and contact photodermatitis.

Treatment

Patients should avoid sunlight as much as possible. Sunscreening creams are sometimes helpful. Oral beta carotene is sometimes helpful as a photoprotective agent.

Hepatic porphyrias

Acute intermittent porphyria is not considered here because it rarely if ever affects the skin.

Porphyria variegata

This is the common type of porphyria in South Africa with a frequency of 0.3 per cent and all affected individuals can be traced to two people who married there in 1688. It is inherited as an autosomal dominant. There is overlap chemically with acute intermittent porphyria (AIP) and porphyria cutanea tarda (PCT). Porphyrinogen is increased in both AIP and variegata (but returns to normal in the latter with remission of acute attacks). In variegata porphyria urinary coproporphyria exceeds uroporphyria whereas in PCT the reverse is true.

Clinical features

Bullae, ulcers, erosions occur with minimum trauma and photosensitivity is combined with abdominal pain and peripheral neuropathy or psychosis. Varied clinical signs are common within families. Barbiturates, sulphonamides, alcohol and certain anaesthetics can precipitate attacks.

Treatment

General measures include relief of abdominal pain with antihistamines or Largactil. Intravenous glucose infusion is helpful in acute attacks. The drugs listed above should be avoided as should exposure to sunlight.

Porphyria cutanea tarda *(see Figure 16.1)*

This is perhaps the commonest form of porphyria being of late onset and usually associated with alcoholism. The inheritance is uncertain.

Biochemically, urinary uroporphyrin is markedly raised and coproporphyrin may be. Faecal porphyrins are usually normal and ALA and PBG levels are normal.

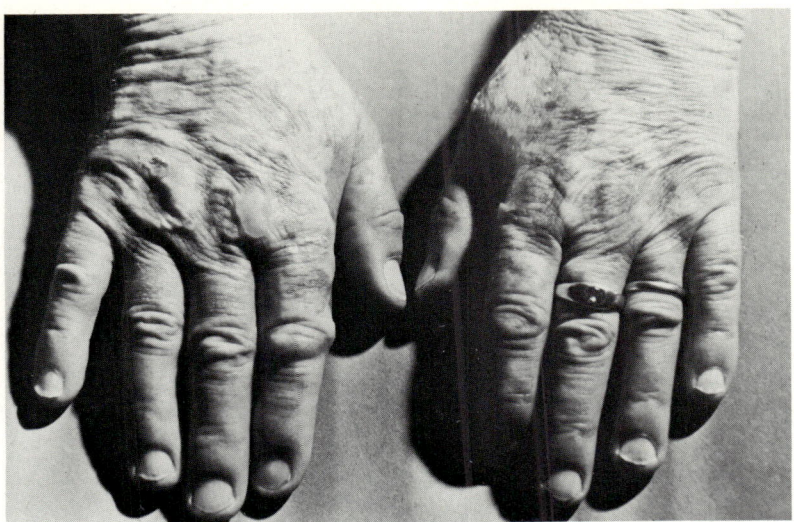

Figure 16.1 *Porphyria cutanea tarda*

Clinical features

Widespread blisters occur especially over the fingers and wrists, but also the forehead and face. Photosensitivity is rare but the blisters follow sun exposure. Chronic lesions may be so fibrotic as to resemble scleroderma. Hyperpigmentation and hypertrichosis are typical.

Treatment

Alcohol should be forbidden, and venesection until the haemoglobin falls below 12 g and the serum iron to 50–60 μg can be helpful. Chloroquine can be helpful but must be used with great caution as acute hepatic porphyrin release can be precipitated.

Hyperlipidaemias

Plasma lipoproteins are separable by centrifugation into four fractions—chylomicrons, very low density lipoproteins (VLDL), low density lipoproteins (LDL) and high density (HDL). These correspond in electrophoresis to origin, pre-beta, beta and alpha fractions.

Triglycerides are largely distributed as chylomicrons and VLDL, and cholesterol mainly as LDL with intermediate amounts of pre-beta and alpha components. There are five types of inherited hyperlipidaemia, all of which may show cutaneous xanthomatous deposits.

Type I hyperlipoproteinaemia

This is an autosomal recessive trait with a lipoprotein lipase deficiency and accumulation of chylomicrons. It presents in childhood with abdominal pains, hepatosplenomegaly, pancreatitis, eruptive xanthomas and lipaemia. Plasma triglycerides are excessively high. Chylomicrons are markedly elevated, but only faint alpha and beta bands are present. Cardiovascular disease is uncommon. Dietary restriction of saturated and unsaturated fats is essential.

Type IIa hypercholesterolaemia

This is an autosomal dominant trait with much increased LDL (beta fraction). Fasting serum is clear and hypercholesterolaemia and sometimes hypertriglyceridaemia occur. Tendon, tuberose xanthomas, premature corneal arcus and xanthelasma and coronary artery disease are common in middle age. The rare homozygotes die in adolescence.

Reduced saturated fats, polyunsaturated fat and bile acid binders are helpful (cholestyramine 30 g/day). Nicotinic acid and clofibrate 2 g daily can be useful. Topical trichloroacetic acid is cosmetically effective in eyelid xanthelasma. Most cases are normocholesterolaemic.

Type III hyperlipoproteinaemia

Here there is pre-beta VLDL accumulation with palmo-plantar and occasionally eruptive xanthomas. The VLDL is abnormal being arginine rich with more cholesterol and less triglyceride than normal. Combined hypercholesterolaemia and triglyceridaemia occurs. Peripheral vascular disease and ischaemic heart disease can occur.

A reduction of carbohydrate and cholesterol is helpful, and normal amounts of fat can be taken. Clofibrate 2 g daily is helpful if diet fails to control lipid levels.

Type IIb and IV hyperlipoproteinaemia

Here there is accumulation of VLDL and insulin resistance. Decreased breakdown and increased synthesis are likely and insulin resistance is associated with weight gain. If the LDL are elevated then Type IIb is diagnosed.

Patients often develop ischaemic vascular disease. Eruptive xanthomas and pancreatitis can occur.

Treatment includes dieting (low calories, low carbohydrates). This reduces the VDLD and the LDL can then be reduced with cholestyramine or nicotinic acid.

Type V

Fat and carbohydrate induced hyperlipoproteinaemia disappear on dieting. Often the cholesterol and triglycerides are very high and the VLDL (pre-beta) fraction is raised. Abdominal pain, hepatosplenomegaly and pancreatitis occur. Cardiovascular problems are not especially common, and treatment consists of a low carbohydrate, low fat diet.

Sarcoidosis

Sarcoidosis is a systemic disease showing multisystem involvement with sarcoid granulomas for which no causative agent is found. The term sarcoidosis, therefore, carries no aetiological connotation although no doubt with more refined diagnostic methods some cases now designated sarcoidosis will be shown to be caused by specific agents. The diagnosis is based solely on histological and immunological criteria when a diligent search has excluded a causative agent.

Aetiology

Acute disease is usually seen under the age of 30 whereas the slow onset chronic disease is commoner in the 30s and 40s. Familial cases are reported. Sarcoidosis is common in the Negro and Bantu, the lesions being more tumid and necrotic than those seen in other races.

The pathomechanism for sarcoidosis is unknown but the basis of the disease might be:

(1) A disorder of suppressor T lymphocytes causing defective cell mediated immunity (type IV) with consequent compensatory B cell proliferation.
(2) A primary reticuloendothelial disorder with lymphoreticular proliferation causing 'T cell failure' and delayed granuloma formation as evidenced by the Kveim test. Such delayed granulomatous sensitivity is seen with beryllium and zirconium sensitivity.
(3) A particular form of granulomatous reaction perhaps histiocyte mediated independent of cell mediated immunity.
(4) A symptom complex syndrome comparable to erythema nodosum caused by an infective or non-infective agent. Mycobacteria (*M. tuberculosis*, anonymous mycobacteria, etc.) and as yet unidentified organisms are incriminated. The low solubility and low potency of the bacterial antigen may determine the slowly developing sarcoid granuloma.
(5) A syndrome from the interaction of an unknown specific agent in an individual with a genetically defective T cell response. This concept postulates a specific agent combined with a 'sarcoid diathesis'.

At present the evidence is equally divided in favour of each of these hypotheses.

Histopathology

Sarcoid granulomas in the dermis comprise foci of epithelioid cells surrounded by a narrow mantle of lymphocytes (the so-called 'naked tubercles'). Central caseation is rare. Other epithelioid granulomas with foreign body giant cells, lymphocytes and fibrosis are also seen.

Hypodermal nodules are seen in the Darier–Roussy type of cutaneous lesion and a diffuse epithelioid infiltrate in the papillary zone of the dermis is found in the uncommon erythrodermic sarcoidosis. Sarcoid granuloma from specific causes must be excluded (*see Table 16.4*); sections are examined for mycobacteria, fungi, etc.

Clinical features

The disease may begin acutely with fever, arthralgia, generalized lymphadenopathy and erythema nodosum. Sometimes respiratory and ocular symptoms are present. In mild disease erythema nodosum and bilateral hilar lymphadenopathy are the only findings. In the acute cases spontaneous remission is usual.

In the more chronic course the skin changes are more torpid and include lupus pernio (*Plate 16.3*), and show persistent nodules or plaques (*Plate 16.4*). Less commonly miliary facial plaques, subcutaneous nodules (Darier–Roussy type) and erythrodermic plaques are seen.

Lupus pernio affects the nose, cheeks, ear lobes, fingers and toes. The affected skin shows diffuse infiltration with swelling and red-violet discoloration. A variant with marked telangiectasia and soft tumid swellings is termed *angiolupoid*. Underlying bone involvement is usual with this chronic type of sarcoidosis affecting the skin. The nasal bones are involved and the phalanges shows 'lattice-like' rarefactions. The commonly seen papules, plaques and nodules are round or oval with a slightly irregular edge. The size ranges from 0.5–5 cm and they are pink, brown or purple brown and may show superficial scaling. Diascopy unmasks clusters of fawn macules within the lesion resembling the 'apple jelly' nodules of lupus vulgaris. The nodules and plaques of chronic sarcoidosis are bilateral although rather asymmetrically disposed; the limbs are affected more than the trunk. On the forehead annular lesions are common while in the scalp sarcoidal infiltration causes patchy hair loss.

The rare *miliary sarcoidosis* consists of grouped dusky red papules 0.1–0.5 cm across on the forehead, sides of the nose and chin. The differential diagnosis from acne agminata often depends on histological examination.

Multiple plaques and nodules are usually associated with pulmonary involvement which often proceeds to fibrosis.

An important diagnostic sign in early sarcoidosis is transient infiltration of pre-existing scars. Similarly the sites of needle puncture or skin testing may show significant infiltration. More persistent skin infiltration is commonly seen with chronic sarcoidosis. Occasionally sarcoidal infiltration appears in one of the coloured areas of a tattoo.

Associated findings indicating multiorgan involvement in individuals with cutaneous sarcoidosis include lymphadenopathy, hepatosplenomegaly, iridocyclitis, lacrimal and salivary gland enlargement, and nerve palsies.

Table 16.4 Differentiation of sarcoidal tissue reactions

	Sarcoid granuloma confined to skin	Sarcoidal granulomatosis	Sarcoidosis
Pathogenesis	Silica, beryllium, mercury, zirconium	Inhalation of beryllium; viral, bacterial, fungal, parasitic disease	Unknown
Relevant history	Often occupational	Sometimes geographical	Occasionally familial
Skin	Nodules confined to inoculation site	Widespread lesions	Widespread lesions
Systemic involvement	None	Localization determined by source and spread of responsible agent	BHL*, liver, spleen, eyes, lymph nodes
Investigations			
Chest x-ray	Normal	May be abnormal	BHL*, pulmonary infiltration
Blood changes	None	May be hypergamma-globulinaemia; calcium normal	Usually hypergamma-globulinaemia; calcium often increased
Tuberculin reaction	Normal	Normal	Depressed or negative
Kveim reaction	Negative	Negative	Positive
Patch test	Often positive 4–6 weeks	Often positive 48 hours	Negative to many antigens
Intradermal test	Often positive	Positive in leprosy and zirconium	Negative
Treatment	Remove cause	Specific chemotherapy	Steroids sometimes indicated
	Intralesional steroid	Steroids contraindicated	

* BHL: Bilateral hilar lymphadenopathy

The immunological characteristics of sarcoidosis are:

(1) depressed cell mediated immunity,
(2) excessive proliferation of B cells producing immunoglobulins,
(3) delayed granulomatous reaction as elicited by Kveim reaction.

A negative tuberculin test is found in a high proportion of patients and non-reactivity extends to many antigens (*Candida albicans*, mumps, etc.) and chemicals that normally sensitize the skin. BCG either fails to produce tuberculin conversion or produces only temporary sensitization. The immediate Type 1 sensitivity remains intact and the development of immunity to tetanus toxoid, diphtheria antigen, etc. is normal.

Investigations

The prime aim is to exclude tuberculosis, sarcoidal granulomatosis (e.g. syphilis, leprosy). Skin biopsy reveals sarcoid granulomas. Stains and culture for acid fast bacilli exclude mycobacterial infection. PAS stain excludes fungal infection. Urine and sputum should be examined for acid fast bacilli. Blood examination shows an increase in gamma globulin and in active and extensive disease hypercalcaemia is usual. Chest x-ray reveals hilar node enlargement or pulmonary involvement. Radiological changes in the fingers are characteristic; cystic rarefactions are seen in the subcortical and periarticular regions and 'lace-like' rarefactions are common in the shaft of the phalanges. Liver, scalene node, muscle or conjunctival biopsy may be required to confirm systemic involvement.

Prognosis

Acute cases usually resolve spontaneously within a year. The chronic lupus pernio type which has associated pulmonary involvement is usually persistent and the pulmonary lesions may progress to fibrosis.

Differential diagnosis

The skin lesions may mimic lupus vulgaris, lymphocytoma, eosinophilic granuloma, Jessner's lymphocytic infiltrate, tuberculoid leprosy and syphilis. In the Negro and Bantu tumid and ulcerative lesions closely resemble lepromatous leprosy.

The differential diagnosis from other sarcoidal granulomatoses is shown in *Table 16.4*.

Treatment

Acute sarcoidosis with erythema nodosum usually responds well to butazolidin or corticosteroids. The chronic skin lesions are helped by antimalarials. However, chloroquine is not usually favoured in view of the risk of serious ocular complications. Intralesional steroid injection usually clears a localized nodule or plaque. With widespread chronic lesions, particularly in the presence of ocular or pulmonary involvement, corticosteroid therapy is essential. Prednisolone 15 mg daily is usually effective in controlling the disease.

17 Lymphoreticular and myeloproliferative disorders

R. J. Cairns

The initial concept of the reticuloendothelial system (RES) as a widespread phagocytic system proved useful for many years and diseases arising from these tissues were designated as reticuloses. These included diseases originating from specialized cells in the marrow, lymph nodes, liver, spleen and skin. Later the term reticulosis was dropped and lymphoma substituted; this term was employed to designate malignant disease of lymphoid elements in the RES.

Difficulties then arose with the designation of histiocytic and non-lymphocytic disorders. The terms lymphoreticulosis is currently in favour. Like the original reticuloses the lymphoreticuloses comprise disorders arising in the lymph nodes, spleen, liver, lungs, bone marrow, as well as the skin. The two main families of cells involved are the macrophages (histiomonocytic cells) and lymphocytes. Lymphocytes are subdivided into two major groups: the T lymphocyte derived from the thymus and the B lymphocyte of bone marrow origin. It is still convenient to refer to neoplasia of lymphoreticular tissue as either lymphoma or histiocytosis according to the cell of origin. Neoplasia arising from myeloid tissue is referred to as myeloproliferative disease or myelopathy. These latter include granulocytic leukaemia, myelomatosis and the lymphatic leukaemias. Mast cell disease and Kaposi's sarcoma whilst not fitting into any classification of lymphoreticular disease are considered in this chapter.

Lymphoreticular disease is now classified in relation to the histological appearance of a biopsy usually in the lymph node or skin. Such a biopsy may show one of four basic changes, all deviations of normal growth:

(1) Hypoplasia: this is rare and found in immunodeficiency states—it is not discussed further here.
(2) Reactive hyperplasia: with a variable and even dominant inflammatory component. The process may be diffuse or nodular in the affected organs. Cells are well-differentiated without anaplasia and the proliferation represents stable clonal growth.

(3) Low grade malignancy: the cellular infiltrate may show a few bizarre anaplastic cells and a variable inflammatory component may be present. Some of these disorders involute; others persist or progress to frankly malignant disease.

(4) Malignant or highly malignant neoplasia: anaplastic cells sometimes with a few inflammatory cells are present. The growth is progressive and may finally show circulating malignant cells (leukaemia).

The classification of reticuloendothelioses is further based according to the presumed cell of origin. However, the histiogenesis of some disorders is controversial because the appearance of cells change according to their rate of growth. Most lymphomas probably represent deviant cell growth of one or more cell lines or stated another way *these disorders probably represent cell deviation with abnormal clonal growth from a single point in a particular cell line.* Another important consideration is the anatomical compartment that is first affected. This may be the skin, lymph nodes or internal organs. Thus mycosis, fungoides and Sezary lymphoma are primary cutaneous lymphomas. Another consideration with lymphoreticular disease is the resultant disorder of function.

Three major functional components of the original RES are recognized:

(1) Scavenging and antigen processing by histiocytes and Langerhan's cells.

(2) Surveillance—the initiation and continuation of cell mediated immunity by thymus dependent lymphocytes (T lymphocytes).

(3) The myeloid compartment which is concerned with 'seeding' the blood with erythrocytes, neutrophils, eosinophils, basophils and platelets. B lymphocytes arise from plasma cells which are concerned with immunoglobulin production.

The aetiology of lymphoreticular disease is largely unknown. However, certain factors which may be relevant are:

(1) Viral infection. Certainly the Burkitt's lymphoma represents infection of B lymphocytes with the Epstein–Barr virus with associated T cell proliferation.

(2) Failure of cell mediated immunity. Failure of antigen processing or suppressor T cells may allow proliferation of B lymphocytes and other lymphoreticular cells.

(3) Chromosomal abnormalities. Bloom's syndrome and Down's syndrome both show an increased incidence of leukaemia.

(4) Mutation, maturation arrest or loss of feedback control are other possible mechanisms causing abnormal lymphoreticular proliferations.

(5) Neoplasia may begin *de novo* or from progressive unstable growth arising from a reactive process.

Inflammatory lymphoreticular disease

The diverse clinico-pathological entities encountered in clinical practice depend on the particular cells undergoing reactive hyperplasia (*Table 17.1*). There is some variability in the pattern of cellular response and the designation of the disease is usually based on the predominant cell type seen under the microscope. The physician is often able to make a provisional diagnosis on clinical grounds based on the evolution, appearance and distribution of the eruption. Frequently the exact diagnosis is only reached by histological examination of the skin, lymph nodes, marrow and other tissues.

Table 17.1 Inflammatory (reactive) disorders with stable clonal proliferation

Cell of origin	Terminology	Example
Histiocyte	Reticulogranuloma	Histiocytoma, juvenile xanthogranuloma
	Macrophage granuloma	Lepromatous leprosy Leishmaniasis
Lymphocyte (B, T or other types)	Lymphoplasia	T—lymphadenosis cutis benigna,
	Pseudolymphoma	some lymphocytomas Jessner's infiltrate
		B—plasma cell reaction
Probable mixed histiocyte and lymphocyte	Lymphocytoma	Some lymphocytomas Lymphomatoid granulomatosis
Other cells		
Eosinophil	Eosinophilic granuloma	Granuloma faciale Parasitic granulomata
Mast cell		Mast cell naevus Urticaria pigmentosa

Reticulum cell (histiocyte)

Hyperplasia of reticulum cells is referred to as a reticulogranuloma. Because the reticulum cell is potentially phagocytic certain reticulogranulomas contain ingested iron and fat.

Histiocytoma (fibroma en pastille) (*Plate 17.1*)

This is a fairly common granuloma. The lesion appears as a firm painless nodule measuring 3 mm to 3 cm across. The colour varies according to the stored material—from skin colour, yellow (fat) to golden brown or black (haemosiderin). The tumour is usually solitary although it sometimes erupts suddenly in large numbers. The important differential diagnoses include xanthoma and nodular malignant melanomas.

Juvenile xanthogranuloma

Juvenile xanthogranuloma is a variant of histiocytoma seen in early childhood, usually resolving spontaneously before puberty. Yellow papules or small nodules with an erythematous halo appear on the face and scalp. Occasionally an intraocular xanthogranuloma coexists with skin lesions. Foam cells and foreign body giant cells are conspicuous in histological sections.

Multicentric reticulohistiocytosis *(Plate 17.2)*

This is a rare disorder affecting the skin and joints, and is sometimes associated with internal malignancy. The skin and the joints show focal areas of infiltration with histiocytes. When unassociated with malignancy the disorder may be self-limiting.

Histiocytic granulomas

Histiocytic or macrophage granulomas are encountered with lepromatous leprosy and dermal leishmaniasis, and Wegener's granulomatosis.

Lymphocyte

Recently two major categories of lymphocyte have been delineated and various lymphocytic processes are currently classified according to T cell hyperplasias and B cell hyperplasias. The small T lymphocyte is produced in the paracortical zone of lymph nodes in the adult and carries cell bound antibodies.

T lymphocytes

T lymphocytes are normally present in the dermis and in small numbers in the epidermis. These cells are the mediators of cell-mediated immunity. In diverse inflammatory processes T cells are increased in the skin. They are present in the erythemas, lichen planus and lupus erythematosus in the dermis, and in the epidermis and dermis in eczema.

Jessner's lymphocytic infiltrate

Jessner's lymphocytic infiltrate is a nodular infiltrated eruption predominantly affecting males. The face is the site of predilection although other areas especially the scapular region may be affected. Differential diagnosis is from lupus erythematosus, insect bite reaction and nodular lymphocytoma.

Miliary and nodular lymphocytomas

Miliary and nodular lymphocytomas appear as grouped papules in the central area of the face, particularly the forehead and cheeks. Certain cases show light sensitivity with exacerbation of the eruption in sunny weather. Localized lesions are effectively treated by intralesional triamcinolone.

B lymphocytes

B lymphocytes are derived from bone marrow in the adult. The plasma cell is of the same lineage and produces immunoglobulin. Certain granulomatous disorders show a predominance of plasma cells. This is particularly noted with granulomas affecting the face, mouth and nasopharynx. Likewise syphilitic granulomas are characteristically rich in plasma cells. A reactive myeloid plasmocytosis is seen from chronic immunological stimulation. The resulting abnormal protein in these cases of 'benign plasmocytosis' is sometimes deposited in the skin and other tissues as amyloid.

Mast cells

These cells are situated in the dermis particularly in relation to smaller blood vessels. They have three major secretory products: heparin, hyaluronidase and histamine. The *mast cell naevus* is one of the rarer naevi seen in children and forms a raised brown nodule measuring 1 to 3 cm in diameter showing urtication from minor trauma. In some instances trauma or even exposure to sunlight causes blister formation. The release of histamine from the lesion may cause a transient generalized flush in children that causes alarm to onlookers.

Urticaria pigmentosa (*Plate 17.3*)

This usually appears as a pigmented, macular or maculopapular eruption in childhood. Occasionally only a few brown macules are present and these simulate the café au lait patches of neurofibromatosis. However, the pigmented lesions of urticaria pigmentosa urticate with stroking, after a hot bath or with friction from clothing. A variant of urticaria pigmentosa seen in later life shows telangiectatic patches rather than pigmented areas. This form of the disease should be viewed as a potentially systemic disorder. About 20 per cent of all cases of urticaria pigmentosa in the adult show bone lesions and hepatosplenomegaly or intestinal pathology. In this event the disease is more correctly designated as *systemic mast cell disease*. There is no effective treatment although antihistamines are useful to relieve itching. With systemic disease cytotoxic drugs are employed.

Eosinophils

These cells appear in the peripheral blood in Type 1 hypersensitivity reactions and in parasitic disease.

Granuloma faciale

Granuloma faciale is sometimes termed the eosinophilic granuloma of the erythema elevatum diutinum type. It appears as a red, orange or purple tumid nodule, most commonly on the face. The primary basis is probably vascular with a secondary eosinophilic infiltrate. Differentiation from nodular lymphocytoma is usually only possible by microscopy. Rarely multiple eosinophilic granulomas are found in perioral and perianal regions without any systemic disease. Similarly granulomas with heavy eosinophilic infiltration are sometimes seen with insect bites and the parasitic infestation trichinosis. Granuloma faciale often responds to intralesional injections of triamcinolone or cryotherapy.

Neoplastic lymphoreticular disease

Hodgkin's disease

An uncontrolled proliferation of histiocytes and T lymphocytes with varying degrees of anaplasia. Whether the prime disorder is that of T lymphocytes, histiocytes or both cells is controversial. A well-differentiated group is sometimes termed Hodgkin's paragranuloma while the more anaplastic classic Hodgkin's disease with primitive histiocytes and relatively few lymphocytes merges into the highly malignant histiocytic lymphoma.

Aetiology

The cause of Hodgkin's disease is unknown. One theory is that an oncogenic virus infects T cells.

Histopathology

Groups of histiocytes, a variable number of lymphocytes and inflammatory cells are characteristic. Sternberg–Reed cells are usually present.

Clinical features

Cutaneous signs are not uncommon but only rarely are they the initial finding. On p. 213 are listed some of the general clinical features which may herald the onset of the disease. An atrophic ichthyosiform dermatosis is occasionally seen with Hodgkin's disease; it is rare with other lymphoreticuloses. Infiltrative tumorous and ulcerative lesions are mostly features of advanced disease;

pruritus, however, may appear early. Immunological depression of cell-mediated immunity is commonly encountered.

Treatment

Antipruritic drugs are sometimes helpful. Accurate staging of the disease and the combination of chemotherapy and radiotherapy have greatly improved the prognosis in recent years.

Mycosis fungoides *(Plate 17.4)*

This is an uncommon lymphoma with neoplastic and inflammatory cells including T lymphocytes, neutrophils and eosinophils. It is a primary cutaneous lymphoma although visceral lesions are sometimes found at post mortem. The name derives because earlier clinicians likened the tumours to mushrooms.

Histopathology

The so-called mycosis fungoides cells (Lutzner cells) and T lymphocytes are found grouped in the epidermis and constitute the Pautrier microabscess. The dermis is infiltrated with inflammatory cells which in the later stages infiltrate the mid and lower dermis between the collagen fibres.

Clinical features

Five clinical stages are recognized:

(1) erythematous stage with pruritic erythematous plaques (parapsoriasis en plaques) and poikiloderma,
(2) the infiltrative stage when the infiltrated plaques become palpably indurated and show a range of colours,
(3) the tumour stage with large nodules which may ulcerate,
(4) disseminated disease affecting the lymph nodes, liver and spleen,
(5) the visceral stage with leukaemia.

Sometimes the first two stages are absent and there may be sudden onset of tumours; in other instances the eruption remains for many years in the erythematous stage resembling a banal eczema.

Treatment

Early erythematous patches often respond to topical steroids. Superficial x-ray, Grenz ray and electron beam therapy and more recently PUVA are sometimes used; chemotherapy (methotrexate, cyclophosphamide, bleomycin and procarbazine) is used for radio-resistance lesions or in visceral dissemination. Systemic corticosteroids are indicated for generalized erythroderma. Recently staging of the visceral disease by lymphangiography and laparatomy have been employed in the hope of producing more effective therapeutic regimens.

Colour Plate Section

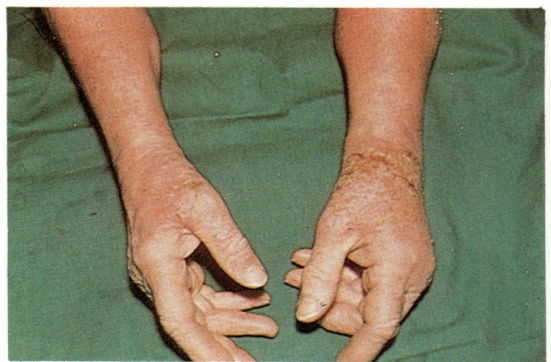

Plate 5.1 Contact dermatitis—cumulative insult (detergent and rubber gloves)

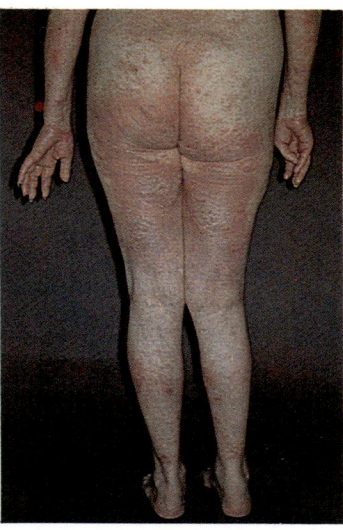

Plate 5.2 Contact dermatitis from suspenders—secondary sensitivity to rubber and nickel

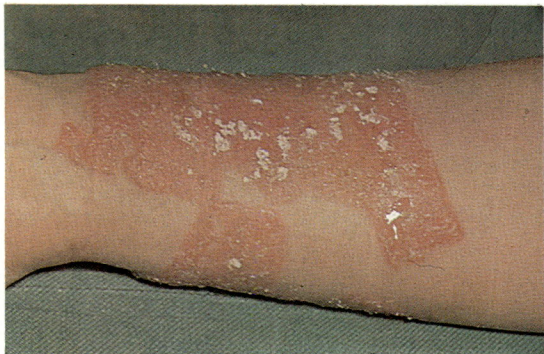

Plate 5.3 Contact dermatitis—elastoplast

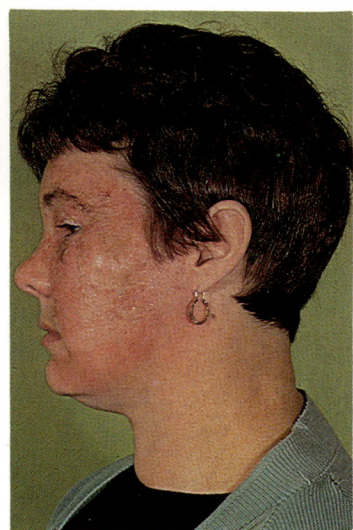

Plate 5.4 Contact dermatitis—Savlon

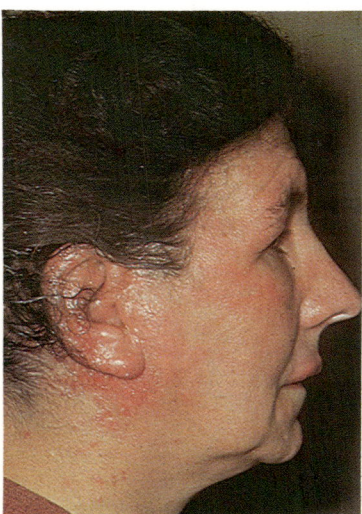

Plate 5.5 Contact dermatitis—
PARA hair dye

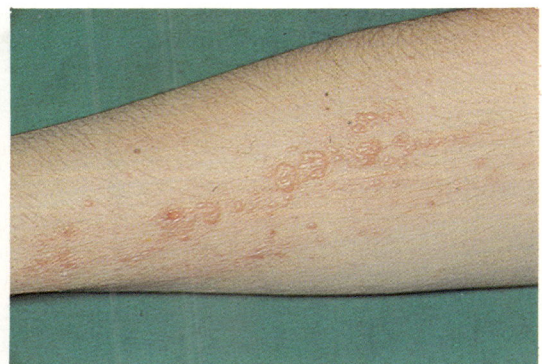

Plate 5.7 Primula dermatitis—linear vesicular eruption

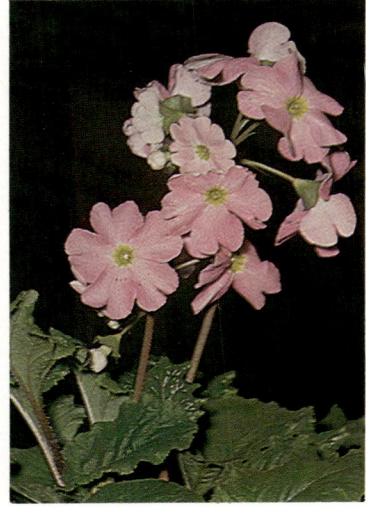

Plate 5.6 Primula obconica

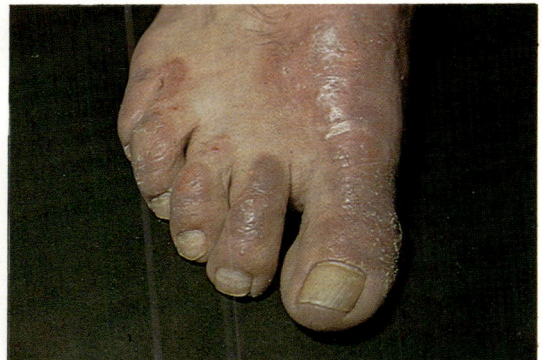

Plate 5.8 Contact dermatitis—shoes

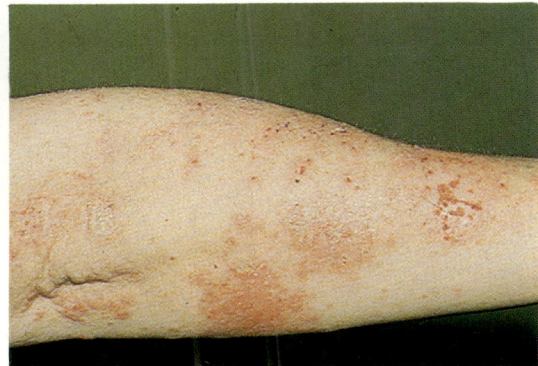

Plate 5.9 Discoid eczema

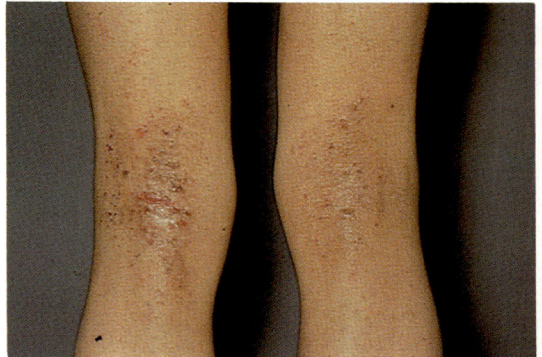

Plate 5.10 Atopic dermatitis

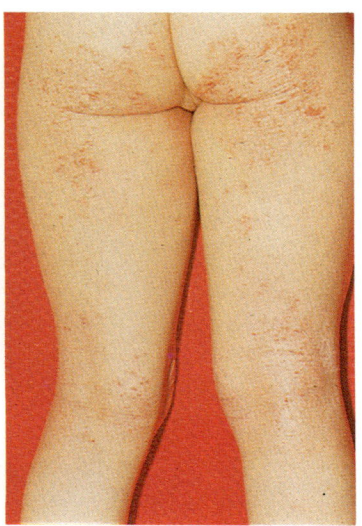

Plate 5.11 Atopic dermatitis

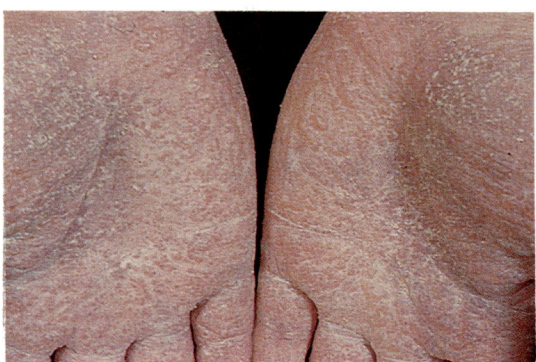

Plate 5.12 Pompholyx palms—vesicular eczema

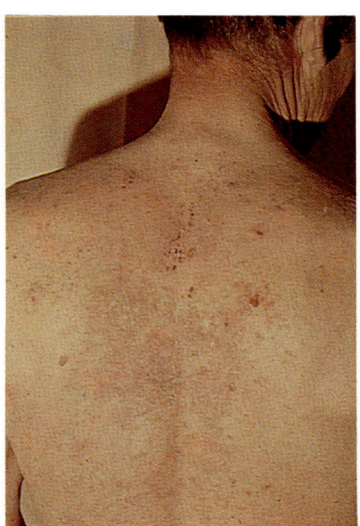

Plate 5.13 Seborrhoeic dermatitis

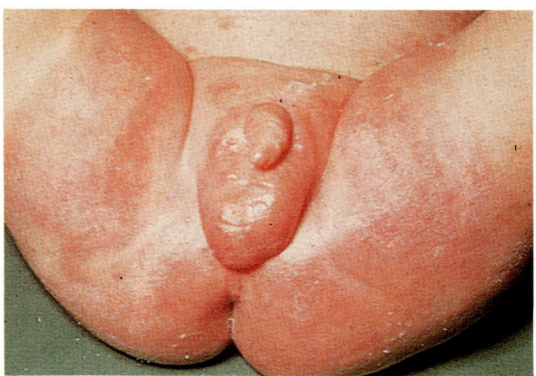

Plate 5.14 Napkin dermatitis aggravated by plastic pants

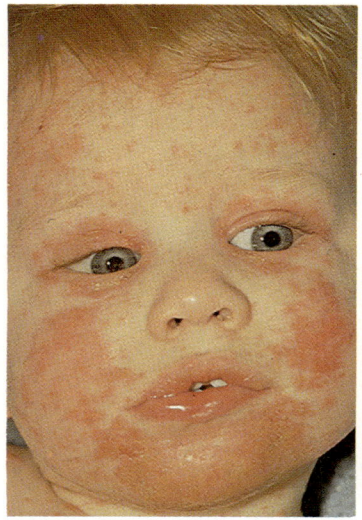

Plate 5.15 Infantile eczema face secondary to napkin dermatitis

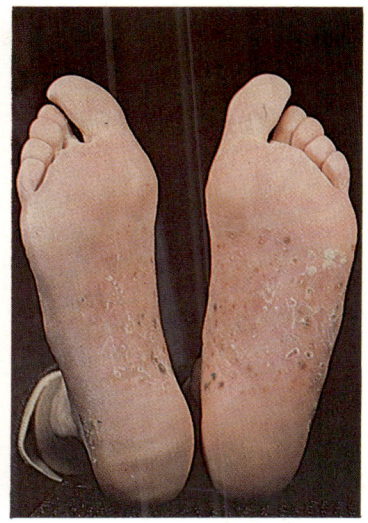

Plate 5.16 Recalcitrant pustular eruption soles

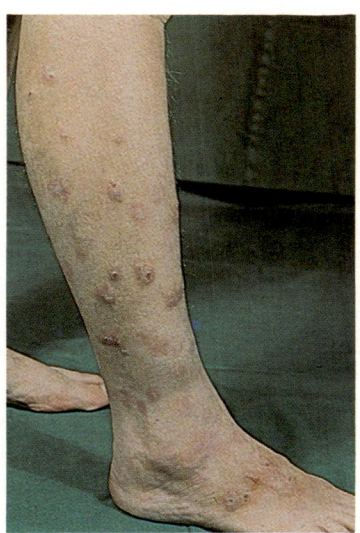

Plate 5.17 Prurigo nodularis

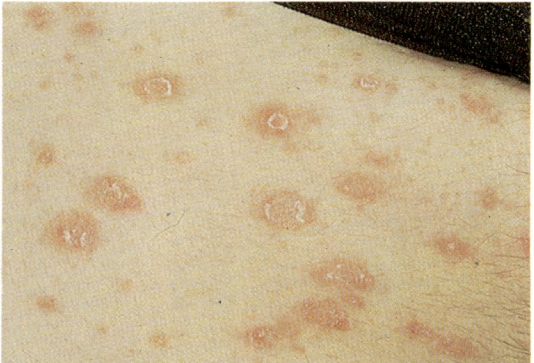

Plate 5.18 Pityriasis rosea

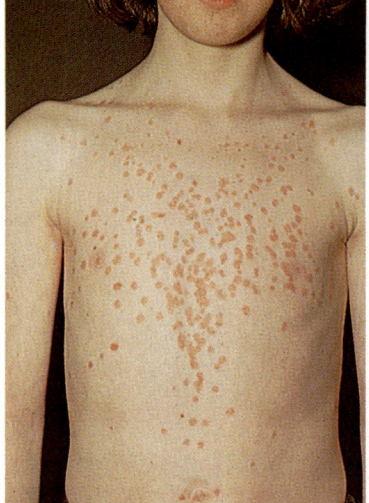

Plate 6.1 Guttate psoriasis

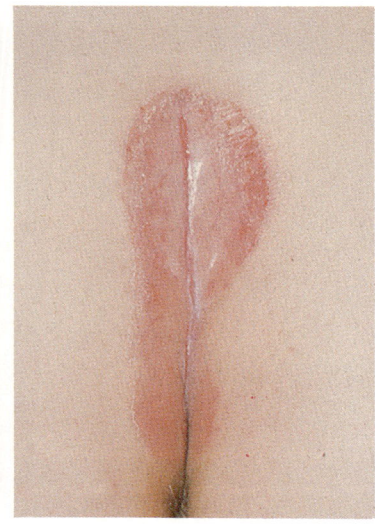

Plate 6.2 Flexural psoriasis

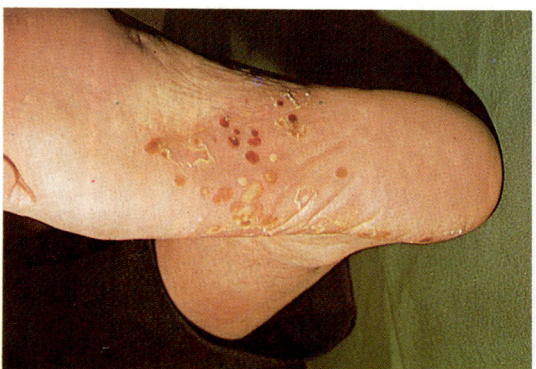

Plate 6.4 Pustular psoriasis on soles of feet

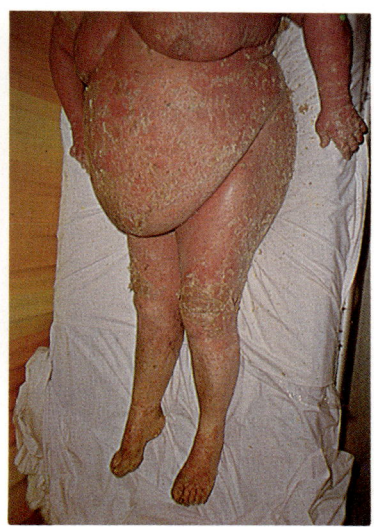

Plate 6.3 Erythrodermic psoriasis
(exfoliative dermatitis)

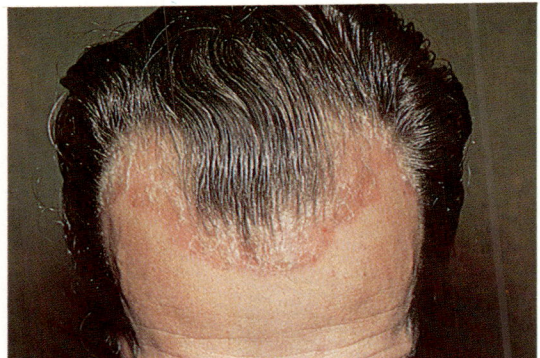

Plate 6.5   Psoriasis on scalp

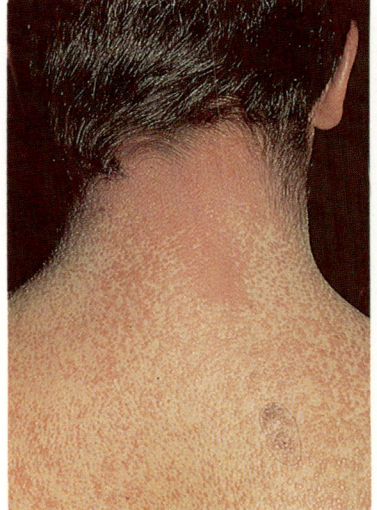

Plate 6.6   Pityriasis rubra pilaris

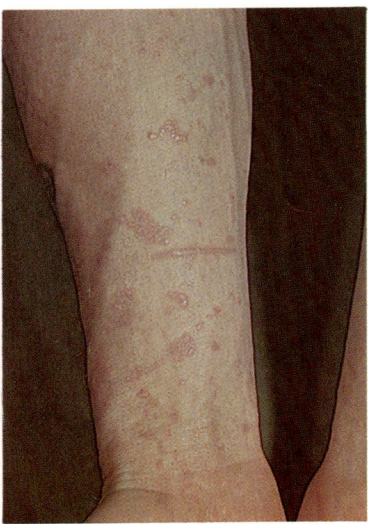

Plate 6.7   Lichen planus

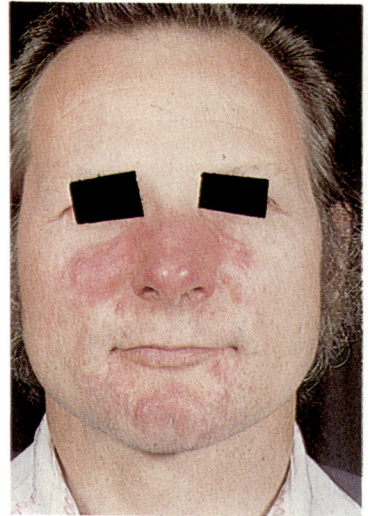

***Plate* 7.1**   Rosacea

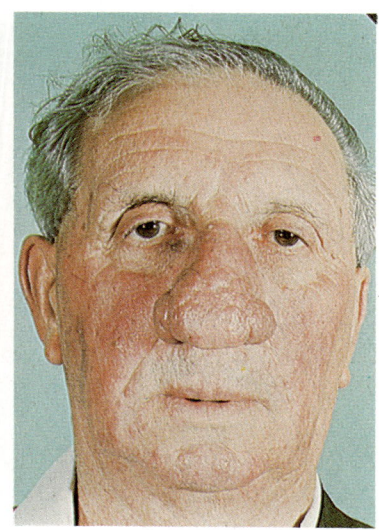

***Plate* 7.2**   Rhinophyma

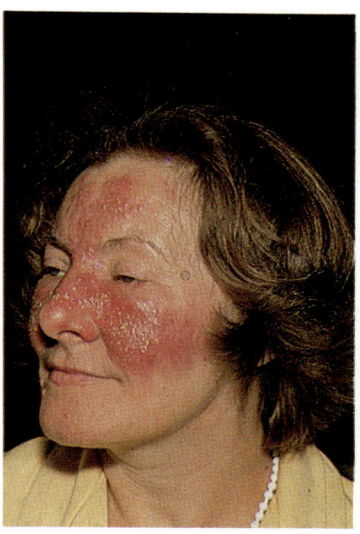

***Plate* 7.3**   Steroid cream induced rosacea

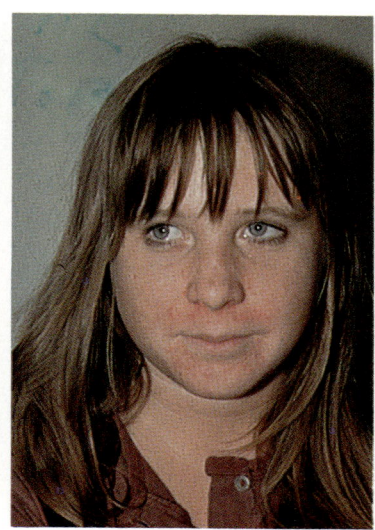

***Plate* 7.4**   Perioral dermatitis

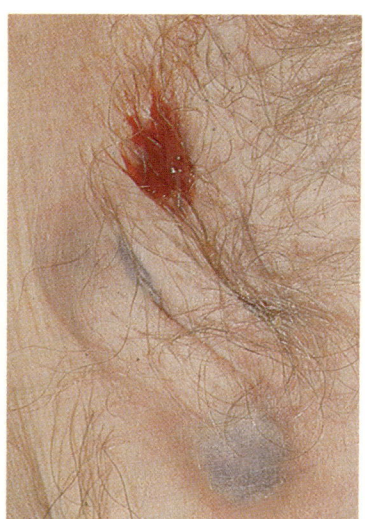

Plate 8.1 Hidradenitis suppurativa

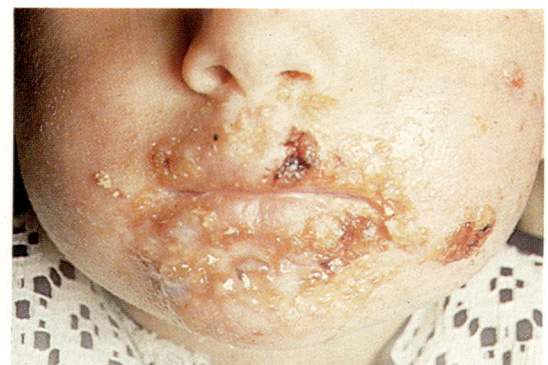

Plate 8.2 Impetigo on face

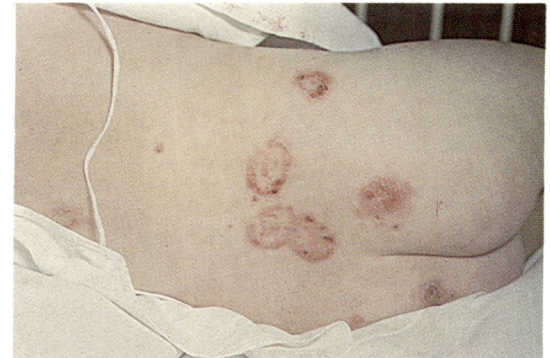

Plate 8.3 Impetigo on trunk

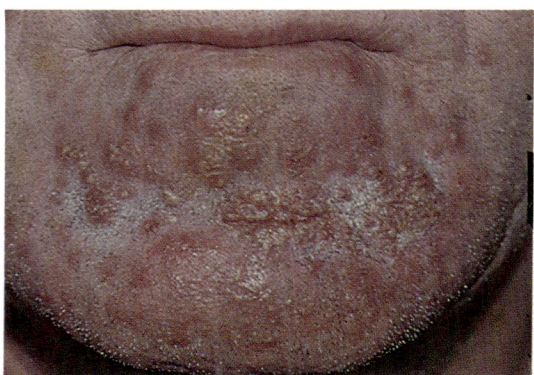

Plate 8.4 Sycosis barbae

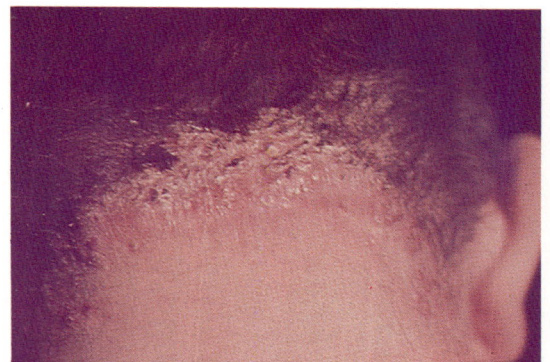

Plate 8.5 Acne keloid

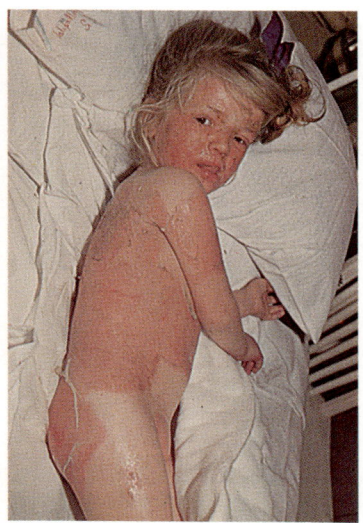

Plate 8.6 Toxic epidermal necrolysis (TEN) due to staphylococcus Type 71

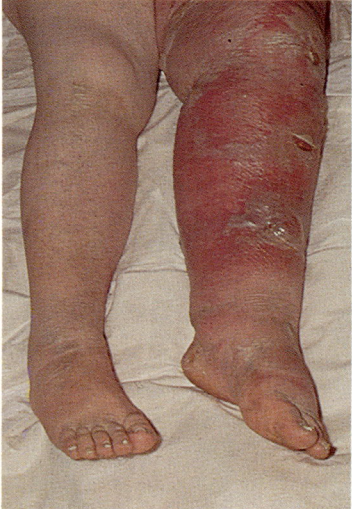

Plate 8.7 Cellulitis on leg with bulla formation

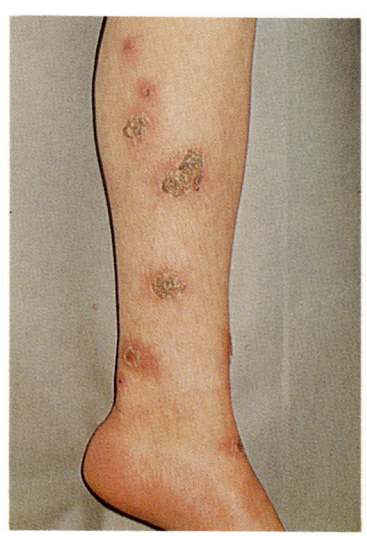

Plate 8.8 Ecthyma

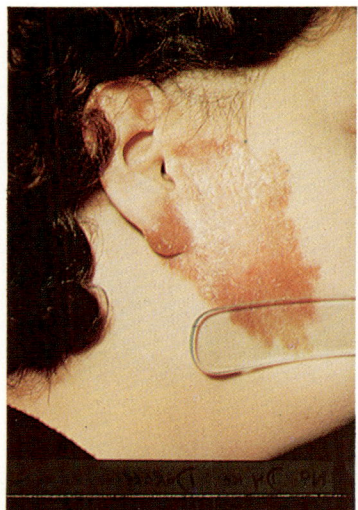

Plate 8.9 Lupus vulgaris (diascopy to show 'apple jelly' nodules)

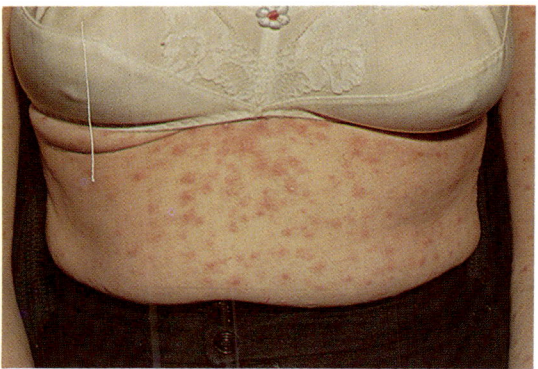

Plate 8.11 Secondary syphilis

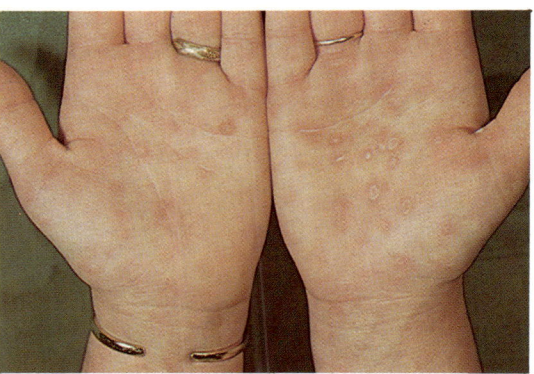

Plate 8.12 Secondary syphilis on palms

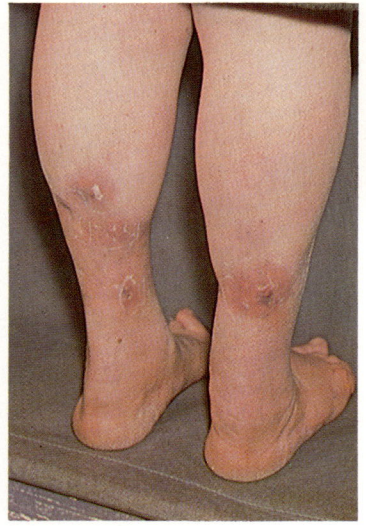

Plate 8.10 Erythema induratum (Bazin's disease)

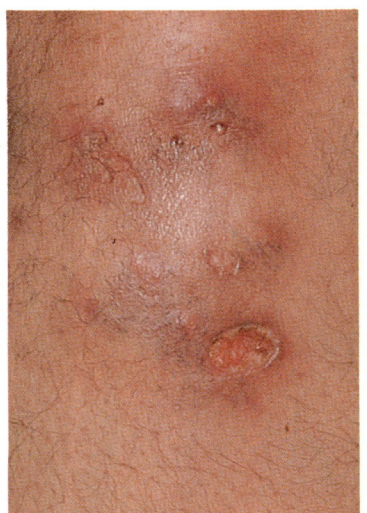

Plate *8.13* Tertiary syphilis—dermal gummata

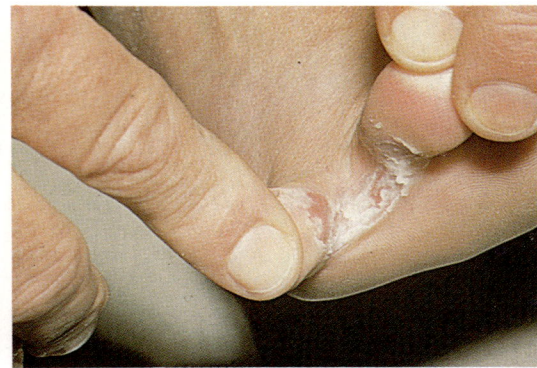

Plate 9.1 Tinea pedis

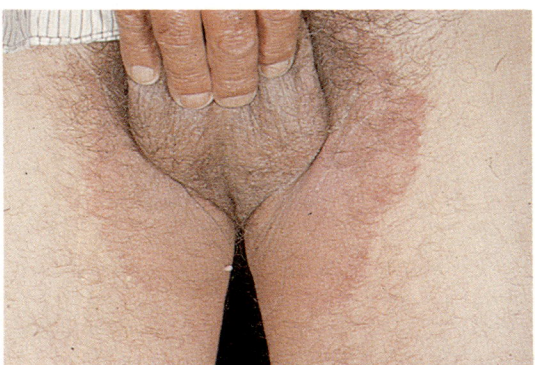

Plate 9.3 Tinea cruris

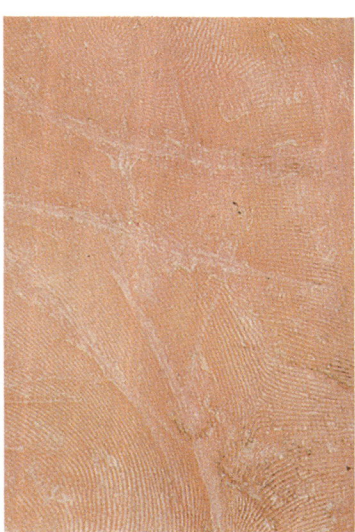

Plate 9.2 Tinea manuum

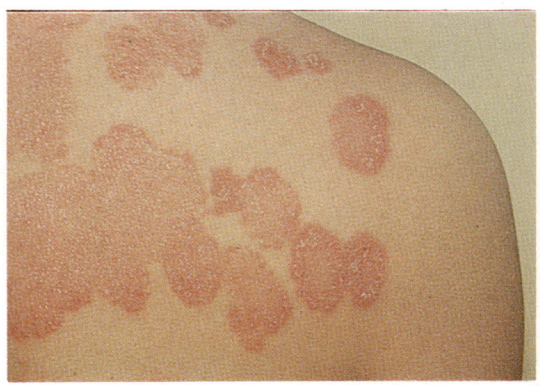

Plate 9.4 Tinea corporis

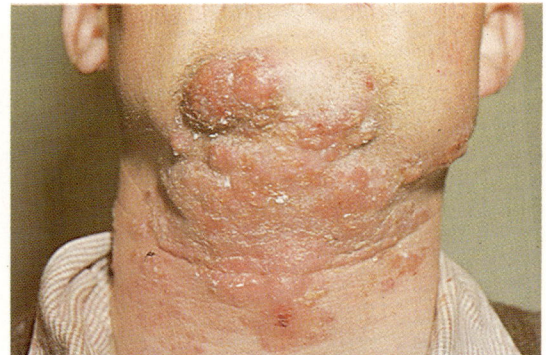

Plate 9.5 Cattle ringworm—beard

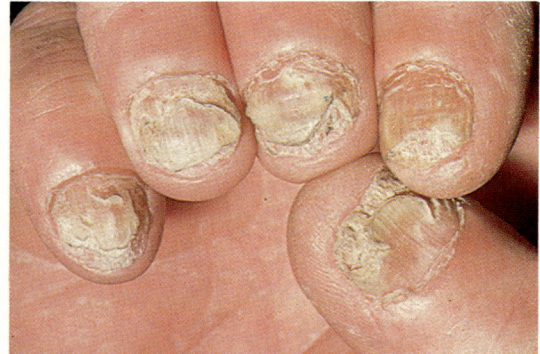

Plate 9.6 Tinea unguium

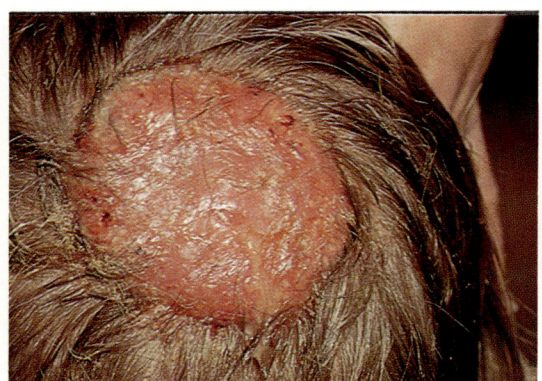

Plate 9.9 Kerion scalp

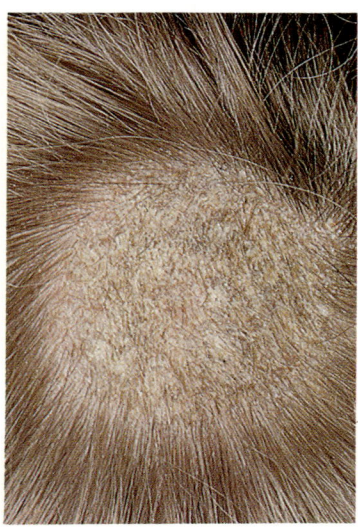

Plate 9.7 Tinea capitis (*M. canis*)

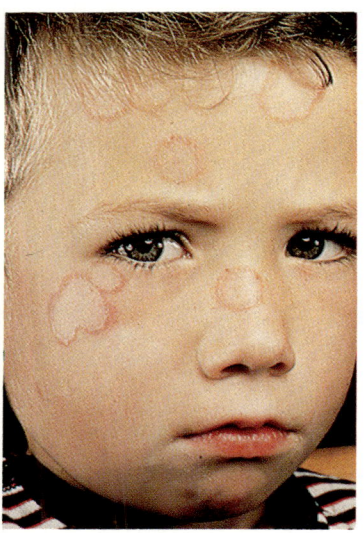

Plate 9.8 Tinea on face (*M. canis*)

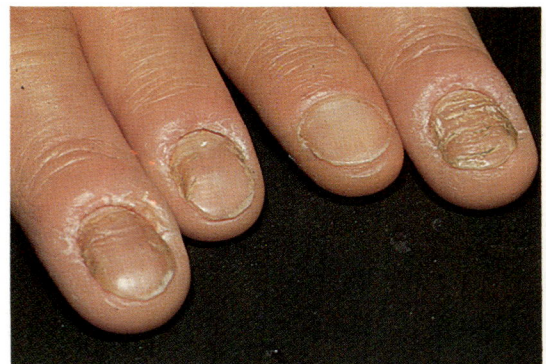

Plate 9.10   Candidal paronychia

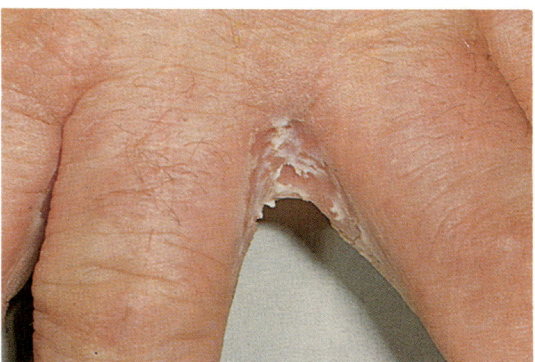

Plate 9.11   Erosio interdigitalis blastomycetica

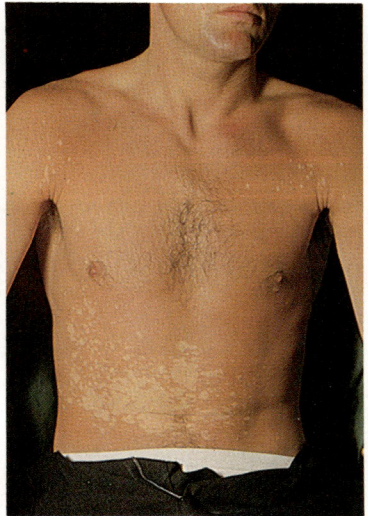

Plate 9.12   Tinea versicolor

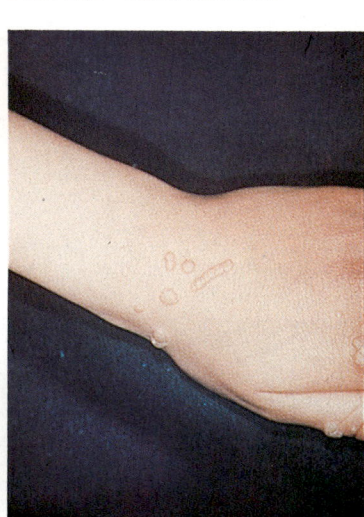

Plate 10.1   Common warts showing isomorphic phenomenon

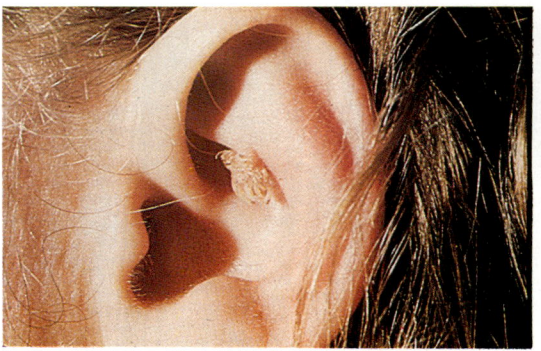

Plate 10.2   Filiform wart ear

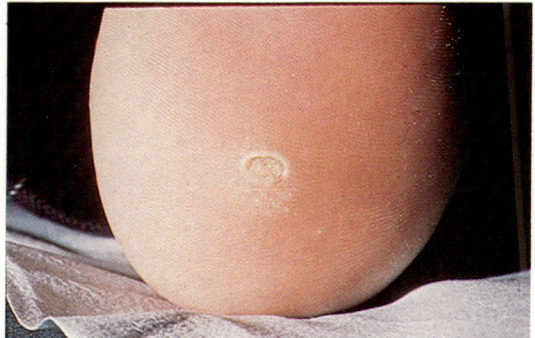

Plate 10.3   Plantar wart

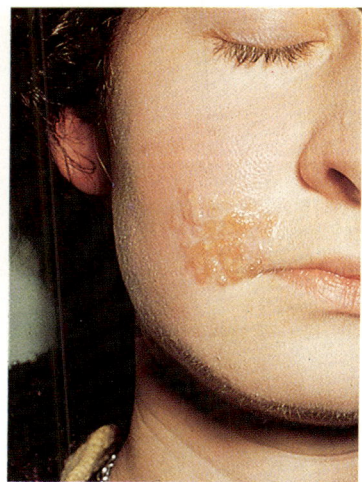

Plate 10.6   Herpes simplex

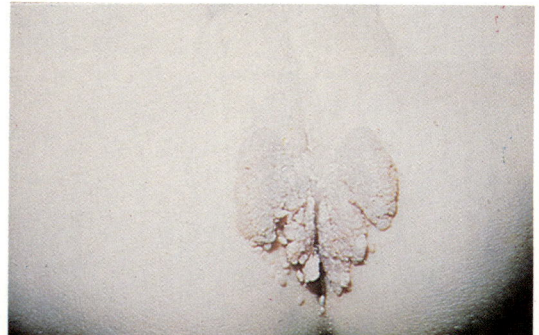

Plate 10.4   Acuminate warts

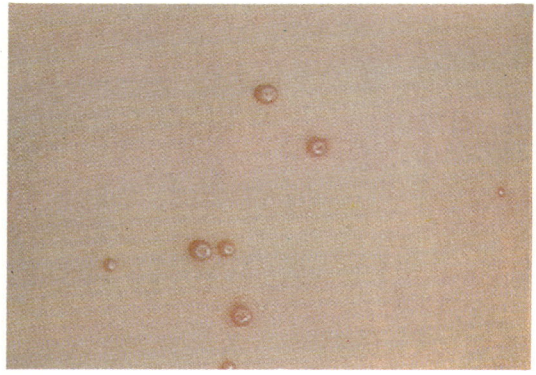

Plate 10.5   *Molluscum contagiosum*

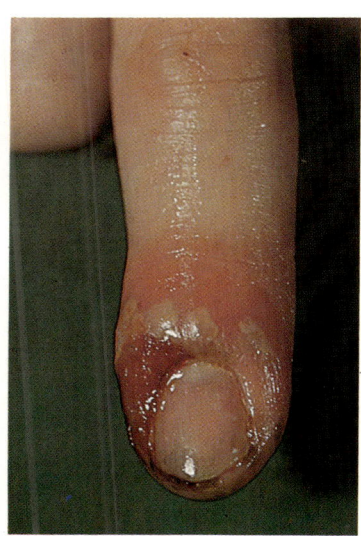

Plate 10.7   Herpetic whitlow

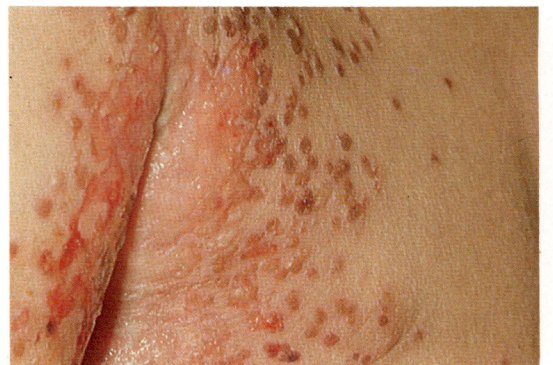

Plate 10.8   Kaposi's varicelliform eruption

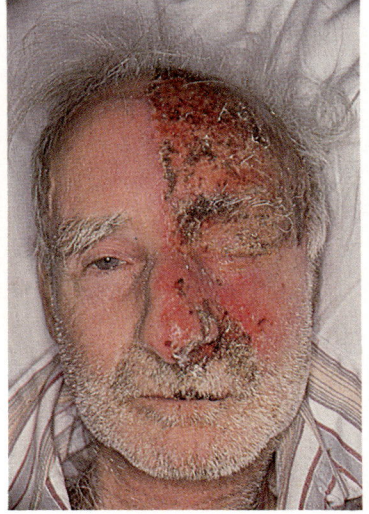

Plate 10.9   Herpes zoster

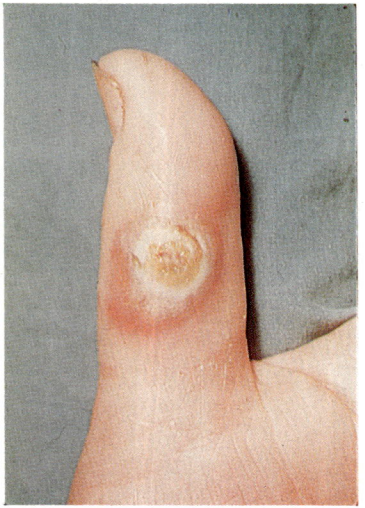

Plate 10.10   Orf

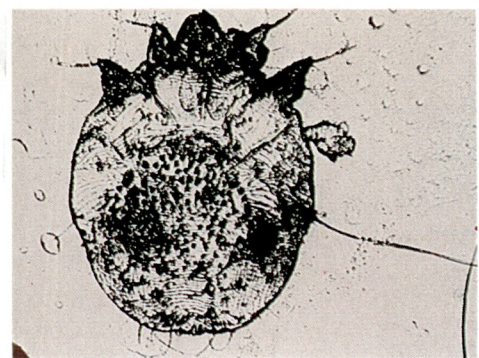

Plate 11.1   Acarus (scabies)

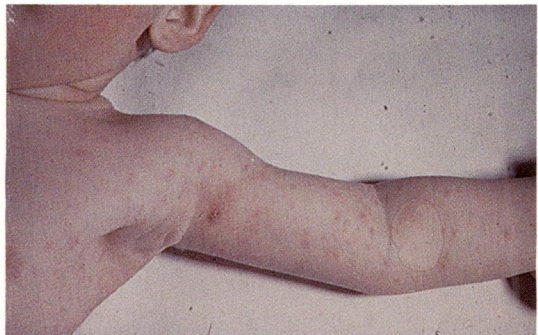

Plate 11.2 Scabies—infant

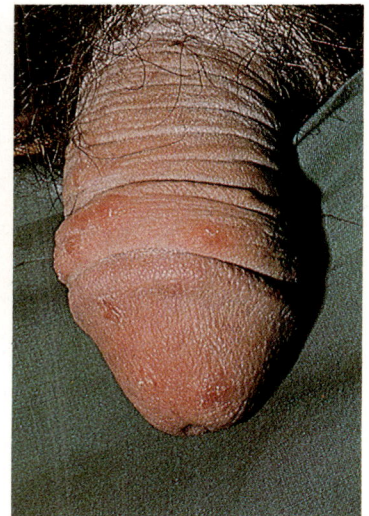

Plate 11.3 Scabies—penile lesions

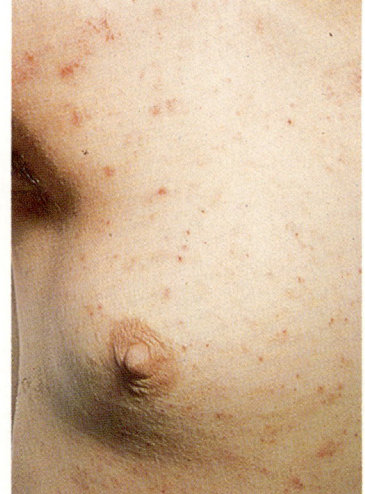

Plate 11.4 Scabies—trunk

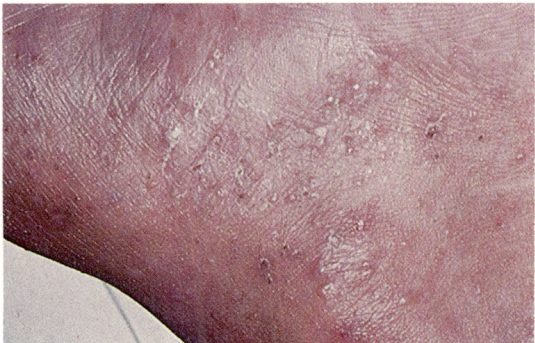

Plate 11.5 Scabetic burrows medial side foot

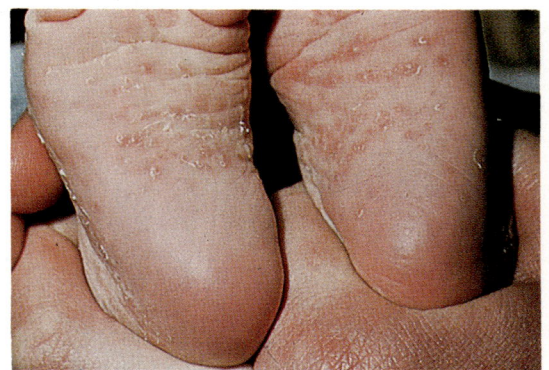

Plate 11.6 Scabies—soles

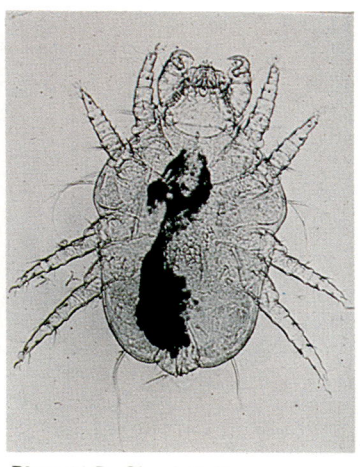

Plate 11.7 Cheyletiella spp.

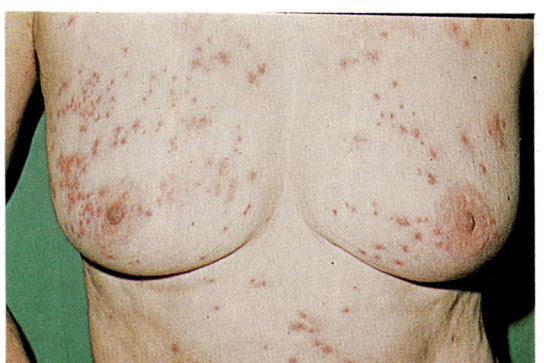

Plate 11.8 Papular urticaria due to cheyletiella

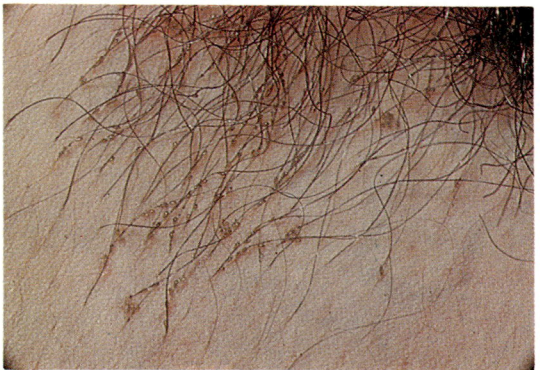

Plate 11.9 Phthirus pubis

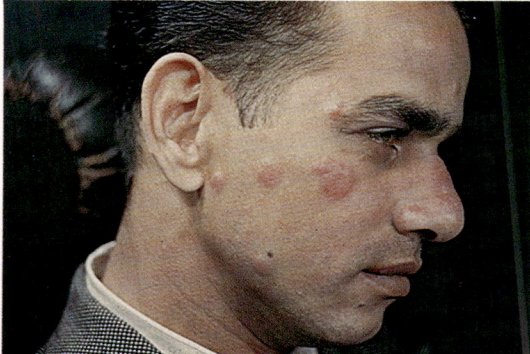

Plate 12.1   Tuberculoid leprosy

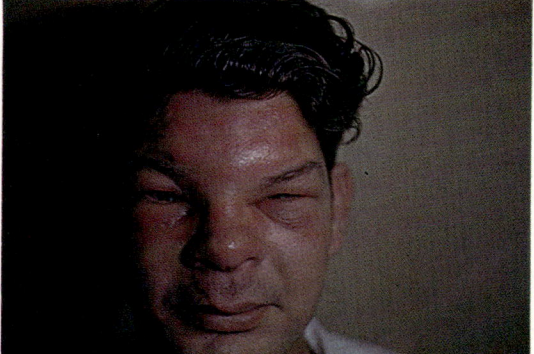

Plate 12.2   Lepromatous leprosy

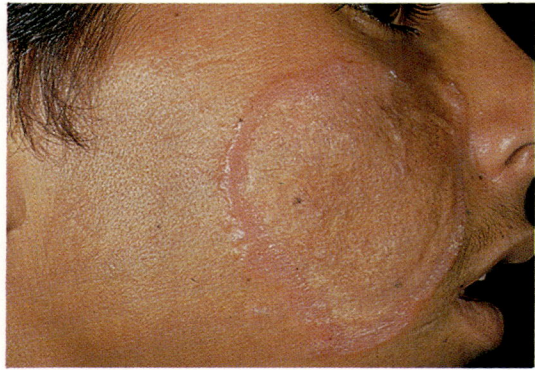

Plate 12.4   Chronic cutaneous leishmaniasis

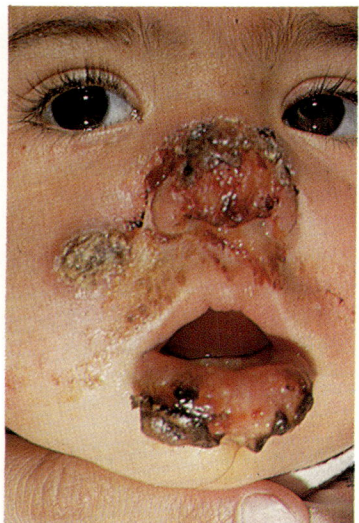

Plate 12.3   Acute cutaneous leishmaniasis

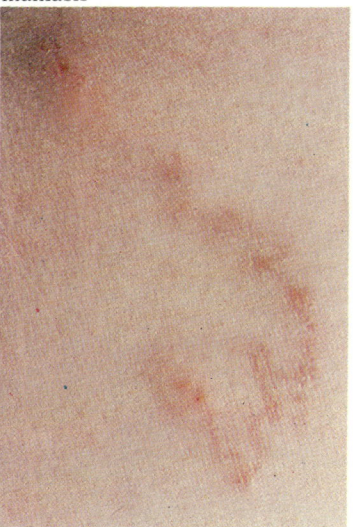

Plate 12.5   Larva migrans (St.
John's Hospital for Diseases of
the Skin)

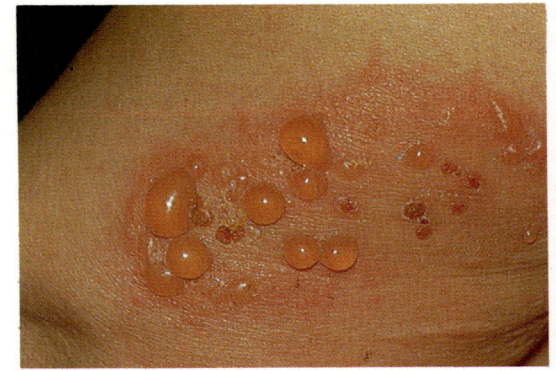

Plate 13.1   Bullous pemphigoid

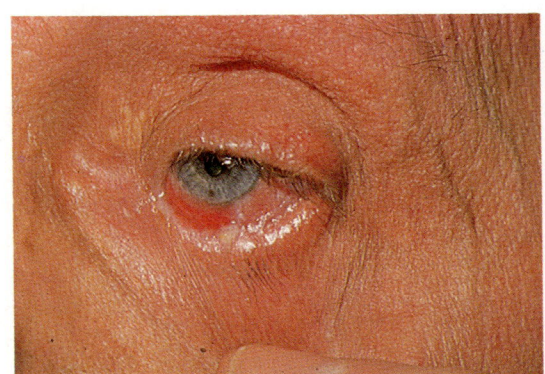

Plate 13.2   Cicatricial pemphigoid with conjunctival scarring

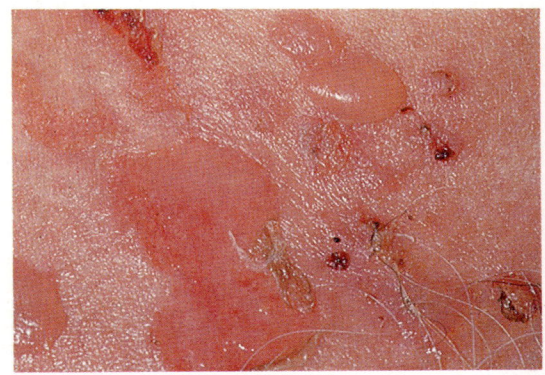

Plate 13.3   Pemphigus vulgaris

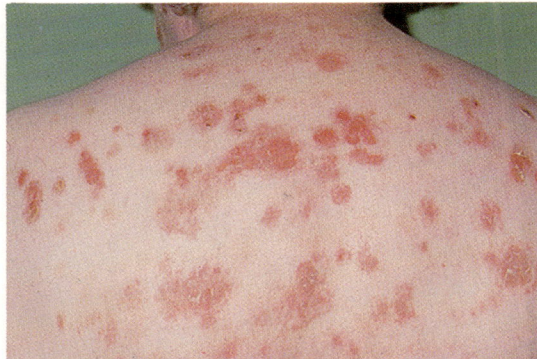

Plate 13.4   Pemphigus foliaceus

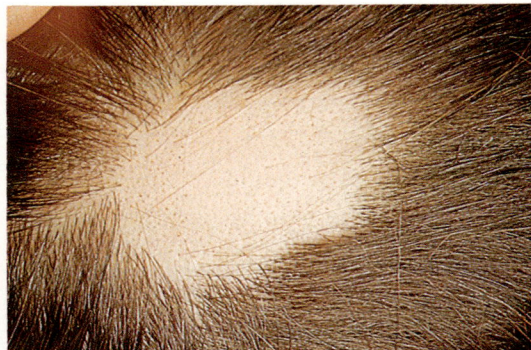

Plate 14.1   Alopecia areata

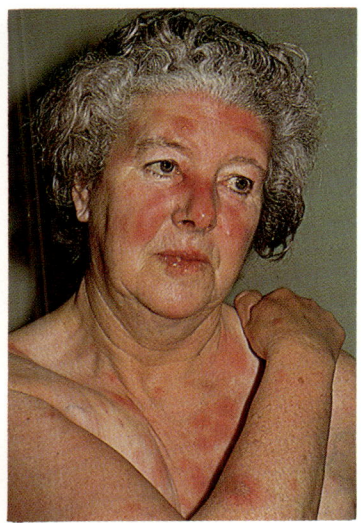

Plate 13.5   Stevens-Johnson syndrome—acute erythema multiforme

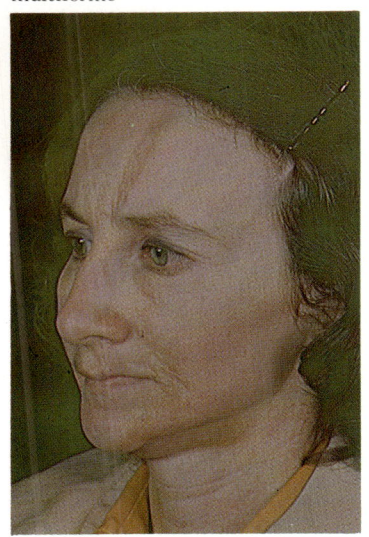

Plate 14.2   Localised scleroderma (Coup de sabre)

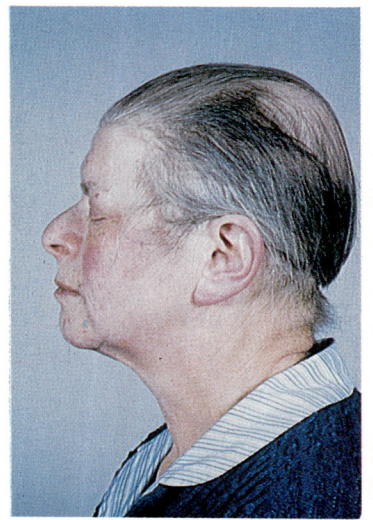

Plate 14.3 Postmenopausal alopecia

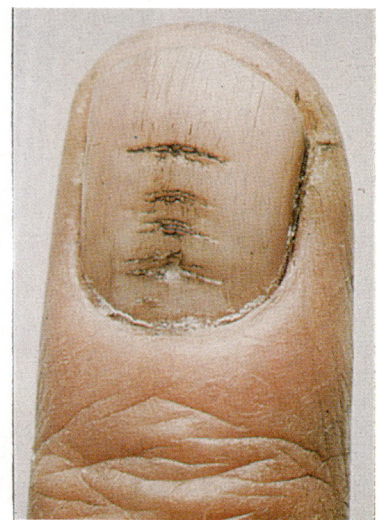

Plate 14.4 'Laddering' of nail

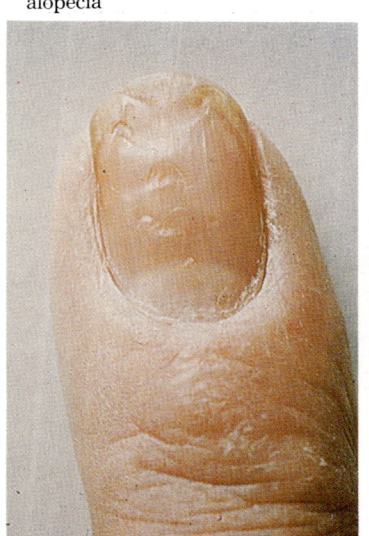

Plate 14.5 Eczematous nail dystrophy

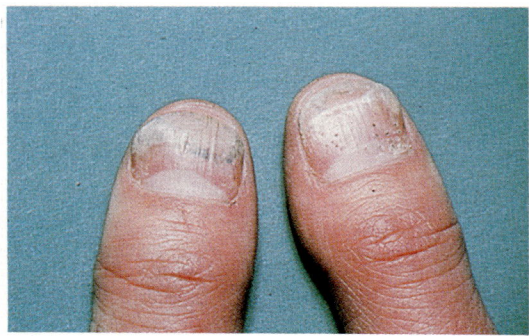

Plate 14.6 Pitting seen in psoriasis

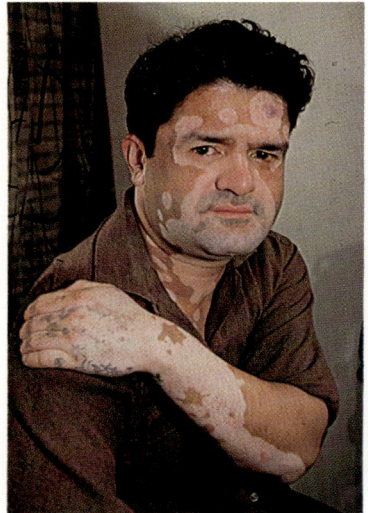

Plate 15.1   Vitiligo

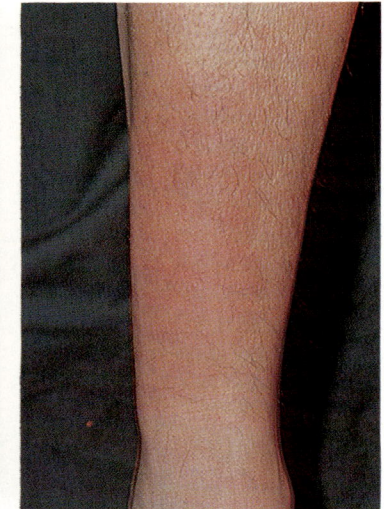

Plate 16.1   Pretibial myxoedema

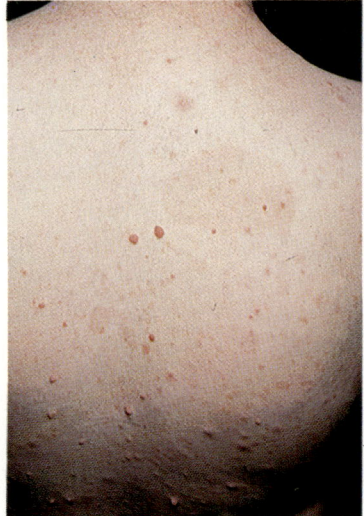

Plate 15.2   Café au lait
pigmentation in
neurofibromatosis

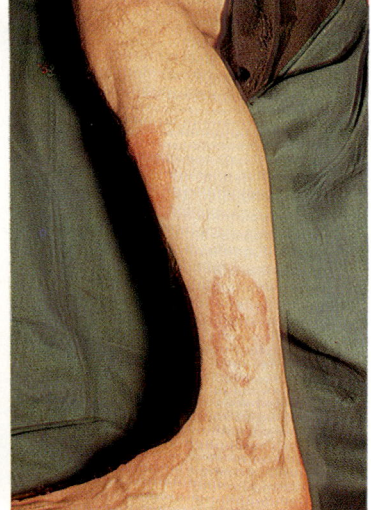

Plate 16.2   Necrobiosis lipoidica

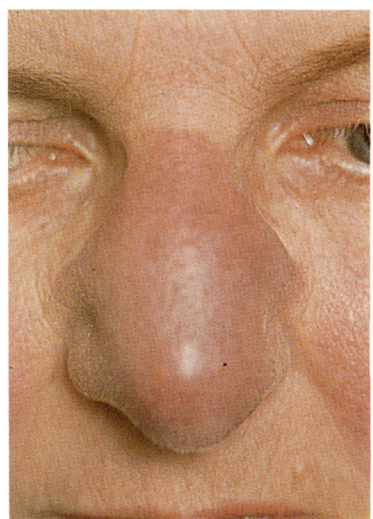

Plate 16.3   Lupus pernio
(sarcoidosis)

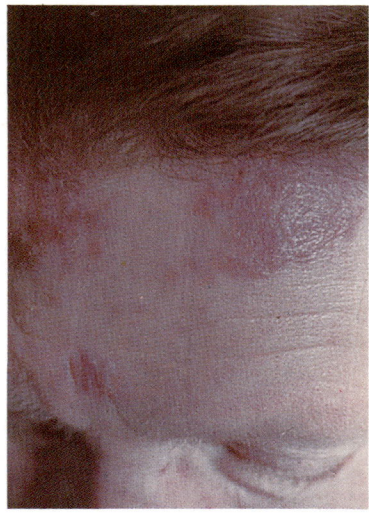

Plate 16.4   Sarcoidosis

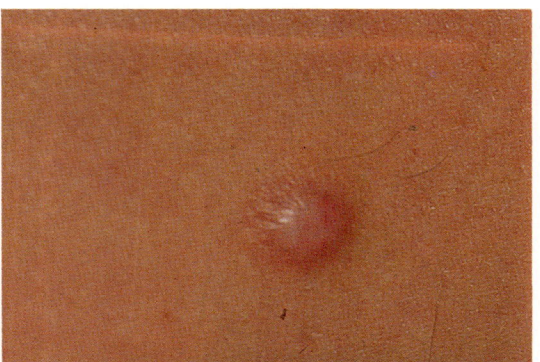

Plate 17.1   Histiocytoma

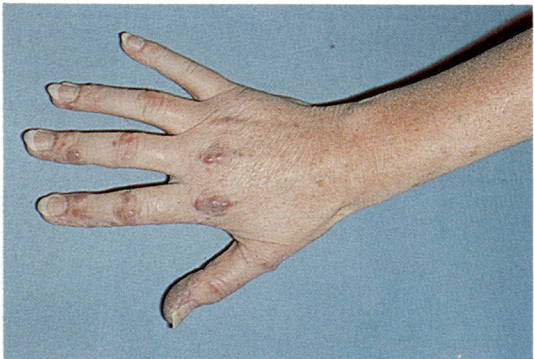

Plate 17.2   Multicentric reticulohistiocytosis

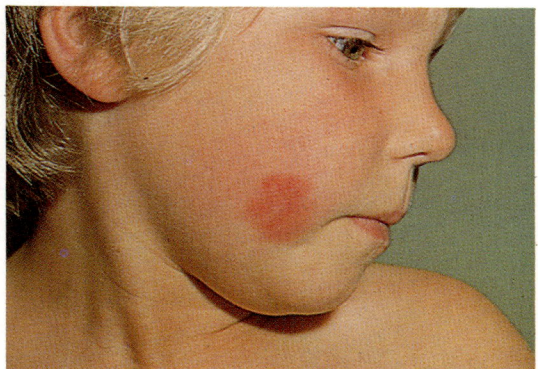

Plate 17.3   Mast cell naevus (urticaria pigmentosa)

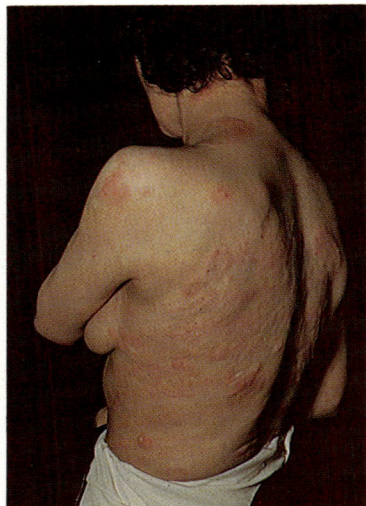

Plate 17.4   Mycosis fungoides

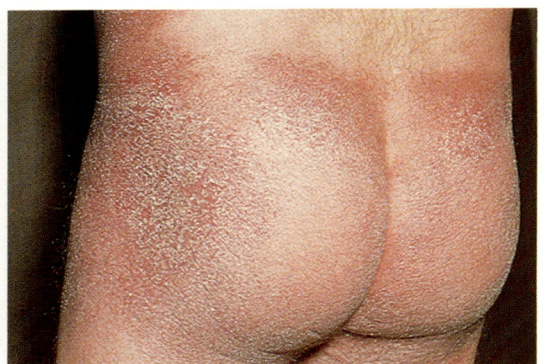

Plate 17.5   Poikiloderma vascularis atrophicans

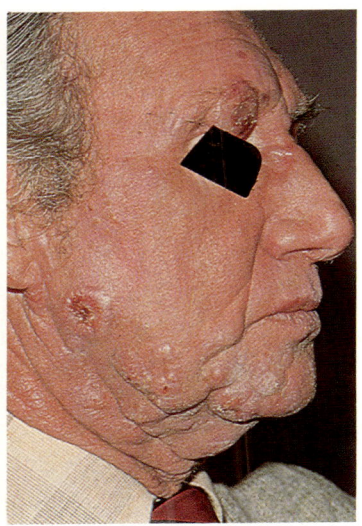

Plate 17.7   Pilar mucinosa—
malignant lymphoma

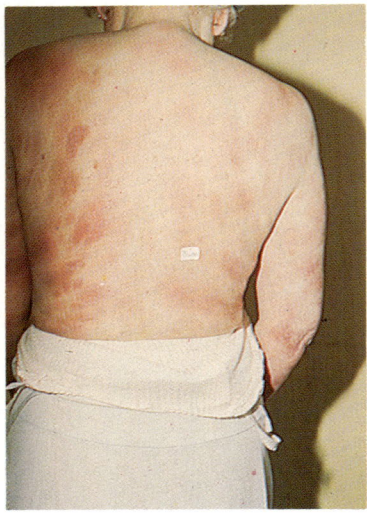

Plate 17.6   Parapsoriasis en plaque

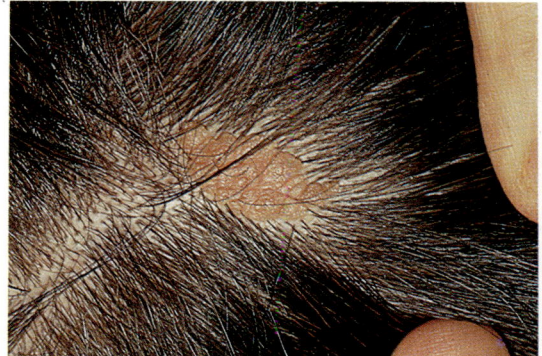

Plate 18.1   Naevus verrucosus scalp

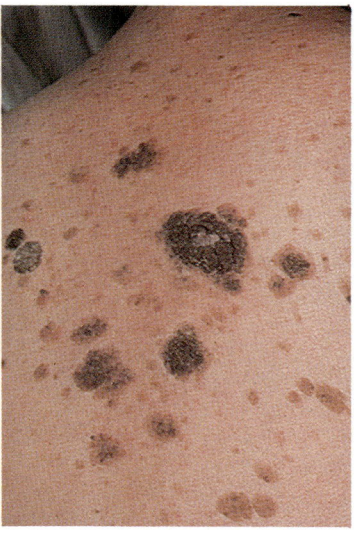

Plate 18.2   Seborrhoeic warts

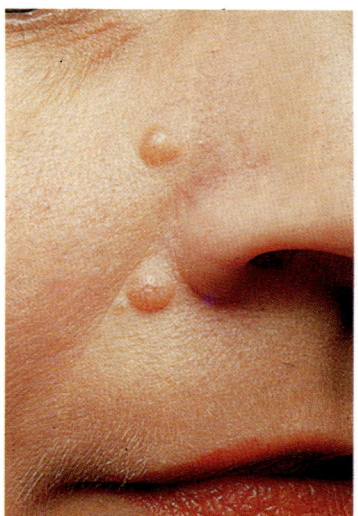

Plate 18.3   Cellular naevi

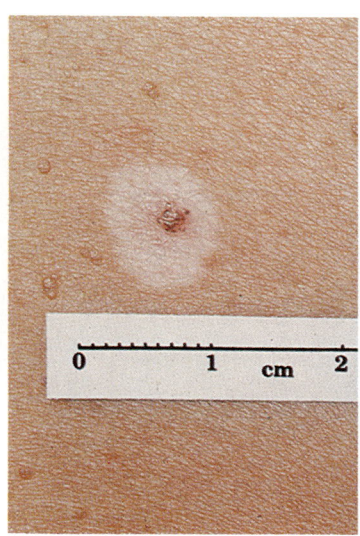

Plate 18.4   Halo naevus

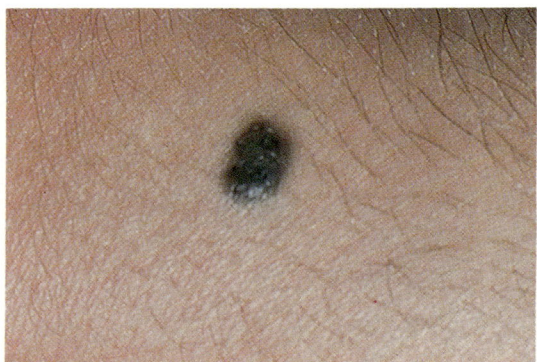

Plate 18.5   Blue naevus

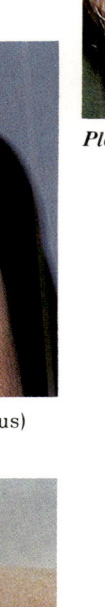

Plate 18.8   Actinic keratoses

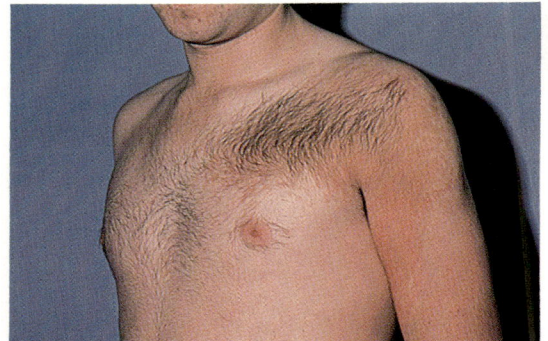

Plate 18.6   Naevus spilus tardus (Becker's naevus)

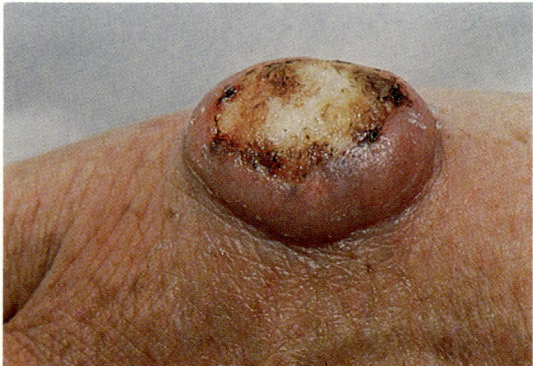

Plate 18.7   Keratoacanthoma

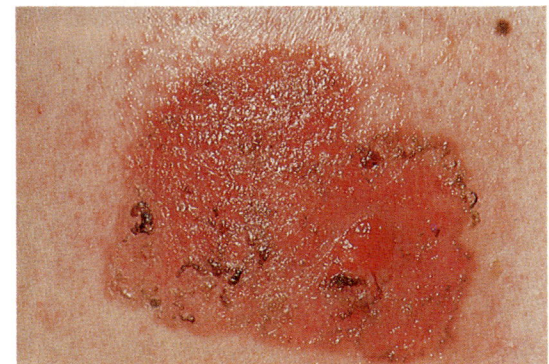

Plate 18.9 Bowen's disease

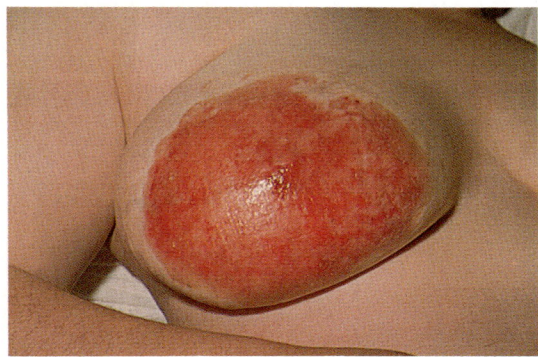

Plate 18.10 Paget's disease of breast

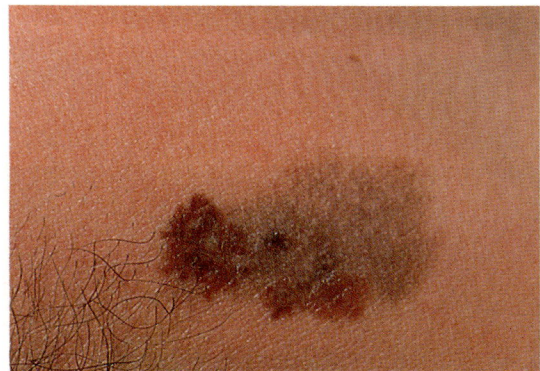

Plate 18.11 Lentigo maligna

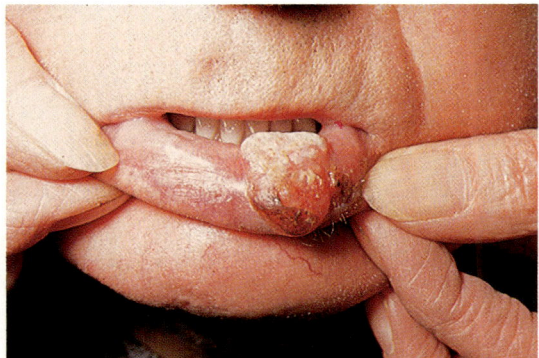

Plate 18.12   Squamous cell carcinoma lip

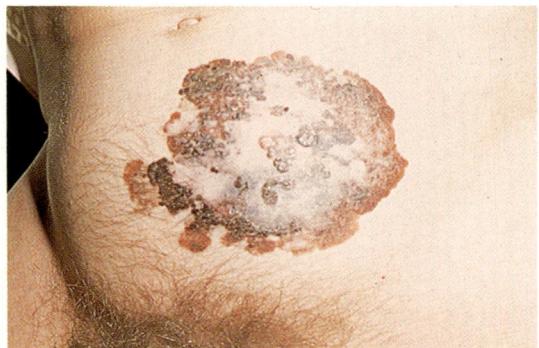

Plate 18.13   Malignant melanoma—superficial spreading

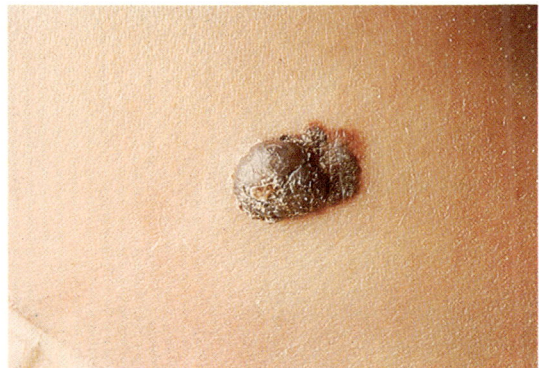

Plate 18.14   Malignant melanoma

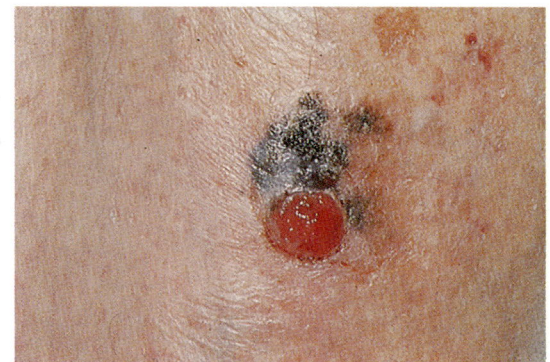

Plate 18.15   Malignant melanoma—lower pole
fungating

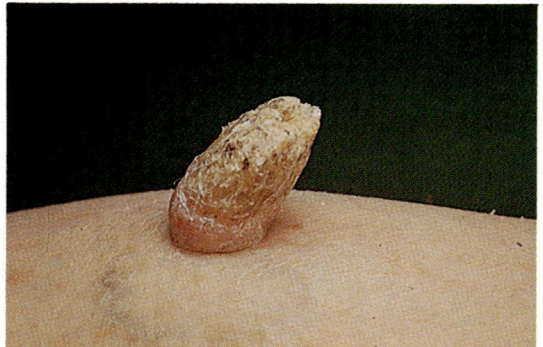

Plate 18.16   Cutaneous horn

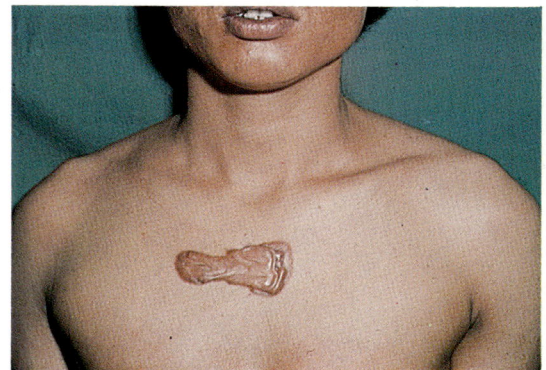

Plate 18.17   Keloid

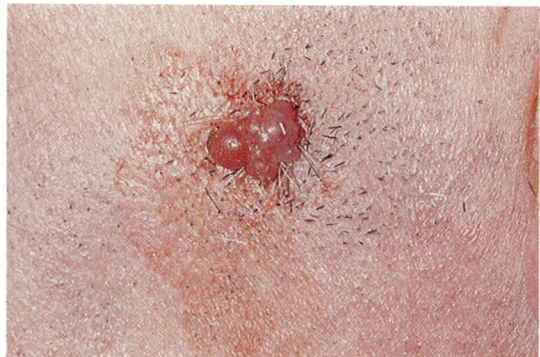

Plate 18.18   Pyogenic granuloma

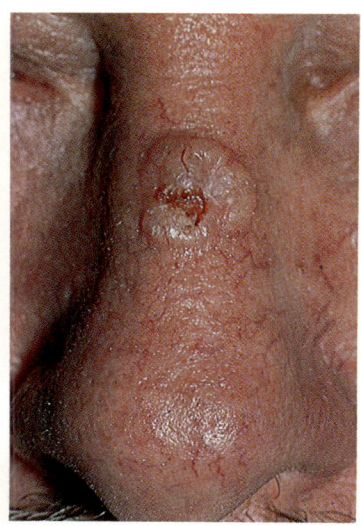

Plate 18.19   Basal cell epithelioma

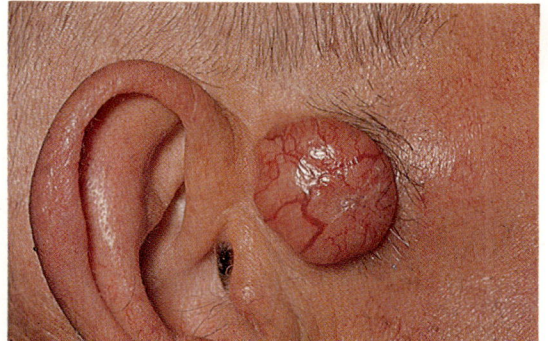

Plate 18.20   Nodulo-cystic basal cell epithelioma

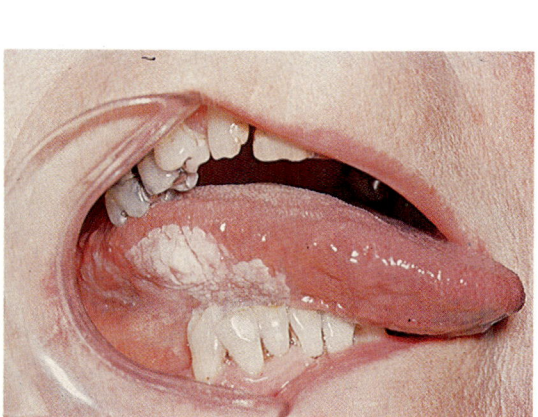

Plate 18.21   Leukoplakia of tongue

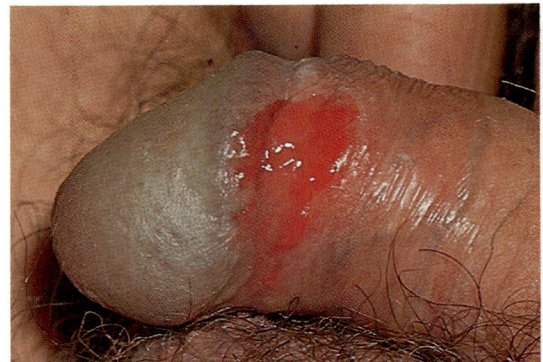

Plate 18.22   Erythroplasia of Queryat

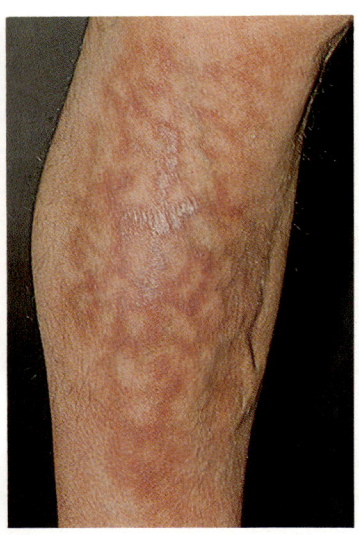

Plate 19.1   Erythema ab igne

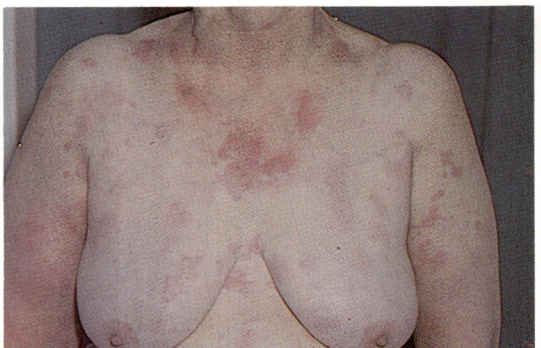

Plate 19.2   Urticaria

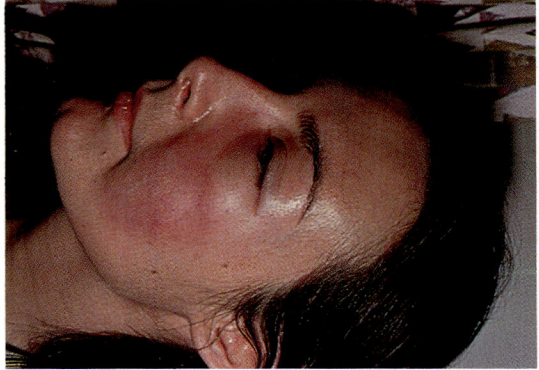

Plate 19.3   Angioedma

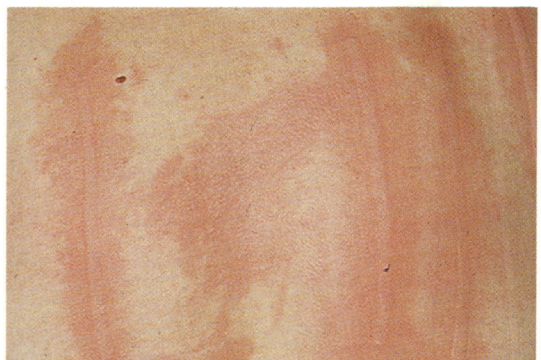

Plate 19.4   Dermographism

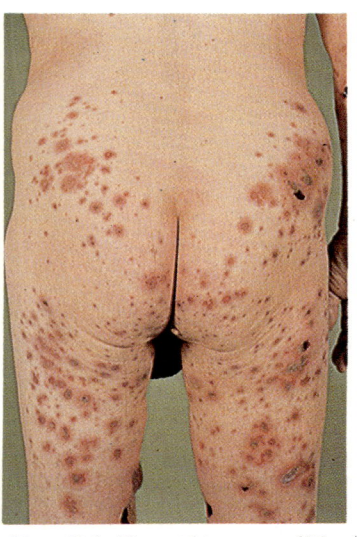

Plate 19.6   Necrotising vasculitis

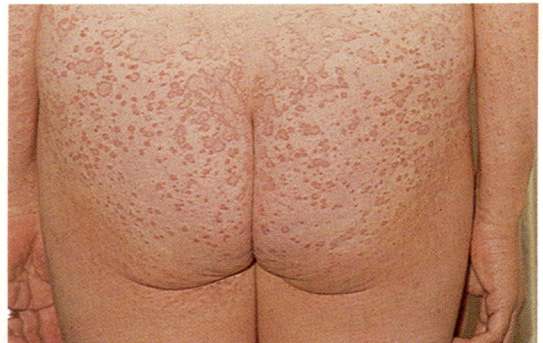

Plate 19.5   Henoch-Schönlein purpura

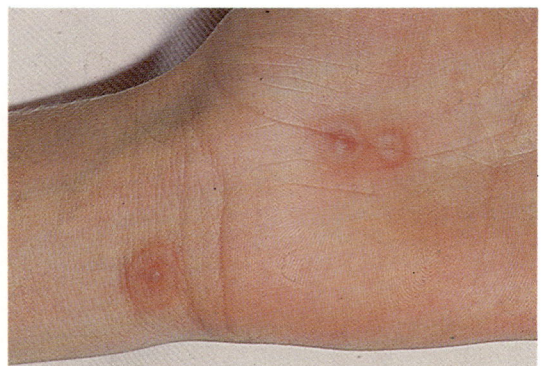

Plate 19.7   Erythema multiforme

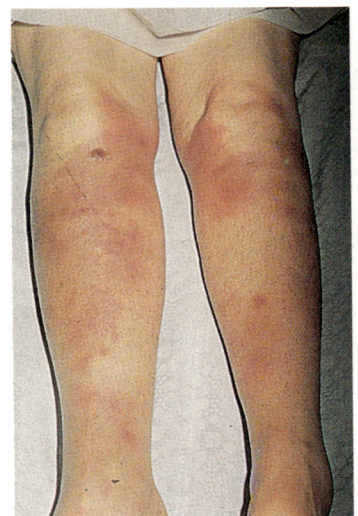

Plate 19.8   Erythema nodosum

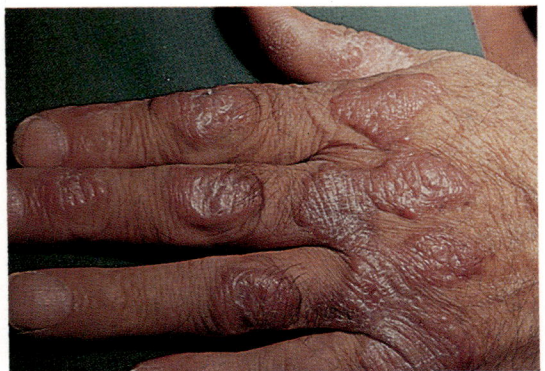

Plate 19.9   Erythema elevatum diutinum

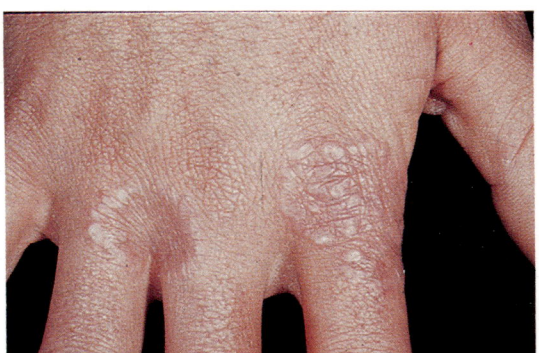

Plate 19.10   Granuloma annulare

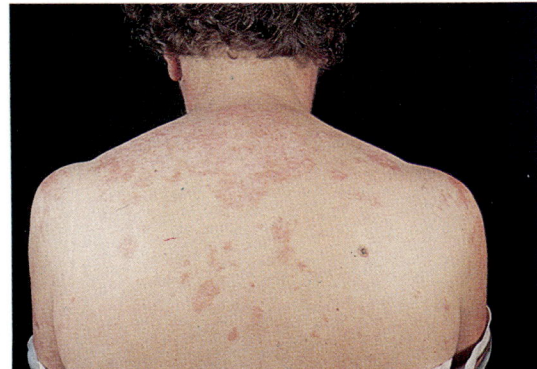

Plate 19.11   Systemic lupus erythematosus

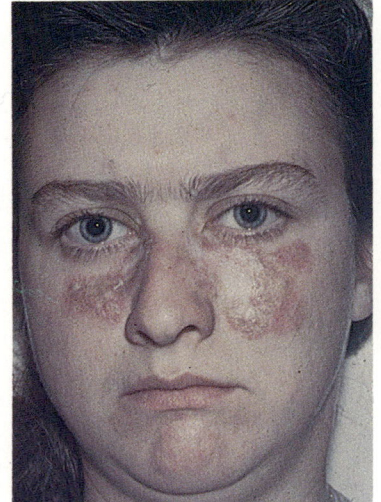

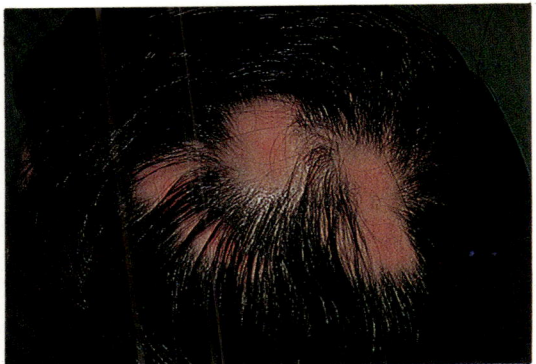

Plate 19.13   Lupus erythematosus scalp

Plate 19.12   Discoid lupus
erythematosus

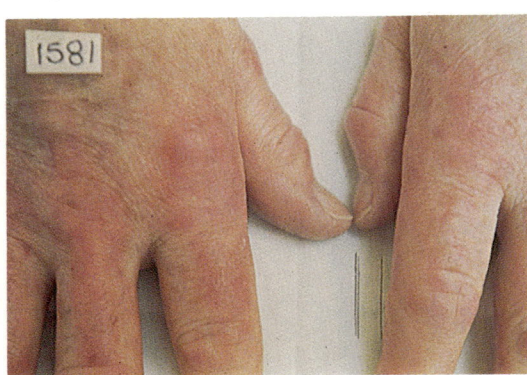

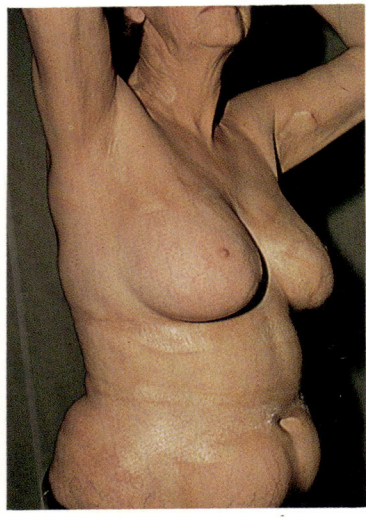

Plate 19.15   Morphoea (localised
scleroderma)

Plate 19.14   Dermatomyositis (Gottron's spots)

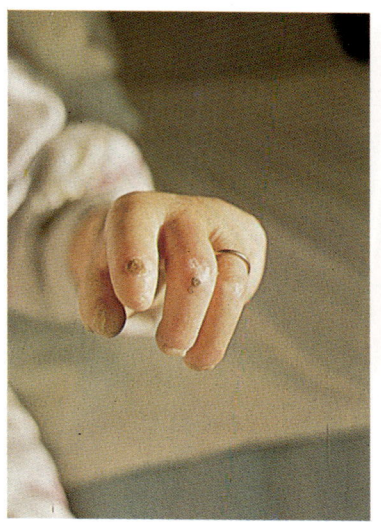

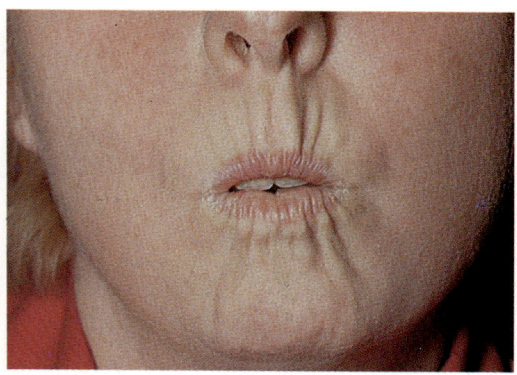

Plate 19.17 Systemic scleroderma showing purse-string mouth

Plate 19.16 Fingers in advanced systemic scleroderma

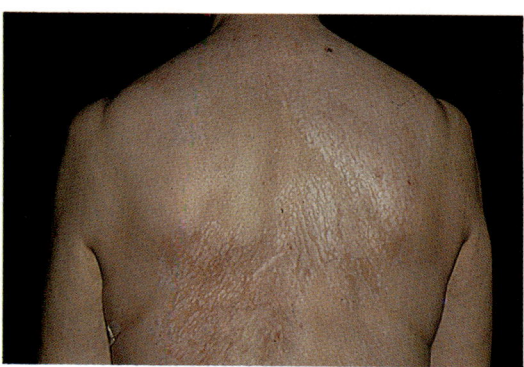

Plate 19.18 Lichen sclerosus et atrophicus

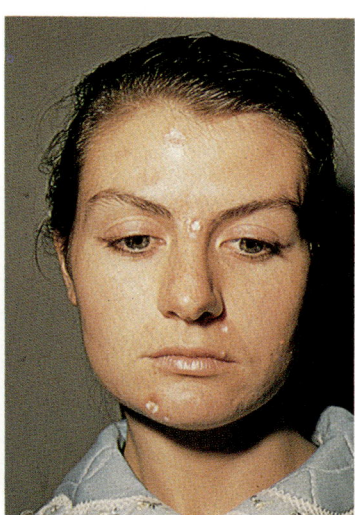

Plate 20.1 Dermatitis artefacta

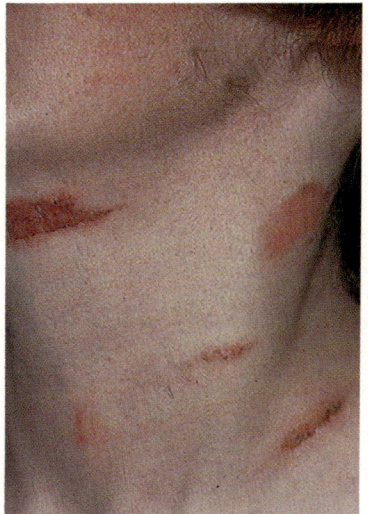

Plate 20.2 Dermatitis artefacta

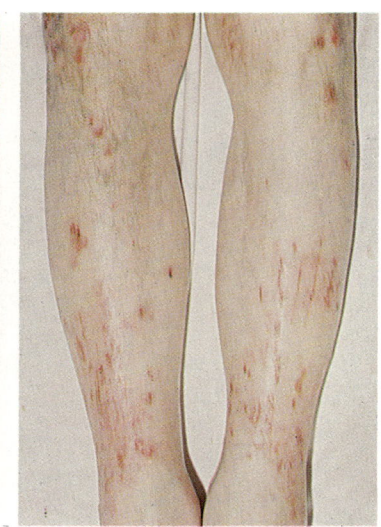

Plate 20.3 Neurotic excoriations

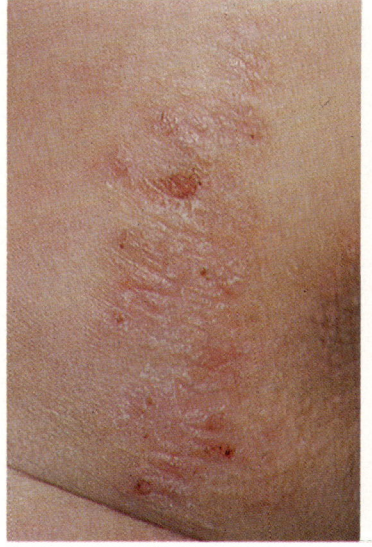

Plate 20.4 Lichen simplex
chronicus

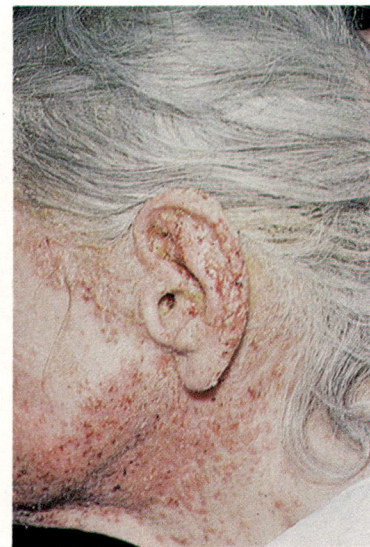

Plate 21.1 Darier's disease

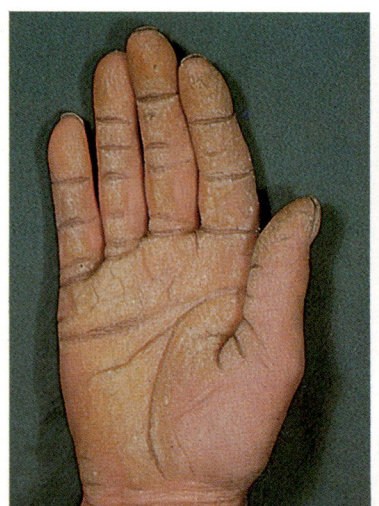

Plate 21.2 Palmoplantar hyperkeratosis (tylosis)

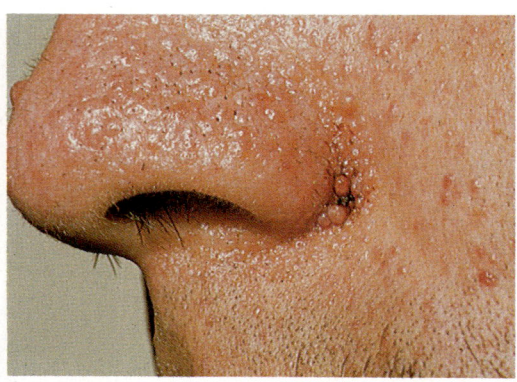

Plate 21.4 Tuberose sclerosis

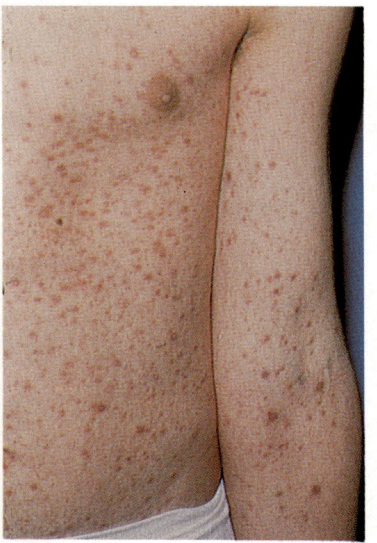

Plate 22.1 Pityriasis lichenoides

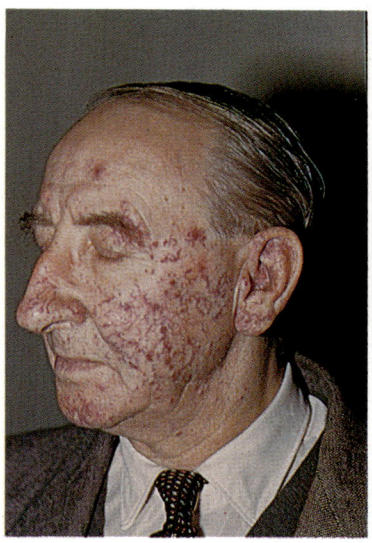

Plate 21.3 Hereditary haemorrhagic telangiectasis

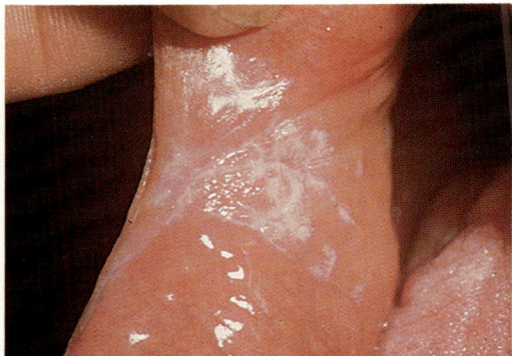

Plate 22.2   Buccal lichen planus

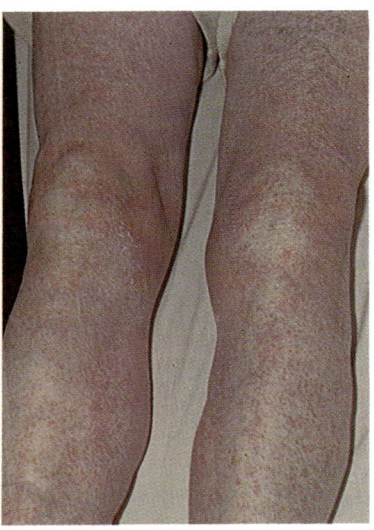

Plate 23.1   Purpuric rash due to carbromal

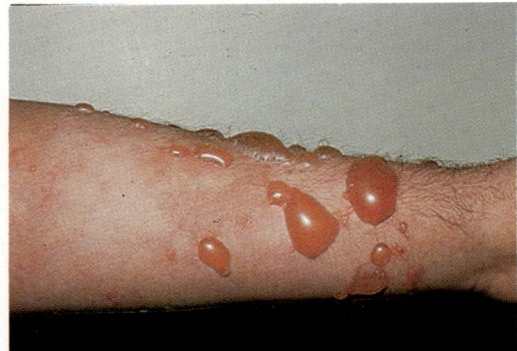

Plate 23.2   Bullous photoreaction to nalidixic acid

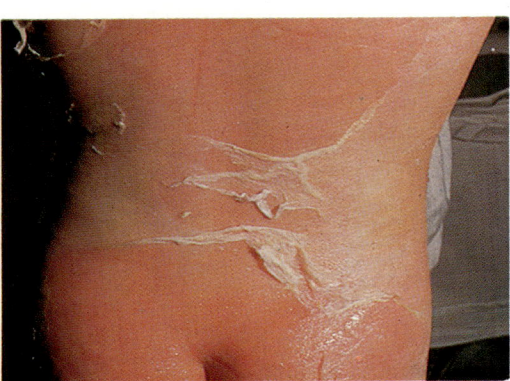

Plate 23.3   Toxic epidermal necrolysis due to cotrimoxazole

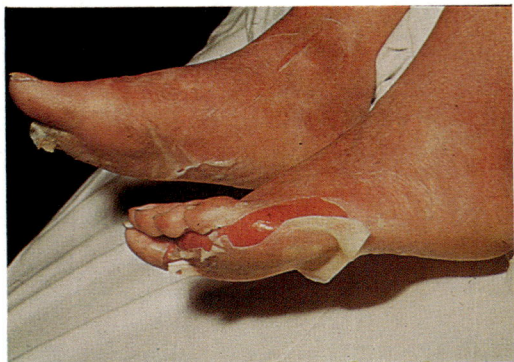

Plate 23.4 Toxic epidermal necrolysis due to sulphonamide

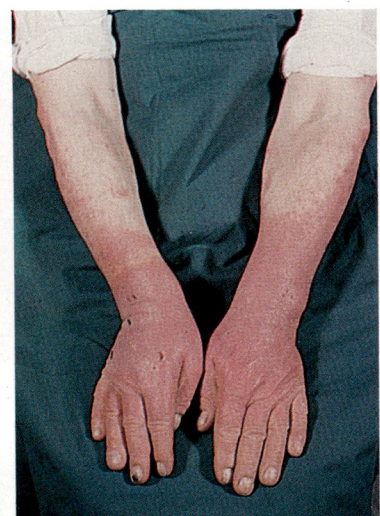

Plate 23.5 Photosensitivity to hydrochlorothiazide

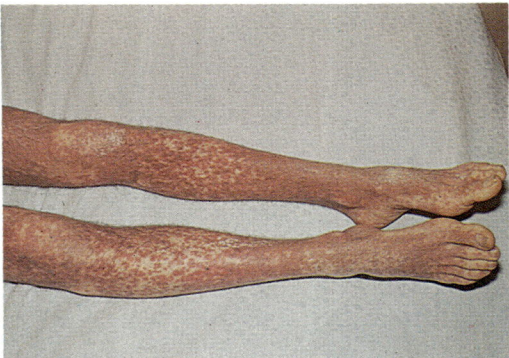

Plate 23.6 Ampicillin rash in infectious mononucleosis

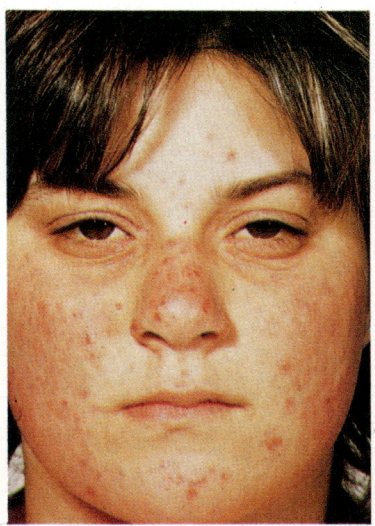

Plate 24.1 Actinic prurigo

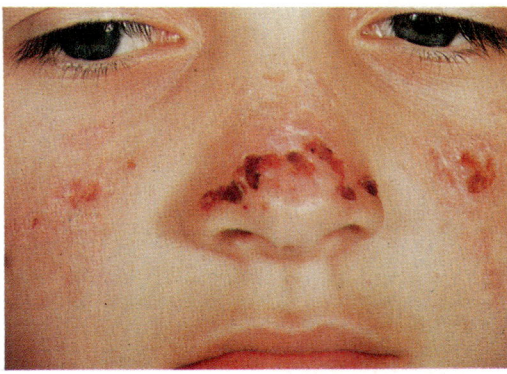

Plate 24.2 Hydroa vacciniforme

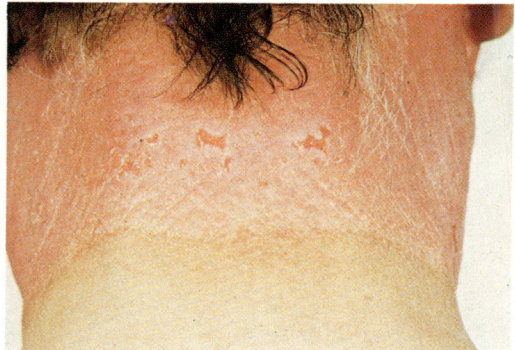

Plate 24.3   Photosensitivity dermatitis

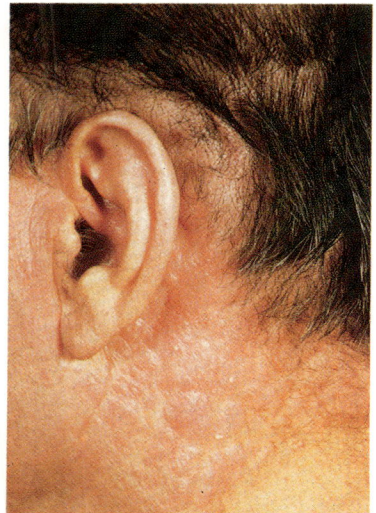

Plate 24.4   Actinic reticuloid

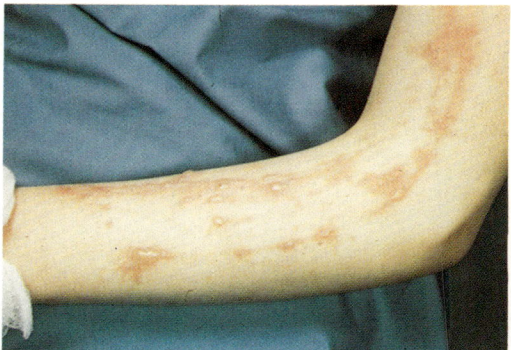

Plate 24.5   Phytophotodermatitis (giant hogweed)

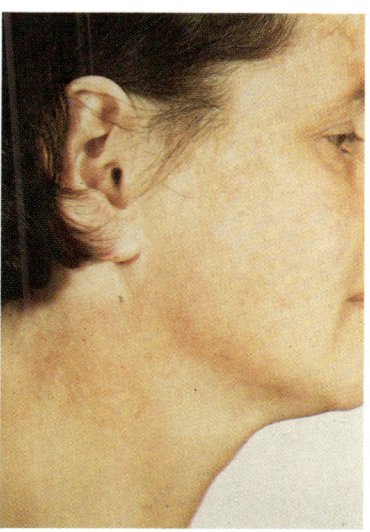

Plate 24.6   Poikiloderma of Civatte

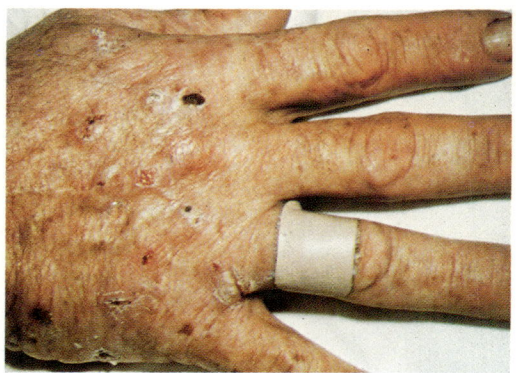

Plate 24.7   Hepatic porphyria

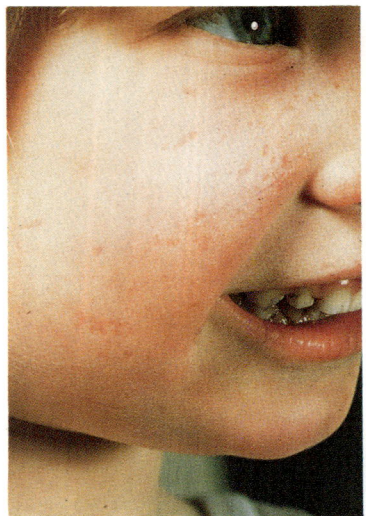

Plate 24.8 Erythropoietic photoporphyria

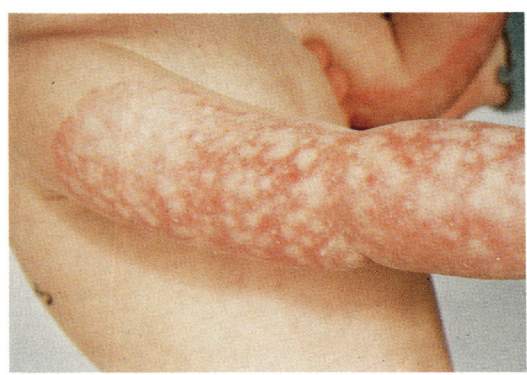

Plate 24.10 Rothmund-Thomson syndrome

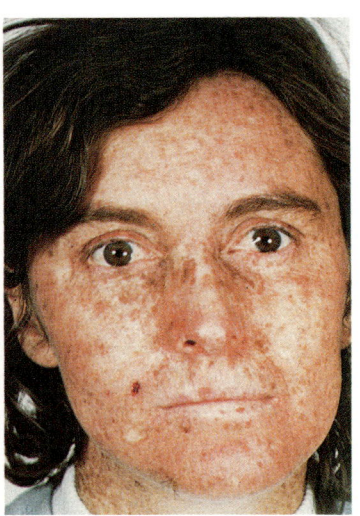

Plate 24.11 Xeroderma pigmentosum

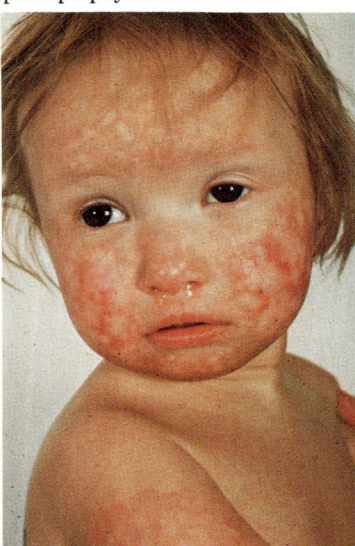

Plate 24.9 Rothmund-Thomson syndrome

Kaposi's sarcoma

This is a neoplastic process of debatable histogenesis. Histologically endothelial proliferation occurs in lymphatics and capillaries. Neovascularization is seen with proliferation of pericytes and fibrosis.

Males are more commonly affected than females (10:1). Three main groups of patients are seen:

(1) young Africans with skin and lymph node lesions,
(2) older Sepharic Jews who exhibit a high incidence of other lymphomas including Hodgkin's disease, mycosis fungoides and chronic lymphatic leukaemia, and
(3) immunosupressed subjects—renal transplant recipients—and long-term steroid patients.

The initial manifestations are usually in the lower limb with oedema and ecchymoses. Following this inflammatory stage angiomatous nodules appear which tend to remain indolent. Occasionally lesions regress spontaneously. In other instances spread to lymph nodes and the gastrointestinal tract is noted. Rarely frank angiosarcomatous changes occur.

The differential diagnosis is from Stewart–Treves syndrome which is commoner in the upper limbs and from angiolymphatic hyperplasia commoner in the head and neck.

General clinical features of the lymphomas

The cutaneous manifestations common to the lymphomas can be classified under three headings:

(1) The pre-lymphomatous eruption

At this stage the cutaneous eruption is non-diagnostic and often closely simulates some of the commoner dermatoses. In some instances this stage lasts for many years. The non-specific or pre-lymphomatous cutaneous manifestations come under the following, as adapted from Bluefarb:

Pallor: due to anaemia.

Pruritus: an early symptom of a lymphoma especially Hodgkin's disease or indeed any visceral neoplasm.

Prurigo-like papules: the result of continued rubbing and scratching, the 'prurigo lymphatica' of older physicians.

Pyoderma: the result of scratching and diminished resistance to infection.

Pigmentation: widespread melanosis seen notably in Hodgkin's disease.

Pemphigoid and other bullous lesions: these are uncommon even in leukaemia where the blister fluid sometimes contains leukaemic cells demonstrable by microscopy.

Pityriasis rubra (Hebra), now termed exfoliative dermatitis: an uncommon mode of presentation of lymphatic leukaemia, Hodgkin's disease and mycosis fungoides. The brick red 'homme rouge' is characteristic of the lymphoblastic erythroderma of Sequeira and Panton.

Poikiloderma (*Plate 17.5*): these patches which resemble radiodermatitis show telangiectasia, macular pigmentation and depigmentation papules and atrophic macules. Poikiloderma when appearing with large plaques of parapsoriasis usually signifies transformation of the disease into mycosis fungoides.

Posterior ganglionitis commonly called zoster: the cause is direct pressure on the dorsal root ganglia, e.g. from lymphoma deposits, or depression of the normal immunological responses of the patient. A haemorrhagic zoster should suggest the possibility of lymphatic leukaemia whilst zoster with aberrant vesicles especially in an elderly subject should lead to the suspicion of a lymphoma such as Hodgkin's disease. Recurrent varicella-zoster disease strengthens the suspicion of immunological defect with an underlying lymphoma.

Phlebitis: thrombophlebitis and particularly thrombophlebitis migrans suggests either a visceral neoplasia (especially pancreatic) or a lymphoma.

Periodontal swelling and buccal ulceration: both primary and secondary agranulocytosis and monocytic leukaemia may present with spongy bleeding gums or less commonly mucosal ulceration (agranulocytic angina).

Protein disturbance: the presenting clinical features of lymphocyte and plasma cell disorders are often the result of either a decrease or increase in circulating proteins. Dysproteinaemia usually affects immunoglobulins. Abnormal proteins found in the circulation include cryoglobulins, macroglobulins and immunoglobulins. The associated cutaneous findings include purpura, amyloid deposits and rarely xanthomata. When the immunological proteins are deficient resistance to infection, both fungal and bacterial, is impaired. Granulopenia is sometimes another factor predisposing to infection.

Perivasculitis: any malignant process—presumably because the cells are 'foreign'—may evoke an abnormal immune response in some individuals, i.e. an autoimmune reaction which shows nonspecific nodules and erythemata. Such lesions are often persistent and resemble erythema nodosum, erythema annulare or erythema multiforme.

Parapsoriasis en plaques (*Plate 17.6*): this appears with large red scaly patches resembling psoriasis which after a variable time (one to 30 years) increase in number and become pruritic. Other changes heralding transformation into mycosis fungoides are palpable infiltration, increased redness or a range of coloration from red to dusky violet, sharper definition, a spread to enclose islands of normal skin and spread to the face, hands and feet. A further important change indicating evolution of the larger plaques of parapsoriasis into a lymphoma is the appearance of patches of poikiloderma.

Pilar mucinosis: extensive infiltrated areas of follicular mucinosis on the trunk signal this early lymphomatous change in the skin. Whereas a localized follicular mucinosis on the scalp, face or neck is frequently self-limiting and not neoplastic, the presence of widespread plaques particularly on the trunk are signs of existing lymphoma. Alopecia mucinosa is more correctly designated early lymphoma rather than lymphoma (*Plate 17.7*). Gelatinous material can be expressed from the hair follicles in many instances and appropriate staining of histological sections shows characteristic mucin deposits in the hair follicle wall.

(2) Infiltrative stage

The appearance of infiltrative plaques on either existing parapsoriasis patches or *de novo* on previously unaffected skin.

(3) Tumour stage

This may result from progression through an infiltrative stage or occasionally there will be frank tumours from the onset. Ulceration can occur over large areas whilst nodules and ulceration on the scalp may result in alopecia.

Investigations

After full clinical examination with particular attention to enlarged lymph nodes, liver and spleen the following investigations are required in order to make an accurate diagnosis:

(1) Skin biopsy—several lesions may require investigation. Cyto-diagnosis has its advocates in establishing a rapid diagnosis.
(2) Blood count, differential and smear examination.
(3) Marrow—sternal marrow or iliac crest biopsy.
(4) Lymph node biopsy.
(5) Serum proteins, electrophoresis to detect abnormal proteins, urine for abnormal proteins.
(6) X-ray of chest and bony skeleton.
(7) Exploratory laparotomy.

Treatment

A solitary reactive or granulomatous lesion is treated by excision, cryotherapy or radiotherapy.

Unfortunately definitive treatment of many lymphomas is unsatisfactory. Fractional small doses of superficial radiotherapy give symptomatic relief in the lymphomatous and early infiltrative dermatoses. Likewise potent topical steroids enhanced by polythene occlusion will relieve pruritus and ultraviolet light sometimes induces a temporary remission. Cytotoxic agents such as cyclophosphamide may be useful in the early infiltrative stage. However there is no evidence that early vigorous treatment modifies the subsequent course of the disease; indeed it may do harm. Sequential treatment, rather than combined treatment by cytotoxic drugs and radiotherapy, is generally advisable commencing with superficial x-ray therapy with cytotoxic drugs being used if recurrent lesions show signs of becoming radioresistant; later the lesions may become radiosensitive again. In widespread cases of Hodgkin's disease and mycosis fungoides electron beam therapy is used.

Other dermatological features of lymphomas and myeloproliferative diseases are shown in *Table 17.2*.

Table 17.2 Dermatological presentations of lymphomas and myeloproliferative disorders

Skin changes	Disorder
Early:	
Pallor	Leukaemia, Hodgkin's disease
Pruritus, prurigo	Hodgkin's disease, leukaemia, polycythaemia
Erythematous patches	Mycosis fungoides
Erythematous papules	Lymphomatoid papulosis
Poikiloderma	Mycosis fungoides
Purpura	Myelomatosis, leukaemia
Erythroderma	Hodgkin's disease, mycosis fungoides, Sezary's syndrome, leukaemia
Melanosis	Hodgkin's disease, mast cell disease
Skin infections	Mycosis fungoides, Hodgkin's disease, leukaemia
Rare manifestations:	
Xanthoma disseminatum	Histiocytosis X
Xanthoma planum	Myelomatosis
Pyoderma gangrenosum	Polycythaemia, leukaemia, myelomatosis
Pemphigoid	Leukaemia, mastocytosis
Pilar mucinosis	Mycosis fungoides
Amyloid	Myelomatosis
Buccal ulcers	Monocytic leukaemia
Late:	
Plaques, nodules, ulcers, vegetating lesions	Mycosis fungoides, Hodgkin's disease, lymphosarcoma, polycythaemia, leukaemia, reticulum cell sarcoma

18 Tumours of the skin

R. J. Cairns

The adult skin represents a cellular mosaic of diverse embryonic origin. Some cells are concerned with renewal and replacement—dividing, maturing and shedding throughout life; others are concerned with pigment, grease, sweat and hair production.

A single cell from any of these diverse functional groups can undergo mutation and divide continuously giving rise to a colony of daughter cells. Such cellular growth is termed clonal proliferation and it may occur as a temporary phenomenon or as a permanent process. When proliferation is stable a naevus or benign tumour results, but when unstable with uncontrolled proliferation, malignancy ensues.

A great variety of malformations and tumours of the skin are derived from cell lines differentiated into ecto- and mesodermal structures. Like tumours affecting other organs, skin tumours comprise the heterogeneous group that closely resemble the features of tumours elsewhere.

The histogenesis of skin tumours is best understood if abnormal cellular growth is regarded as arising from aberrant division occurring at a point along the embryonic path towards full differentiation or maturation. The result of further division of an abnormal single cell depends upon

(1) its line of descent, which largely determines its capabilities,
(2) the point along the path towards differentiation or maturation at which aberration began, and
(3) the severity of upset to the replication mechanism of the cell.

The distinction between malformation, benign and malignant neoplasia is more difficult to define in relation to skin disorder than with neoplasms encountered in other organs.

The following are some of the important terms used in relation to skin tumours.

Tumour

The term tumour is used to designate a localized excessive growth of tissue and in this sense it includes malformations as well as benign and malignant neoplasms.

Naevus

Any localized malformation of the skin is traditionally called a naevus and such a cellular overgrowth may be designated as a tumour although it does not qualify as a neoplasm in the ordinary sense. Malignant neoplasia, however, will sometimes develop as a secondary phenomenon in a naevus.

The term naevus is also, unfortunately, applied to a particular type of developmental lesion, namely a tumour characterized by the presence of naevus cells, cells closely related to melanocytes. This melanocytic naevus represents a benign tumour with a characteristic natural evolution and it would be illogical to classify it simply as a malformation.

In summary then the term naevus is used as a general term for any localized malformation due to overdevelopment (sometimes under-development) of one or several of the normal cellular components of the skin. It comprises relatively stable mature tissue, is often present at birth although it can arise in later life, and is a developmental anomaly. The second designation of the term naevus is for a particular tumour containing naevus cells.

Hamartoma

The term hamartoma is often used as a substitute for the general term naevus as defined above. However, because the suffix -oma implies neoplasia this causes confusion and the term hamartoma is, therefore, generally avoided in cutaneous pathology.

Phakoma and phakomatosis

The same objection applies to these terms which are sometimes used to designate widespread genetically determined disorders with developmental lesions in the skin, eye and nervous system. Some phakomatoses represent multifocal proliferations of cells derived from a single embryonic tissue. Thus neurofibromatosis and Sipple's syndrome arise from cells of neural crest origin. All are developmental malformations affecting scattered adult tissues and malignant change sometimes occurs as a later complication in these developmental abnormalities.

Malignant neoplasia

The hallmarks of malignancy are based on certain histological criteria—cellular pleomorphism, multiple mitoses and the tendency of a proliferating cell to invade, to destroy tissue structures, and to metastasize.

Malignant cells have escaped the control of the normal regulatory processes of the organism and they therefore proliferate excessively. Malignancy is probably the result of a multistage process arising from the mutation of a single or several somatic cells. This event is followed by a combination of events which then permit the development of unstable clonal growth.

Embryonic differentiation

In the course of normal embryonic development from the fertilized ovum an irreversible process occurs whereby cells become differentiated into adult tissue and organs. Naevi are malformations resulting from a disorder of tissue differentiation.

Cellular maturation

The epidermis resembles other renewable cell systems such as the bone marrow and intestinal epithelium and undergoes rapid and continuous proliferation throughout life. Disorders of maturation can arise from either mutation of maturating cells or from a block along the pathway to full maturation.

Clonal proliferation

Clonal growth represents proliferation from a single mutant cell. Such growth may be stable and restrained or unstable and progressive. Stable growth is limited in extent and the cell mass shows cells of uniform morphology. With unstable clonal proliferation exponential growth, multiple mitoses and various cell types are characteristic. When clonal growth deviates in several directions many subclones may appear within a single tumour. In this situation several cell types exist side by side although within each group of cells the cytology is uniform. Such growth is characteristic of an organoid naevus.

Skin tumours are discussed under the following major headings:

    Occupational and environmental skin cancer
    Epidermal naevi and benign tumours
    Reversible proliferations
    Neoplasia *in situ*
    Frankly invasive proliferations
    Some special skin 'tumours'
    Metastatic skin tumours
    Neoplasia of mucous membranes
    Summary and guidelines

Occupational and environmental skin cancer

It has been known for many years that exposure to coal tar and its derivatives, petroleum oil, ultraviolet and x-radiation, and inorganic arsenic renders the individual unduly liable to skin cancer (*Table 18.1*).

Exposure to petroleum oils and arsenic carries an additional risk of certain types of internal cancer.

Table 18.1 Effects of radiation on the skin

Radiation	Source	Occupational and other hazards	Premalignant skin changes
Gamma	Radioactive substances, including isotopes	Atomic plant operatives, research workers	Atrophy, alopecia Telangiectasis Keratosis Poikiloderma
X-ray	Medical: diagnostic and therapeutic Industrial	Radiologists, radiographers, patients, metallurgists	Atrophy, alopecia Telangiectases Keratosis Dyschromia
Ultraviolet	Sunlight	Outdoor workers 'sun addicts'	Atrophy, elastosis, keratosis, lentigines Keratoacanthoma
Infrared	Carbon arc Furnace Earthenware pot (kangri)	Arc welders Stokers, braziers	'Weathered' skin Erythema ab igne Dermal elastosis
	Domestic heaters, open fires	'Shin toasters' (women)	Keratosis

Coal tar

A number of polycyclic hydrocarbons based on the phenanthrene ring are carcinogenic by selectively disrupting DNA in the cell nucleus. The molecular structure of these substances is arranged as flat monoplanar plates of 3, 4, 5 or 6 benzene rings. These damaging hydrocarbons are among the less volatile products of tar distillation and have a boiling range of between 270–400 °C. Some are encountered in the creosote fraction, many in the anthracene fraction and some in the pitch residue. 'Tar oils', particularly creosote, anthracene oils and pitch are used extensively in industry, and constitute a well-known skin hazard. Exposure to tar occurs in coke oven operatives, cable makers, road repairers and shipwrights. Creosote used as a wood preservative is a hazard to railway plate layers, linesmen, etc.

Exposure to pitch is seen in floor, roof, road workers, lens grinders and during the manufacture of pitch pipes.

Soot, a condensative tar oil, was formerly responsible for the high incidence of scrotal carcinoma in chimney sweeps. Similarly, lamp black and carbon black from the burning of tar oils have caused skin cancer.

The light and middle tar distillates act as skin irritants and cause cumulative irritant dermatitis.

Petroleum oils

These complex mixtures are formed by pyrolysis and geochemical synthesis from decaying vegetation. They comprise long chain hydrocarbons (paraffins) and a small proportion of polycyclic compounds ('aromatics'). The 'aromatics' are stable clustered benzene rings with a structure similar to the carcinogens found in coal tar. The distillation of crude petroleum oil gives a series of fractions—the lower molecular weight and more volatile compounds coming off first. As with tar distillation the higher fractions and residues from distillation contain the carcinogenic substances.

The carcinogenic 'aromatics' comprise about 15 per cent of the distillate of the fraction 370–535 °C and are found in impure diesel, fuel and lubricating oils. Exposure to lubricating oils occurs in tool setters, lathe operatives, drillers, and automatic bar operators in the engineering industry. Unrefined cutting oils are particular skin hazards.

Bitumen, the residue from distillation, is a hazard to builders, roof and road workers, etc.

Polycyclic hydrocarbons from both tar and petroleum oils produce folliculitis and phototoxic dermatitis with marked melanosis. The lighter hydrocarbons—petrol, white spirit and kerosene—cause cumulative irritant dermatitis.

Radiation

X-ray, gamma, ultraviolet and infrared radiation have a damaging effect on the skin (*see Table 18.1*).

Chronic repeated exposure to any of these forms of radiation causes subtle cumulative skin damage which is liable to result in malignant change. It has been shown that x-ray photons cause DNA damage and this facilitates the appearance of a mutant cell with malignant potential. Similarly, it has been demonstrated that DNA is the principal target for UVB photons (290–320 nm) causing genetic damage that blocks normal cell replication.

The development of skin cancer from sun exposure depends on the long-term total exposure and partly on the extent to which the exposure to UVB is maintained throughout the year. Thus places further than 30 degrees from the equator do not receive enough ultraviolet radiation in the winter to contribute significantly to the development of skin cancer.

The initial changes seen in the skin from excessive sun exposure constitute epidermal atrophy and dermal elastosis. This 'weathering' of the skin is seen in outdoor workers and particularly in fair skinned individuals resident in sunny climates. The light exposed areas—the face, dorsa of hands, back of the male neck—are especially affected. Additional changes on sun-damaged areas include multiple benign lentigines (liver spots) and actinic keratoses.

On special sites certain variants of sun damage are encountered: on the neck cutis rhomboidalis, ('sailors' neck', 'farmers' neck') is seen; on the forehead severe elastosis causes a lemon yellow discoloration 'peau citrine'; over the zygomatic region a combination of elastosis, comedones and cysts may be noted (Favre–Racouchoud syndrome).

Similar skin changes are seen in the skin in tar, pitch and oil workers after a relatively short period of sun exposure due to the complementary damaging effect of polycyclic hydrocarbons and ultraviolet radiation.

Excessive and cumulative exposure to x-rays results in skin atrophy or 'radiation dermatitis' which shows many of the features of actinic damages. Epidermal atrophy, alopecia, keratoses and

Table 18.2 Discovery of environmental causes of skin cancer

Agent	Date	Discoverer
Soot	1775	Pott
Arsenic	1822	Paris
Coal tar	1875	Volkmann
Shale oil	1876	Bell
Petroleum oil	1879	Haerting and Hess
Arsenic (medicinal)	1880	Hutchinson
Sunlight	1885	Thiersch
Pitch	1892	Butler
X-rays	1902	Frieben
Shale oil	1910	Wilson
Radium	1920	Sequeira
Creosote oil	1920	O'Donovan
Petroleum lubricating oil	1930	Heller

fissures are evidence of chronic exposure to x-ray radiation and within such areas basal and squamous cell carcinoma may develop. Acute over-exposure to x-rays is less liable to induce later development of epitheliomata although basal cell epithelioma of the scalp is reported appearing several decades after x-ray depilation for ringworm. The discovery of environmental carcinogens spans two centuries (*Table 18.2*).

Arsenic

Inorganic arsenic resembles the carcinogenic activity of tar and petroleum oils in that an increased incidence of skin and visceral malignancy is encountered. Liver, lung and intestinal carcinoma show increased incidence. Multiple epitheliomata are common and the range of malignant skin change in any one particular patient can be extensive, including buccal leukoplakia, Bowen's disease, basal cell and squamous cell epitheliomata.

Epidermal naevi and benign tumours

Acanthotic naevus

An uncommon warty tumour (naevus verrucosus) usually present at birth and commonly situated on the scalp (*Plate 18.1*). Microscopically epidermal thickening is seen without the characteristic vacuolated cells of viral warts. Sometimes keratotic cells resembling the 'corps ronds' of Darier's disease are seen. Treatment is surgical excision.

Seborrhoeic wart (*Plate 18.2*)

Seborrhoeic warts are benign keratotic tumours occurring as raised plaques on the trunk and less commonly on the face. They remain benign and represent the most common tumour seen in the older age group.

Aetiology

Seborrhoeic warts are seen in both sexes usually over the age of 40. No specific factors have been identified in the pathogenesis, but eczematous inflammation may stimulate rapid growth, the lesions becoming exuberant.

Histopathology

A retiform acanthosis lies above the surface. The thickened epidermis is composed of sheets of basaloid cells forming an irregular anastomosing network which encloses projections from the surface and the dermal papillae. 'Squamous eddies' or 'pseudo-cell nests' are sometimes seen. Dermal round cell infiltration results from trauma.

Clinical features

Seborrhoeic warts are usually multiple and may be extensive in some cases. Favoured locations include central areas of the body such as the chest, back and abdomen. Distribution is usually bilateral and symmetrical.

Individual seborrhoeic warts are raised, often projecting entirely above the surface and having a 'pasted on' appearance. Size ranges from a few millimetres to 2–3 cm across. The surface is often flat, waxy; sometimes convoluted and cracked. The lesions are friable and colour ranges from fawn to brown and almost black. Characteristic of older and larger seborrhoeic warts is the lobulated surface with keratin plugs giving the appearance of a raspberry. They may catch on clothing and bleed when abraded.

Local variation in the clinical appearance of seborrhoeic warts is frequently noted. Lesions on the trunk tend to be large and grey, whereas in intertriginous areas maceration produces exuberant lesions. Facial seborrhoeic warts are usually dry and those on the eyelids and neck commonly pedunculated. Special variants include 'dermatitis papulosa nigra' on the face of Negroes and multiple flat seborrhoeic warts on light exposed areas, e.g. bald scalp, face, dorsa of hands.

Seborrhoeic warts sometimes erupt in large numbers and when itching is present the possibility of visceral malignancy (especially of the gastrointestinal tract) should be excluded (Laser–Trélat sign). When features of acanthosis nigricans are found with multiple pruritic seborrhoeic warts the existence of internal malignancy becomes more probable.

Prognosis

Seborrhoeic warts remain benign, but are unlikely to disappear without treatment.

Differential diagnosis

Seborrhoeic warts may be mistaken for viral warts, multilobulated cellular naevi or patches of Bowen's disease. Deep black or brown-black mushroom-like protuberances are sometimes mistaken for nodular malignant melanoma, whilst plaque-like seborrhoeic warts are confused with superficial spreading melanoma.

Treatment

Shave excision or curettage, followed by diathermy to the bleeding base, is a simple and effective treatment. Alternatively, moistening with trichloracetic acid or freezing with liquid nitrogen is effective. Pedunculated lesions are treated with diathermy desiccation. Excision and suture is not indicated except for histological study when the diagnosis is in doubt.

Skin tags (acrochordon)

Skin tags are common fibro-epithelial polyps which usually appear in middle life. They are often mistaken for warts, are more frequent in women and seen particularly in obese subjects. They appear as multiple skin-coloured to light brown fleshy tags, on the neck, upper chest, axillae, submammary or inguinal regions. The only symptoms are due to local trauma when an occasional lesion becomes twisted and infarcted.

Apart from obesity, skin tags are a feature of epiloia, acromegaly and acanthosis nigricans.

Treatment

Electro-desiccation or galvano-cautery.

Lentigo *(see Figure 21.7, p. 312)*

Lentigines represent a localized proliferation of melanocytes with thickening of the epidermal rete pegs. They appear as multiple small dark brown lesions. Juvenile lentigines appear in childhood on any part of the skin surface.

The rare cardiomyopathic lentiginoses (Moynahan syndrome) show generalized lentigines; in Peutz–Jeghers syndrome lentigines are present on the lips, central face and palms of hands, in association with intestinal polyposis (*Figure 21.6*, p. 309).

Cellular naevus (synonym: naevus cell naevus, melanocytic naevus) *(Plate 18.3)*

These naevi are the commonest tumours in man. Cellular naevi represent a localized combined hyperplasia of melanocytes and Schwann cells, whereas the intradermal naevus comprises purely dermal cellular hyperplasia.

Aetiology

They are seen in both sexes. A few may be present at birth, but a majority appear in young adult life and may regress in later life.

Histopathology

Proliferation of melanocytes forms groups of cells (naevus cell nests) in the deeper epidermis. These proliferating cells in the junctional region drop into the dermis below. Such naevus cell proliferation, segregation and migration is often accompanied by a Schwann proliferation in the underlying deeper dermis. Other features include epidermal hyperplasia, pilar and connective tissue changes which combine to produce the composite structure of the *compound naevus*.

In certain naevi following regression of the junctional activity only dermal changes remain—the resting *intradermal naevus*. So long as junctional changes persist cellular naevi have the capacity for malignant transformation, although such a change is an extremely rare event. A melanocytic naevus with junctional change without dermal migration is termed a *junctional naevus*, (*see* p. 230)

Clinical features

Cellular naevi may be flat, slightly elevated, dome-shaped, polypoid or papillomatous. Size ranges from pinhead to 1 cm or more. They are solid, non-compressible and can be skin coloured, yellow-brown or black. A purely intradermal naevus is usually skin coloured, without pigmentation. Most naevi first appear in children and young adults, appearing sometimes in crops and increase in size occurs only in relation to the growth of the child. In adult life coarse hairs may project from the surface—the hairy cellular naevus. Naevi appear anywhere on the skin, including the palms, soles and genitalia. The development of a depigmented halo around a cellular naevus usually heralds the onset of spontaneous involution (*see* halo naevus p. 226). Cellular naevi, junctional naevi and lentigines commonly darken at puberty, during pregnancy or with the onset of Addison's disease.

Prognosis

The vast majority remain benign; furthermore, there is no evidence that treatment encourages malignant changes. However, the presence of junctional change implies capability for malignant change and the early tell-tale features of malignant transformation are listed in *Table 18.4*, p. 231.

Differential diagnosis

Small neurofibromas resemble cellular naevi, but are compressible, with a pillow-like consistency. A small dome-shaped naevus may simulate a nodular basal cell epithelioma. Pigmented cellular naevi have been confused with nodular malignant melanoma. When diagnosis is in doubt a biopsy should be taken or referral made for expert opinion.

Treatment

The vast majority do not require treatment; if they catch on clothing or become infected electro-desiccation or shave excision under local anaesthesia often gives a better cosmetic result than simple excision.

Halo naevus (Sutton's naevus) *(Plate 18.4)*

The halo naevus is an uncommon lesion with a depigmented macular halo surrounding a central pigmented naevus. Halo naevi usually appear in children and young adults. Some patients have an

226

associated vitiligo. The process of halo formation and involution is probably dependent on immunological factors with the production of antimelanocyte antibodies.

The presence of halo naevi should alert the physician to the possible coexistence of autoimmune disease, e.g. diabetes, hypo- or hyperthyroidism or pernicious anaemia. Halo naevi have appeared after surgical excision of malignant melanoma.

Blue naevus and Mongolian spot *(Plate 18.5)*

The Mongolian spot is the commoner and is present in the infants of many Oriental races. It shows as a dark blue patch over the sacral region, usually clearing during the second year of life. Aberrant Mongolian spots are not uncommon in Negro children.

The blue naevus is an intradermal naevus composed of spindle cells containing large melanin granules. A particular variant is Ota's naevus affecting the eye and peri-orbital region. Blue naevi are best excised.

Juvenile melanoma (Spitz tumour)

A dome-shaped pink or brown tumour which usually occurs on the face of children. A distinctive histological picture with giant naevus cells and spindle cells may be confused with malignant melanoma. The majority of lesions eventually clear spontaneously. Treatment is total excision.

Naevus spilus tardus (Becker's naevus) *(Plate 18.6)*

This naevus only appears in late childhood as a light brown uniform hairy patch. It commonly appears in the pectoral region and is harmless.

Capillary cavernous haemangioma *(Figure 18.1)*

The lesions are not usually present at birth but appear within the first month or two of life, growing for a year or so and often reaching a size of 3–4 cm in diameter before showing signs of involution, which in most cases is complete by the age of seven or eight. They appear as soft, tumid, reddish-brown nodules, compressible and often blanching completely on pressure. Central ulceration may occur, with subsequent fibrosis. Haemorrhage may follow trauma; this is easily controlled by light pressure.

In the majority of cases no treatment is required. In general the cosmetic result is more satisfactory when the lesion is left to take its natural course. However, in those rare instances where a massive

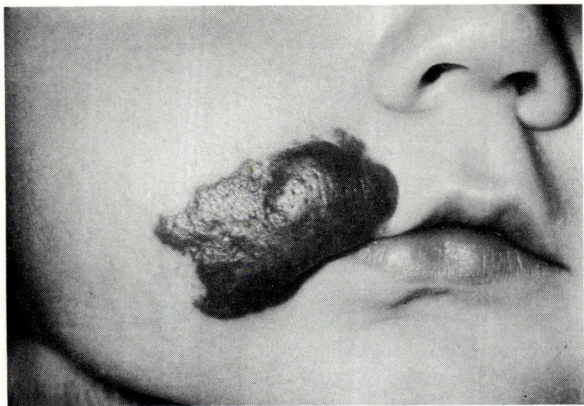

Figure 18.1   *Capillary cavernous haemangioma*

lesion shows rapid growth the opinion of a plastic surgeon should be sought. Systemic steroids or cryotherapy are possible alternative forms of treatment.

Capillary haemangioma (naevus flammeus or port-wine stain)

Flat red patches, usually present at birth, that grow only in proportion to the growth of the child. They do not undergo spontaneous resolution and treatment is unsatisfactory. Cosmetic covering creams are useful in obscuring the lesion.

One clinical capillary defect has somewhat surprisingly an inherited accumulation of glycolipid because of impaired degradation: Fabry's disease. In other types primary vessel wall abnormalities are likely; possibly collagenous or muscular. Localized developmental abnormalities such as Sturge–Weber and Klippel–Trenauney–Weber syndrome are not discussed, although capillary haemangiomas can sometimes accompany the Osler–Weber–Rendu syndrome.

Reversible proliferations

Keratoacanthoma (KA) *(Plate 18.7)*

A common skin tumour which grows rapidly and usually regresses spontaneously within three to four months.

Aetiology

KA is uncommon before middle age, half of all patients are over the age of 60 and males are more commonly affected than females. Many of the patients are fair skinned. Exposure to sunlight, tar, pitch and petroleum oils are important predisposing factors. 'Tar mollusca' and 'pitch warts' represent variants of keratoacanthoma. The sites of origin correspond to areas of sun exposure, but not necessarily to visibly sun-damaged skin. The skin of albinos and individuals with xeroderma pigmentosum is prone to develop keratoacanthomata at an early age and immunosuppressed patients show increased incidence. A virus aetiology has been suggested but never confirmed.

Histopathology

An origin from follicular or sebaceous epithelium is suspected. During the growth phase a marked pseudo-epitheliomatous hyperplasia is found with some cellular anaplasia, mitotic figures and invasion of the dermis, although this never reaches below the level of sweat glands. Marked dermal cellular infiltration is noted as involution proceeds.

Clinical features

The most important characteristic of this tumour is rapid growth. It begins as a small papule which in the course of three to four weeks becomes a shiny skin coloured or pink hemispherical nodule about 1 cm across. It is freely mobile over the underlying tissues. The fully developed lesion at six to eight weeks shows a yellow depressed cornified plug; some weeks later this horny mass separates causing the sides of the lesion to fall in and flatten. Ultimately after some three to four months only a thin puckered scar is seen.

Although the above sequence of events is seen in 80 per cent of patients with keratoacanthomata, certain important variations of this 'classical' course can be encountered. Some lesions of KA may attain a considerably greater size (over 5 cm across) and involution may be greatly delayed. Giant keratoacanthomata up to 10 cm across, persisting many months, can pursue an aggressive course with tissue invasion and destruction. Other morphological types include papular non-cornified 'button' keratoacanthomata, verrucous, vegetating and horny variants (cutaneous horn). Sometimes multiple or aggregated lesions are found and familial (Ferguson–Smith type) and mucosal keratoacanthomata are seen.

Prognosis

A minority, probably about 5 per cent of all keratoacanthomata, fail to resolve and show all the clinical and histological characteristics of a low grade squamous cell carcinoma.

Differential diagnosis

The distinguishing features of the classic KA from squamous cell carcinoma are shown in *Table 18.3*. However, the rare adenoid squamous cell carcinoma shows rapid growth, appears on sun-exposed sites and often exhibits early central ulceration.

Other skin lesions which have caused diagnostic problems include the sebaceous cyst, warty dyskeratoma, large molluscum contagiosum and the secondary deposit.

Table 18.3 Distinguishing features of keratoacanthoma and carcinoma*

	Keratoacanthoma	*Squamous cell carcinoma*
Major factors	UVB, tar, pitch	UVB, tar, pitch, x-rays
Age	50–70	60–70
Rate of growth	Weeks	Months to years
Shape	Crateriform	Irregular
Central area	Keratotic plug	Necrotic centre
	No true ulceration	True ulceration
Course	Growth then regression	Progression
Microscopy	Pseudoepitheliomatous hyperplasia and microabscesses	Epitheliomatous and no microabscesses
	Some anaplasia	Marked anaplasia
	Few mitoses	Many mitoses
	Marked keratinization	Less keratinization
	Dermal infiltrate	Less infiltrate
	Often eosinophils	No eosinophils
	Epithelial growth always above sweat gland level	Epithelial growth often below sweat gland level
	Glycogen	No glycogen

* These differences are not absolute

Treatment

When seen in the early growing phase they are best removed by excision/biopsy because keratoacanthomata may become malignant, recur or leave an unsightly scar. However, if growth has ceased curettage and diathermy, cryotherapy or careful observation are alternative measures. Treatment of the rare recurrent multiple keratoacanthomata is unsatisfactory, although methotrexate has proved useful in certain instances.

Junctional naevus

A common brown pigmented macule showing central speckling and pigment strands.

Aetiology

In most instances the junctional naevus represents a transient phase in the early development of a compound cellular naevus and is seen in childhood. However, most adults show one or more of these benign lesions occurring anywhere on the skin surface.

Histopathology

Groups of naevus cells are seen in the deeper part of the epidermis. Increased dermal melanin is found, but inflammatory changes are absent.

Clinical features

Individual lesions are round or oval 0.1 to 1 cm across. The surface is smooth, flat and skin furrows are preserved. Colour ranges from light brown to dark brown-black. The outline is well-defined and the centre shows flecking or streaks of darker pigment. Junctional naevi appear anywhere on the skin surface and mucous membranes, although particularly frequent on the palms, soles and genitalia.

Prognosis

Considering the great frequency of these naevi and the rarity of malignant melanoma the incidence of malignant change in junctional naevi must be very low. The changes suggesting early malignancy are important and listed in *Table 18.4*.

Table 18.4   Ominous features in a naevus

Onset of symptoms—intermittent irritation, smarting or burning
Change in size or shape
Change in pigmentation—multi-coloured, dark, pale, even white areas, charcoal, slate-grey or black pigmentation
      Pseudopods or satellites particularly dangerous
      NB An amelanotic melanoma may arise from a pigmented naevus
Erythema, induration or friability
Haemorrhage, crusting or ulceration

Differential diagnosis

Ephelis (freckle), macular cellular naevus, senile lentigo, flat pigmented seborrhoeic wart and lentigo maligna.

Treatment

It is prudent to remove any junctional naevus on a site liable to be subjected to trauma. Likewise, a lesion on the mucous membranes or ano-genital region should be prophylactically excised. Any suggestion of malignant change requires early biopsy.

Neoplasia *in situ*

The diverse neoplastic processes discussed so far represent either non-progressive proliferations—stable clonal growth as seen with differentiated naevi—or a reversible process having the capability of spontaneous regression, e.g. keratoacanthoma, halo naevus and junctional naevus.

Unfortunately, certain neoplastic proliferations progress beyond a 'point of no return' so that either arrest or regression of the proliferative process becomes impossible. It seems likely that such uncontrolled cellular activity with escape from restraint results from a stepwise sequence of disturbances of cell metabolism. This may be caused initially by damage to chromosomal mechanisms concerned with cell division and differentiation. Malignant change appearing in a cell is not an all or none process, but the result of chromosomal damage, i.e. mutation which allows the establishment of an abnormal cell line. When cellular proliferation escapes from immunological control exponential growth of the tumour is usual and distant metastases ultimately develop.

Within the epidermis such clones of cells with unstable growth show as islands of cells with cellular and nuclear pleomorphism, individual cell keratinization and multiple mitoses.

Selective damage to chromosomes in the nuclei of epidermal cells can be caused, as we have seen, by certain chemicals and radiation. The chemicals include polycyclic hydrocarbons found in tar, soot, pitch and mineral oils, and inorganic arsenic. Such molecules have a special affinity for DNA and photons of the UVB and x-ray light range have the same disruptive effect on the DNA helix. The cumulative effect of such damaging mutations is to produce an increased incidence of intraepidermal and frankly invasive neoplasms.

Actinic keratoses (*Plate 18.8*)

A discrete superficial keratosis seen on light exposed and sun-damaged areas of skin in older individuals. It is the most common premalignant skin tumour and if left untreated shows a low incidence of progression to invasive squamous cell carcinoma.

Aetiology

The incidence in individuals with fair complexion is high, whereas darker races are seldom affected. Males are affected more commonly than women, no doubt due to greater sun exposure. Similarly the greater intensity and duration of sun exposure accounts for the greater incidence and earlier age of onset in lower latitudes and in outdoor workers, i.e. farmers, fishermen, etc. The effect of sun exposure is cumulative, the first lesions only appearing after ten to 20 years, and new lesions continuing to appear for many years after intense exposure has ceased. It has been noted that actinic keratoses become active in immunosuppressed subjects. They are seen at an early age in albinos and in xeroderma pigmentosum.

Histopathology

The composite changes seen in the epidermis in actinic keratoses are characteristic. The interfollicular epithelium shows islands of neoplastic cells which often form bud-like projections below the epidermis, although strictly confined by the basal lamina. Cellular pleomorphism, hyperchromatism and abnormal mitoses characterize the intra-epithelial dyskeratosis. The follicular and sweat duct epithelium undergoes a reactive hyperplasia. Parakeratosis overlies the dysplastic areas and hyperkeratosis is seen above the adnexal epithelium, thereby producing alternating columns of parakeratosis and hyperkeratosis. The dermis shows actinic elastosis and lymphocytic infiltration.

Clinical features

Lesions are commonly multiple and appear on exposed sites. The face, lower lip, ears, bald scalp, dorsa of hands and forearms are most frequently involved. Keratoses range in size from 0.1 to 1 cm or larger. They appear as slightly elevated, dry, hyperkeratotic papules, covered by a fine adherent scale which when removed leaves a bleeding surface. The surface can be flat, rough, conical or verrucous. Rarely the hyperkeratosis is excessive, creating a cutaneous horn (*see* p. 246). The lesions are sometimes better felt than seen, and are painful when pressed. A characteristic of actinic keratoses is an accompanying 'weathering' of the skin with epidermal atrophy, dermal elastosis and 'senile' lentigines (liver spots).

Prognoses

Probably less than 5 per cent of the lesions slowly enlarge, become elevated and progress to invasive squamous cell carcinomata. Signs of supervening malignancy of key importance are increased induration, rapid enlargement, peri-lesional erythema, bleeding and ulceration. The resulting carcinoma is not usually aggressive and distant metastases are rare. However, an occasional complication of solar keratosis is Bowen's disease with metastatic spread.

Differential diagnosis

Verruca vulgaris, seborrhoeic wart and Bowen's disease occasionally cause diagnostic problems. Actinic keratosis on the face may closely resemble a patch of LE and a biopsy may be required to establish the diagnosis.

Treatment

Large inflamed indurated or recurrent lesions should be biopsied to rule out squamous cell carcinoma. It is important that all keratoses appearing on sun-damaged skin are treated. Patients with multiple lesions respond favourably to 5-fluorouracil. The entire areas of involvement are treated daily with 5% cream. The lesions undergo a selective inflammatory reaction which ultimately subsides with resolution of the lesion. Another effective treatment is curettage and electro-desiccation. Cryotherapy with liquid nitrogen or carbon dioxide slush also provides satisfactory results.

Arsenical keratosis (*Figure 23.1,* p. 333)

A corn-like keratosis affecting particularly the palms and soles. It is premalignant and may progress to squamous cell carcinoma.

Aetiology

The effects of exposure to inorganic arsenic may make their first appearance only ten, 20 or more years after medication has ceased. In some instances only short exposure (several weeks) has produced keratoses and squamous cell carcinoma several decades later.

Histopathology

The epidermal changes range from acanthosis, intraepidermal cell dysplasia, to typical Bowen's disease. In contrast to actinic keratoses dermal changes from sun damage are absent.

Clinical features

Small round or oval corn-like hyperkeratoses are seen on the palms and soles. In the early stages they may appear as yellow transparent 'pearls' embedded in the skin. On the dorsa of the hands, limbs and trunk they are usually raised and verrucous. Induration, inflammation and ulceration herald the onset of malignant change.

Important associations, usually signs of chronic arsenic exposure, exist with arsenical keratoses. These include widespread melanosis with 'rain-drop' stippling, multiple Bowen's disease and multiple epitheliomatosis (basal and squamous cell carcinoma). Diffuse plantar/palmar hyperkeratoses and lingual leukoplakia may also be found. Because of the known association with hepatic cirrhosis and liver and lung carcinoma, careful search and regular screening are performed to exclude visceral complications of arsenical medication.

Differential diagnosis

From viral warts, keratosis punctata, keratoses of Cowden's syndrome.

Prognosis

Squamous cell carcinoma arising in arsenical keratoses tends to invade aggressively and metastasize readily to the regional lymph nodes. It follows that because of the inherent phenomenon of latency, once keratoses have appeared it is then too late to prevent further keratoses, basal and squamous cell carcinomata from appearing in the skin.

Treatment

The multiplicity of keratoses often makes excision impracticable. Effective surgery for early malignant lesions, regular follow-up and screening are mandatory.

Bowen's disease *(Plate 18.9)*

An intraepidermal epithelioma originating from cells of the keratinocyte lineage. Although the course is usually chronic and benign, invasion and metastases can occur.

Aetiology

The condition is commoner in older age groups and favours men with a fair complexion. Chronic sunlight exposure is important and exposure to tar, pitch and petroleum oils is sometimes a provocative factor. Eyelid lesions have been seen in oil workers from oil contamination when rubbing the eyelids.

Multiple patches of Bowen's disease on covered skin are a sequel to chronic exposure to inorganic arsenic and usually appear many years after exposure. Thus multiple Bowen's disease may be a marker for visceral malignancy (*see* p. 184). Occasionally localized Bowen's disease appears in an actinic keratosis, but in about two-thirds of patients with solitary patches no cause is apparent.

Histopathology

Large areas of epidermis are transformed by *in situ* malignant process. The cells show anaplastic change with 'speckling'. Abnormal cells show variation in size and shape, loss of prickles and numerous mitotic figures. Bizarre clumped cells, individually keratinized and vacuolated cells are seen. The follicular epithelium may show similar changes. The basement membrane is intact and the dermis shows lymphocytic infiltration.

Clinical features

Bowen's disease appears as small round oval or irregular polycyclic plaques. Slight erythema, infiltration and scaling are usual and patches closely mimic eczema. Such patches are sharply demarcated and often slightly elevated. Nodules, erosions, crusting and melanosis are seen with these slowly growing lesions, spreading by peripheral extension and persisting indefinitely. Solitary lesions are common on the fingers and dorsa of the hands. On mucous membranes they appear as pruritic plaques. A special verrucous variant—multicentric pigmented Bowen's disease—appears in the groin and vulva and resembles condylomata acuminata or seborrhoeic warts.

Prognosis

The incidence of malignant change is low—about 5 per cent. Increased induration, nodules and erosion probably indicate invasive disease. In the absence of a clear relationship of exposure to sun or polycyclic hydrocarbons possible exposure to arsenic should be investigated. Some authors consider that multiple Bowen's disease, even in the absence of arsenic exposure, is commoner with visceral malignancy.

Differential diagnosis

On the hands a patch of Bowen's disease mimics discoid eczema and psoriasis, whereas on the face and trunk pigmented basal cell epitheliomata and seborrhoeic warts may cause diagnostic difficulties. The superficial basal cell epithelioma of the Graham–Little type (benign erythematoid epithelioma) and superficial gummatous syphiloderm closely mimic Bowen's disease.

Treatment

Surgical excision or radiotherapy is the most effective treatment. Local destructive measures such as electro-desiccation, curettage, or cryotherapy, although frequently effective, are often followed by punctate recurrence because of the existence of deep adnexal involvement. Topical 5-fluorouracil is less effective than for actinic keratoses.

Paget's disease (*Plate 18.10*)

A special form of intraepithelial neoplasia (carcinoma *in situ*) originating from ductal cells in the breast and overlying epidermis. Underlying ductal adenocarcinoma is present in most instances.

Aetiology

Paget's disease of the breast is usually found in women over 40 years. Extramammary Paget's disease is found in both sexes, but is more common in women. Two major hypotheses include (1) multifoccal origin with *in situ* change appearing simultaneously in both the epidermis and lactiferous ducts, and (2) metastatic spread into the epidermis from the underlying ductal dysplasia. The latter fails to explain the existence of extramammary carcinoma without any underlying apocrine gland carcinoma.

Histopathology

Islands of Paget cells are seen within the epidermis. They are round, larger than prickle cells, with a large nucleus and abundant pale-staining cytoplasm. Sometimes clefts appear within the dyskeratotic areas. The dermis shows a chronic lymphocytic and plasma cell infiltrate. In the later stages ductal malignancy spreads beyond the boundaries of the duct into the surrounding dermis.

Clinical features

The nipple shows changes which closely simulate eczema. A sharply marginated superficial erythematous plaque or red exudative area with superficial erosion abrades easily. The lesion is restricted to part of the nipple in the early stage; later the nipple retracts or is destroyed and the areola is affected. The underlying breast may already be palpably indurated with carcinoma and a blood-stained discharge may be present.

Extramammary Paget's disease which occurs predominantly in the ano-genital region (*Figure 18.2*) and axillae is sometimes associated with carcinoma of underlying apocrine or eccrine glands.

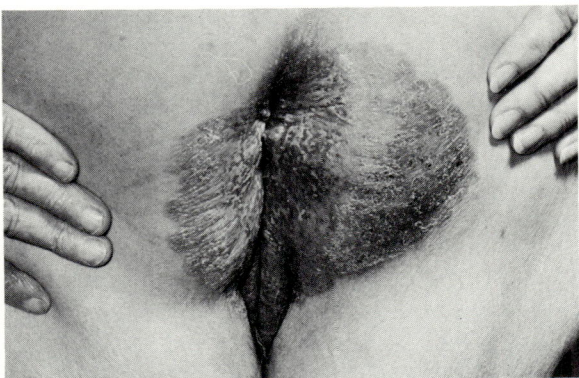

Figure 18.2 *Extramammary Paget's disease anogenital region*

The lesion appears as an infiltrated plaque with erythema, exudation or erosion. It is sometimes pruritic or painful. A rare variant is the vegetating type appearing in the flexures. Extramammary Paget's disease is sometimes associated with distant visceral carcinoma.

Prognosis

The outlook is determined by the extent of the underlying carcinoma at the time of surgical excision.

Differential diagnosis

Eczema of the nipple, mastitis with infective eczema, erosive adenomatosis and Fox–Fordyce disease of the nipple have all been confused with Paget's disease.

Treatment

The only effective treatment is excision of the nipple and adequate removal of the underlying ductal carcinoma; radiotherapy may be palliative. In extramammary disease the appropriate treatment is surgical excision.

Lentigo maligna (Hutchinson's melanotic freckle) *(Plate 18.11)*

An intraepidermal malignant melanoma—the pre-invasive stage of lentigo maligna melanoma (LMM). It is a neoplasia *in situ* arising in cells of the melanocyte lineage.

Aetiology

Lentigo maligna commonly affects older individuals in the sixth and seventh decades. Most lesions occur on sun-exposed areas as solitary pigmented lesions and are more common in males than females.

Histopathology

Active areas of proliferating melanocytes are seen at the dermoepidermal junction. These cell nests of atypical melanocytes are confined above the epidermal basement membrane. An intense band-like dermal lymphocytic infiltrate is characteristic. Evidence of sun damage in the adjoining dermis is usual.

Clinical features

The face is the site of predilection. The lesion begins as a small light to dark-brown macular patch. The radial enlargement at a variable rate causes an irregular outline and some areas may even show spontaneous regression. The patches are usually non-elevated and sometimes slightly scaly. Patchy pigmentation, sometimes with depigmentation, is seen within the affected area. The colour within an individual lesion ranges through tan, dark-brown to grey and black in a mottled or spotty pattern.

After several years of radial growth the lesion develops a nodule, shows verrucous changes or becomes infiltrated and enlarges more rapidly. This heralds the onset of vertical growth and evolution into an invasive LMM.

Prognosis

About 30 per cent of lentigo malignas give rise to invasive malignant melanoma. When this occurs there is fortunately little tendency to metastasize.

Differential diagnosis

A junctional naevus is round or oval and shows no atypical cells or dermal infiltrate. Superficial spreading melanoma (SSM) usually appears on covered sites in younger subjects and shows more variegated colours (*see Table 18.5*). Pigmented basal cell epithelioma occasionally causes diagnostic problems. A senile lentigo (liver spot) shows uniform pale brown pigmentation.

Treatment

Local excision or cryotherapy.

Frankly invasive proliferations

Squamous cell carcinoma *(Plate 18.12* and *Figure 18.3)*

This constitutes a truly anaplastic and invasive neoplasm derived from the cells of keratinocyte lineage and characterized by extension beyond the epidermis. Although the growth rate is variable invasion of the dermis is unrelenting and if untreated it spreads to the regional lymph nodes.

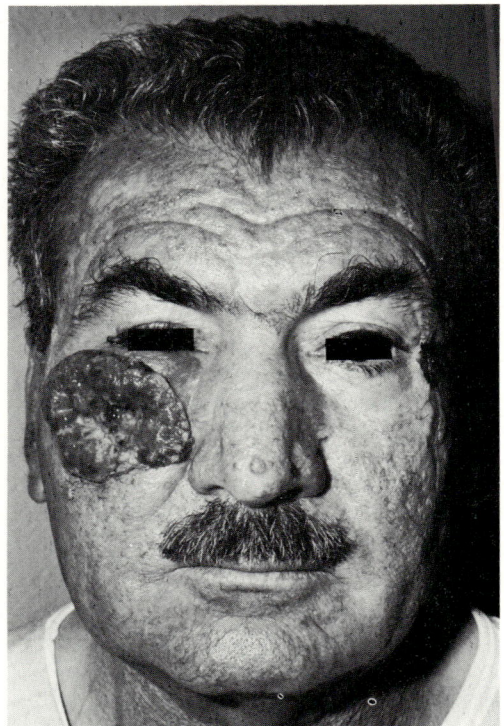

Figure 18.3 *Fungating squamous cell carcinoma right cheek with small basal cell epithelioma nose*

Aetiology

Squamous cell carcinoma sometimes arises from apparently normal skin, but commonly it develops from skin damaged by environmental noxae, in areas of chronic inflammation or in certain genodermatoses. The tumour shows increasing incidence with advancing age. Many diverse aetiological factors are responsible for the development of squamous cell carcinoma on the skin and these may be summarized as follows:

(1) Repeated sun exposure combined with fair skin colour. Individuals of Celtic or Scandinavian stock are particularly prone. UVB light, 290–320 nm, is the carcinogenic waveband which produces cumulative skin damage.

(2) Repeated exposure to the polycyclic hydrocarbons present in tar, pitch, soot and mineral oils. The carcinogenic effect of these chemicals is enhanced by exposure to ultraviolet light.

(3) Repeated exposure to x-rays and repeated subthreshold burn exposure to infrared radiation causing cumulative chromosomal damage.

(4) Certain genetic skin disorders: albinism and the congenital poikilodermas including xeroderma pigmentosum, Rothmund–Thomson syndrome and dyskeratosis congenita. Darier's disease with vegetating lesions may develop squamous cell carcinoma.

(5) Premalignant dermatoses and neoplasia *in situ*: actinic keratoses, arsenical keratoses, Bowen's disease.

(6) Granulomatous disease with pseudoepitheliomatous hyperplasia: lupus vulgaris, syphilis, leprosy, deep fungal infections are occasionally complicated by squamous cell carcinoma.

(7) Mucosal dysplasias, atrophy and hyperplasias: carcinoma *in situ*—leukoplakia, erythroplasia; atrophy—Paterson–Kelly syndrome, lichen sclerosus, lichen planus; hyperplasias—Cannon's naevus.

(8) Chronic ulcers and sinuses: chronic stasis ulcer, hidradenitis suppurativa.

(9) Viral infections under special circumstances: giant condylomata acuminata (Buschke–Lowenstein), epidermodysplasia verruciformis.

(10) Certain epidermal naevi—stable clonal growth becomes disturbed, e.g. porokeratosis of Mibelli.

(11) Regenerative and hyperkinetic epidermal disorders: burn scars, epidermolysis bullosa dystrophica and some of the ichthyosis group of disorders.

Histopathology

Irregular proliferating masses of squamous cells invade the dermis as coherent strands and columns. Epidermal cells show marked pleomorphism (nuclear and cytoplasmic), abnormal mitoses and heterochromatism. In well differentiated lesions keratinized cells and 'horny pearls' are found. Acantholytic squamous cell carcinoma shows malignant dyskeratoses with lacunae and cavities containing degenerating cells. The more anaplastic epidermal cells show little resemblance to normal prickle cells, mitotic figures are more frequent and tumour cells sometimes simulate those seen in a malignant melanoma or sarcoma. The edge of the squamous cell carcinoma may show evidence of a precancerous lesion, eg pseudoepitheliomatous hyperplasia (PEH), actinic keratoses, etc. With PEH invasion penetrates no deeper than sweat glands and microabscesses are found in acanthotic epithelium.

Clinical features

Squamous cell carcinoma favours exposed areas and usually appears on sun-damaged skin, sometimes from a pre-existing keratosis or granuloma. The tumour has three major presentations:

(1) a skin coloured nodule without crust or ulceration,
(2) a red fleshy nodule with a warty surface,
(3) a crust covered crater surrounded by a raised dirty red-yellow indurated margin.

Growth is slow compared with a keratocanthoma, but faster than a basal cell epithelioma. Nevertheless, the rare adenoid squamous cell carcinoma arising *de novo* from normal skin may grow rapidly and ulcerate early thus resembling a keratoacanthoma, yet infiltration and metastatic spread occurs early.

On the lips, genitalia or perianal skin a small fissure or non-healing ulcer may be the initial presentation of squamous cell carcinoma and unfortunately on these sites the tumour often metastasizes early to regional lymph nodes. However, lymphadenopathy may result from infection and is not necessarily an indication of metastatic spread.

Prognosis

The outlook depends on the grade of malignancy, location, depth of invasion and the extent of spread. As a rule squamous cell carcinomata arising in actinic keratoses metastasize late, whereas those appearing in arsenical keratoses invade and metastasize early.

Differential diagnosis

From keratoacanthoma, basal cell epithelioma and granulomas with PEH.

Treatment

In small lesions surgical excision with 0.5 cm clearance is the treatment of choice. For larger and more anaplastic tumours on the face and neck radiotherapy is sometimes preferable. Elderly or debilitated patients who cannot tolerate surgical procedure are best treated by radiotherapy; however radiotherapy is not always effective for lesions on the trunk, extremities or in the ano-genital region. Many centres hold a skin cancer clinic combining dermatologist, plastic surgeon and radiotherapist, as every case requires expert individual assessment.

Malignant melanoma (MM) (*Plates 18.13, 18.14* and *18.15*)

This is a highly invasive neoplasm derived from cells of the melanocyte lineage and can appear anywhere on the skin surface, mucous membranes, subungually or in the eye.

Aetiology

Malignant melanomas are rarely encountered before puberty but can occur at any age, the majority of cases first appearing in the 35–55 age group. The age and sex incidence of each of the three important clinical types of malignant melanoma differ and are shown in *Table 18.5*. When the tumour arises *de novo* from apparently normal skin this melanoma d'emblee is presumed to develop from either cell rests or mutated melanocytes. Sometimes a superficial spreading melanoma (SSM) or a nodular melanoma (NM) arises from the junctional region in an active melanocytic naevus or from a junctional naevus. Much less commonly a malignant melanoma arises within a giant 'bathing trunk' naevus, a blue naevus, or on the sun exposed skin of an individual with xeroderma pigmentosum. In Great Britain there is no particular predilection of this tumour to appear on exposed sites, but in sunny climates actinic exposure is an important provocative factor. Trauma probably accounts for the high incidence of plantar malignant melanoma in Africans.

The existence of familial cases is established, but more important are the racial factors that control skin colour; skin susceptibility to solar damage is high in fair skinned, blue eyed and red headed subjects. The incidence of malignant melanoma is higher in Celts and Scandinavians than in darker skinned races.

Rarely malignant melanoma arises in a scar, e.g. vaccination, burn or tattoo. The relationship between pituitary MSH secretion and the pathogenesis of melanocyte malignancy remains at present undetermined.

Histopathology

The histological features of the major clinical types of malignant melanoma are shown in *Table 18.5*. A common feature of all melanomas is the presence of focal areas of anaplastic cells in the epidermis, the so-called 'cell nests'. Sooner or later malignant cells break through the epidermal basement membrane and invade the dermis to reach the lymphatics. The level of invasion provides an important prognostic guide and five levels of invasion are recognized (Clark and McGovern), (*see Table 18.6*).

Clinical features

The majority of malignant melanomas correspond to one of the three distinctive types shown in *Table 18.5*. A useful guide to prognosis

Table 18.5 Clinical types of malignant melanoma

	Superficial spreading melanoma (Plate 18.11)	Nodular melanoma (Plate 18.12)	Lentigo maligna melanoma (Plate 18.13)
Age—years	35–45	45–55	60–70 +
Sex incidence	F > M	M > F	M > F
Duration	1–5 years	Months–2 years	5–15 years
Colour	Variegated	Uniform	Slight variegation
	Red, brown, grey and black. Pink often	Brown, blue, grey, blue-black or black	Shades of brown and black. Pink rare
Hypopigmentation	Occasional halo	Rare halo	Rarely central (regression)
Texture	Matt or glossy	Glossy	Matt
Size	1–10 cm	0.1–2 cm	1–5 cm
Shape	Irregular, notched, 'crab-like'	Regular, indentations rare	Irregular, notched, 'crab-like'
Margin	Palpable	Palpable	Flat
Growth	Early horizontal, later vertical	Early vertical	Early horizontal, later vertical
Mortality	50%	55%	10%

and management is provided in *Table 18.6*, because each type shows distinctive clinical, histological and ultrastructural features. It is likely that some 20–30 per cent of SSM and NM arise from pre-existing naevi. It follows that recent change appearing in a pigmented lesion—*whether the naevus is recent or long-standing*—should arouse suspicion of malignancy. The suspicious features are shown in *Table 18.4*. There is no conclusive evidence that trauma or treatment of a benign naevus induces malignant change. Nevertheless, when the diagnosis of malignant melanoma is suspected it is prudent to reduce palpation and manipulation of the lesion because of the risk of 'milking' malignant cells into the lymphatics. Likewise, when malignant melanoma is suspected excisional rather than incisional biopsy should be carried out. The staging of malignant melanoma is based on the extent of the disease.

Staging of malignant melanoma

Stage I	*Stage II*	*Stage III*
Skin only	Skin and regional nodes	Skin, nodes and spread beyond
Local invasion only	Lymphatic permeation and embolism	Haematogenous dissemination

Table 18.6   Prognostic guides to malignant melanoma

	Favourable	*Unfavourable*
Clinical type of tumour	Lentigo maligna melanoma	Nodular melanoma
Sex	Female	Male
Endocrine status	Post-menopausal	Pregnancy
Duration	Less than 6 months	Over 6 months
Growth rate	Years	Months
Site	Face and limbs	Trunk
Contour	Flat	Nodular
Surface	Intact	Ulcerated
Bleeding	Absent	Present
Pigmentation	Dark brown	Blue, pink or absent
Margin	Well-defined	Ill-defined
Growth direction	Lateral	Vertical
Satellites	Absent	Present
Stage	I	II or III
Histology		
Invasion	Levels 1 and 2	Levels 3, 4 and 5
Cells	Uniform	Pleomorphic
Melanin	Marked	Moderate or sparse
Mitoses	Few	Many
Lymphocytes	Many	Few
Lymphatics	Not affected	Permeated

Prognosis

With early diagnosis and adequate surgical treatment the five-year survival rate is good. The major factors that determine the prognosis are the clinico-pathological type of tumour, the depth of invasion, the extent of the disease and the features shown in *Table 18.6*.

Differential diagnosis

Melanocytic naevi: pigmented cellular naevi may become trauma-
tized, inflamed or develop impacted hairs, and histological
examination is required to confirm the diagnosis. Active
junctional naevi, juvenile melanomas (Spitz tumours), halo
naevi and senile lentigines may also cause diagnostic problems.
Epidermal tumours: those that cause difficulty include pigmented
basal cell epitheliomas and pigmented seborrhoeic warts. Occasionally subcorneal haemorrhage, 'talon noir' and tinea nigra
may be mistaken for early malignant melanoma.
Vascular lesions: those that sometimes simulate a malignant
melanoma include pyogenic granuloma, haemangioma, angiokeratoma (especially when thrombosed) and Kaposi's sarcoma.
The harmless histiocytoma which is sometimes dark brown is usually easily distinguishable from malignant melanoma.

A subungual melanoma may provide a difficult diagnostic problem when it appears as a brown and imperceptibly enlarging subungual stain. In rare instances a small malignant melanoma is located in the nail bed and the only visible change is a brown linear streak extending longitudinally in the nail plate. A subungal melanoma may be mistaken for a subungal haematoma and chronic paronychia.

Treatment

Treatment depends on the histological findings—the cell type, the level of invasion and the extent of the disease. Accurate staging is based on a complete clinical examination and investigations listed below.

Investigations to stage malignant melanoma

Full blood count	Chest x-ray	Liver scan
Urea	Skull x-ray	Ultrasonogram
Electrolytes	ECG	Brain scan
Liver function tests	Lymphography in leg melanomas	
Urine for melanogens		

Stage I: when malignant melanoma is confined to the skin, i.e. no enlargement of regional lymph nodes is demonstrable.

The following are intended as guidelines to the extent of local excision which should be carried out to the deep fascia. It is usual to follow excision with a complete full thickness skin graft.

Type of melanoma	Level	Minimum margin
Superficial spreading melanoma (SSM)	1	1 cm
	2	2–3 cm
	3–5	5 cm
Nodular melanoma (NM)	1–5	5 cm
Lentigo maligna melanoma (LMM)	1–2	1 cm
	3–5	5 cm

Stage II: with firm rubbery lymph nodes. Excise as in stage I and remove the regional lymph nodes.

Stage III: with regional nodes and haematogenous dissemination. Local excision is combined with various schedules of chemotherapy.

It is now generally agreed that there is no place for the *routine* removal of apparently normal lymph nodes. Likewise, lymph node excision is rarely performed in an area of unpredictable lymph drainage, e.g. mid-back or when the lesion is a considerable distance from regional nodes, e.g. below the knee or elbow or in LMM.

It should be remembered that follow-up forms an important part of the management of these patients. It is particularly important to watch for local recurrences and the appearance of new primary tumours.

Some special skin 'tumours'

Cutaneous horn (cornu cutaneum) (*Plate 18.16*)

This represents a localized and excessive horny overgrowth which in extreme instances produces a horny projection reaching a length of several centimetres.

Aetiology

The clinical lesion of a cutaneous horn is based on several distinct histopathological entities. These include:

Keratoses: actinic keratoses are sometimes accompanied by excessive cornification and such lesions are premalignant.

Viral warts: under certain conditions these growths develop elongation of dermal papillae with extreme thickening of the stratum corneum; they are infectious.

Keratoacanthoma: with excessive elongation of the central horny plug the lesion may acquire a horn-like configuration.

Rarely fibrokeratomas and giant porokeratoses (Mibelli) present as a cornu cutaneum.

Clinical features

The predominant characteristic is a horny projection up to 5 cm in length, firmly attached to the skin.

Treatment

Excision biopsy is essential because without histological study it is impossible to know if the lesion is benign, premalignant or a viral wart.

Painful nodule of the ear (chondrodermatitis nodularis helicis)

This is a rather uncommon but often disabling affection of the pinna that causes sleep loss on account of its extreme tenderness. Although included here this is a reactive process and not a neoplasm.

Aetiology

The disorder occurs almost exclusively in men over the age of 50. Exposure to cold and trauma are probably provocative. Some doubts exist concerning the primary basis of the disorder. One suggestion is that the initial change is degeneration of ear cartilage with associated perichondritis; another is that overgrowth of the vascular tissue comprising an arteriovenous anastomosis (glomus body) is the prime disorder.

Clinical features

A small keratotic papule 1–5 cm in diameter appears on the helix. The lesion is extremely tender and sometimes a small pit exuding serum or pus underlies the crusted cap. Pain on pressure and intermittent seropurulent discharge are the predominant features.

Differential diagnosis

The following lesions should be considered because any of these disorders can affect the pinna: basal cell epithelioma, squamous cell carcinoma, actinic keratosis, gouty tophus, rheumatoid nodule, granuloma annulare.

Treatment

A completely effective treatment is a wedge-shaped excision of the lesion to include a small area of underlying cartilage; this also provides the opportunity for histological confirmation of the diagnosis. Good results are also seen with intralesional injections of triamcinolone.

Keloids (*Plate 18.17*)

A keloid results from excessive fibroblastic response to injury.

Aetiology

Darker races are more susceptible to keloids than those with a fair skin. The upper chest, especially the sternum, shoulders, ears, neck and lower legs are more prone to keloids than elsewhere on the skin surface. Extensive keloids sometime follow thermal burns or severe acne vulgaris. However, many keloids appear spontaneously without any trauma or pre-existing disease. Rarely keloids are a manifestation of widespread connective tissue disorder termed polyfibromatosis. The protean features of this developmental disease include epilepsy, torticollis, thyroid fibrosis, hepatic fibrosis, Peyronie's disease and knuckle pads. Dupuytren's contracture and plantar fibromas complete the clinical picture.

Clinical features

A keloid begins as a small firm red papule which slowly enlarges; often enlargement is eccentric with claw-like extensions. Early lesions are rubbery, pruritic and tender on pressure, whereas mature keloids are firm, asymptomatic and often hyperpigmented.

Differential diagnosis

The following should be considered; infiltrated scars, e.g. sarcoidosis, hypertrophic scars, morphoea, juvenile elastoma, shagreen patches of epiloia.

Treatment

Early treatment with intralesional steroids is sometimes very satisfactory and is probably more effective when combined with compression therapy.

Pyogenic granuloma (granuloma telangiectaticum) (*Plate 18.18*)

A very common 'tumour' comprising an overgrowth of dermal reparative tissue. The term pyogenic granuloma is a misnomer since it is neither pyogenic nor a granuloma although it may be associated with infection.

Aetiology

The lesion usually arises at the site of a scratch, abrasion or ingrowing toe nail. The relative frequency in children probably relates to a higher incidence of minor trauma.

Histopathology

Proliferating capillaries are seen in a loose connective tissue stroma which is usually circumscribed by an epidermal collarette.

Clinical features

A single small sessile or pedunculated lesion grows rapidly and resembles a red to purplish raspberry. Few lesions exceed 1 cm across. With further development they become crusted, eroded, bleed freely and then collapse only to enlarge again. Satellite lesions are sometime found.

Differential diagnosis

The diagnosis should always be suspect in an adult and a biopsy should be performed. Nodular malignant melanoma, especially the amelanotic melanoma, causes diagnostic difficulties. Angiosarcoma, haemangiopericytoma, and on the face and neck a dental sinus, may likewise cause diagnostic problems. The pseudopyogenic granuloma (which is pruritic), the juvenile melanoma (Spitz tumour), milker's nodes and metastatic deposits may closely resemble pyogenic granuloma.

Treatment

Cryotherapy, curettage followed by diathermy, or removal by surgical excision.

Basal cell epithelioma (*Plates 18.19* and *Figure 18.20*)

Basal cell epithelioma is a locally invasive skin tumour which only very rarely metastasizes. Although it grows slowly it can invade the subcutis, bone or any other tissue.

Aetiology

BCE is the most common malignant skin tumour affecting the white population. The most highly susceptible individuals have light hair, blue eyes and fair skins, thus patients of Scandinavian or Irish stock are particularly prone.

The major causative factor is cumulative exposure to sunlight and most lesions appear on sun-exposed skin in adults over the age of 40. This probably accounts for the predominance in the male sex. The sun-exposed skin shows other manifestations of actinic damage, including epidermal atrophy, elastosis, actinic keratoses and 'senile' lentigines. UVB (300–320 nm) is the active wavelength causing cutaneous malignancy.

Exposure to tar, pitch, petroleum oils, all of which are carcinogenic, enhance the effect of ultraviolet radiation on the skin and cause the development of BCEs after a shorter latent period.

X-ray exposure of the skin is a significant factor in some instances. Cumulative exposure to x-rays is associated with chronic radiation dermatitis with atrophy, telangiectasia, dyschromia and keratoses, and an increased incidence of malignancy. Single over-exposure to x-rays is sometimes followed after several decades by multiple BCEs without any associated x-ray damage.

Multiple superficial and often pigmented BCEs may result from the exposure to the carcinogenic effect of arsenic in an earlier decade.

Albinism and xeroderma pigmentosum both predispose to the early appearance of all three types of cutaneous malignancy—basal cell epithelioma, squamous cell carcinoma and malignant melanoma.

The organoid naevus, naevus sebaceous of Jadassohn, shows a high incidence of basal cell epithelioma. The tumour may arise in the naevus before puberty. Several genetic developmental syndromes include basal cell epithelioma among the cutaneous lesions, e.g. Gorlin–Goltz syndrome, Bazex syndrome.

The status and histogenesis of the basal cell epithelioma is uncertain. The epithelial component is probably derived from pluripotent cells in the epidermis. These cells are probably from hair follicle anlage and differentiation of these cells parallels that of the embryonic cells in the primary epithelial germ. The basal cell epithelioma represents incomplete differentiation and constitutes a proliferation showing stable clonal growth. Certain BCEs show differentiation towards one or other hair germ derivatives. Although invasive anaplasia is absent, stromal participation is an integral part of the tumour.

Histopathology

Basal cell epithelioma usually develops a multicentric bud of basaloid cells with basophilic nuclei and scanty cytoplasm proliferating from the undersurface of the epidermis and invading the underlying tissue. The outermost cells of the masses form a palisade layer and are separated from the dermis by a cleft which is an artefact of fixation. Surrounding stroma shows compression and condensation of collagen.

Some BCEs show early differentiation towards follicular (keratotic BCE), sebaceous (cystic BCE) or eccrine (adenoid BCE) tissue. Occasionally tumours show features of squamous and basal cell carcinoma side by side.

Clinical features

Several types of BCE occur, but the nodulo-ulcerative is the most common. The early lesion is a small, glistening, skin coloured papule which enlarges slowly to form a smooth flat nodule. The centre gradually necroses to form an ulcer which is usually covered by an adherent crust. Sometimes the lesion may reach up to 1 cm across without showing ulceration—nodulo-cystic type (*Plate 18.20*).

Enlargement is slow reaching 0.5–1 cm in five to ten years. Intermittent itching is a common symptom.

The usual appearance when first seen is of a small annular plaque with central ulceration and a pearly semitransparent rolled edge. Fine telangiectases cross the surface. If left untreated it maintains the pearly edge as it enlarges by peripheral spread.

Superficial BCEs are often multiple and appear on the trunk as oval or irregular red or lightly pigmented plaques. The slightly elevated threadlike border provides a clue to the diagnosis. Sometimes lesions are eczematous, psoriasiform (Graham–Little type) or resemble lichen simplex. The presence of multiple pigmented and superficial BCEs suggest the possibility of arsenical exposure.

A solitary pigmented basal cell epithelioma may closely mimic superficial spreading melanoma or malignant melanoma (*see* p. 245).

Sclerosing (morphoea-like) basal cell epithelioma is usually seen on the face and neck as a yellow white waxy plaque with an ill-defined border. Growth is usually slow. Microscopic features include dense fibrosis with small groups or thin strands of tumour cells which are easily overlooked by the inexperienced histopathologist. Serial sections may be required to establish the diagnosis.

An uncommon variant with marked stromal participation is the premalignant fibroepithelial tumour of Pincus. It appears as a sessile or pedunculated papule on the trunk; it is non-invasive. By contrast is the rare invasive 'terebrant ulcer' showing little stromal reaction.

Multiple BCEs appear in the basal cell naevus syndrome (Gorlin–Goltz syndrome). This widespread developmental disorder is sometimes familial. It begins in childhood or early adult life with multiple BCEs on the face and trunk. Associated features include dental cysts (which may become malignant), bone cysts, bifid ribs, dysraphic spinal changes and CNS abnormalities which include cerebellar medulloblastoma. Associated skin lesions include milia, keratin cysts, lipomas and fibromas. A diagnostic feature is porokeratotic plantar and palmar pits, 1–3 mm across which are easily overlooked.

Bazex syndrome is a less well-known disorder with multiple BCEs and 'ice-pick' pits (follicular atrophoderma) on the dorsa of the hands.

Differential diagnosis

The nodular variant may resemble a cellular naevus, cylindroma or secondary deposit. The pigmented basal cell epithelioma often mimics a seborrhoeic wart or malignant melanoma. The spectacle-frame acanthoma on the side of the nose, malar or post-auricular region may closely resemble a BCE, but the centre shows fissuring and the pearly thread-like margin of the BCE is absent.

Treatment

Surgical excision of solitary lesions usually presents no problems although large lesions may require extensive skin grafting. Curettage and electrodesiccation give excellent results for lesions up to 1 cm across. Cryotherapy and topical 5-fluorouracil (Efudix) are sometimes employed in selected cases and results are good. Similarly, radiotherapy in expert hands will produce good cosmetic results and has a recurrence rate of only 3–4 per cent.

Special problems arise with sclerosing BCEs since excision may be inadequate because of poorly delineated margin. Likewise, lesions adherent to cartilage or on the eyelids present special problems in relation to surgery or radiotherapy. The naevoid BCEs associated with Gorlin–Goltz syndrome have a particular tendency to scar severely after radiotherapy and they are therefore best treated by surgery or topical chemotherapy.

Metastatic skin tumours

The skin is a relatively uncommon site for secondary deposits from internal carcinoma. The commonest source of the primary tumour is the breast, followed by kidney, lung, stomach and uterus. Nevertheless, carcinomas of virtually any other organ may metastasize in the skin.

Internal carcinoma reaches the skin by haematogenous or lymphatic spread. This implies dissemination of the disease with a poor prognosis. Lesions arising from contiguous spread, e.g. carcinoma erysipelatoides of the breast or from underlying carcinoma, e.g. Paget's disease, are not truly metastatic. Several clinical types of cutaneous metastases exist and can cause diagnostic problems. Often the diagnosis is only reached by histological examination.

The commonest presentation is single or multiple firm indolent nodules in the dermis and subcutis. Colour ranges from yellow to purple and brown. Rarely a fibrotic scleroderma-like patch is seen on the scalp from breast carcinoma. This has been designated 'alopecia neoplastica'.

The erysipelas-like 'carcinoma en cuirasse' arises from spreading dermal lymphatic permeation and associated venular thrombosis.

As a rule cutaneous metastases appear within the vicinity of the underlying tumour, thus urogenital tumours often metastasize over the lower trunk and groin, whilst gastrointestinal and renal tumours metastasize over the abdominal wall. Breast and lung carcinoma often involve the chest wall. Certain tumours, however, favour distant sites and both renal and breast carcinomas sometimes metastasize to the face and scalp.

Neoplasia of mucous membranes

Leukoplakia (*Plate 18.21*)

A special form of epithelial neoplasia *in situ* confined to mucous membranes and appearing as white thickened 'frosted' areas. Semantic problems have arisen concerning the term leukoplakia. Here we define leukoplakia as a leucokeratosis with intraepithelial dysplasia. Some authors include under the heading leukoplakia intraepithelial dyskeratoses without cellular anaplasia.

Aetiology

Two mucosal areas are commonly affected by leukoplakia.

(1) The oral mucosa including the cheeks, tongue, gingiva and lips. On these sites chronic irritation from heavy smoking, ill-fitting dentures or cheek biting are frequent predisposing factors. Syphilitic glossitis (either healed mucous patches or superficial sclerosing glossitis) and the oral lesions of lichen planus may sometimes become leukoplakic. Lingual leukoplakia sometimes has an arsenical basis and leukoplakia of the lower lip is an occasional sequel to chronic actinic cheilitis. However, in many oral leukoplakias no local factor can be demonstrated. Buccal leukoplakia is a feature of several rare syndromes, e.g. dyskeratosis congenita, Howell–Evans syndrome.

(2) Vulval mucosa. Leukoplakia in this area usually arises *de novo* although it sometimes develops in long-standing patches of lichen sclerosus and more rarely as a result of prolonged scratching with lichenification.

Histopathology

The dysplastic epithelium shows varying degrees of anaplasia with thickening and downward proliferation of abnormal epidermis. The lower border of the epithelium is irregular 'jagged' and 'fringed'. The dermis shows a lymphocytic infiltrate which often invades the epidermis. Cellular pleomorphism and mitotic figures constitute the hallmark of leukoplakic change.

Clinical features

The affected mucosa is white, thickened, verrucous and often fissured. Early lesions appear as small 'candle wax' patches and the colour ranges from white to grey. Large patches appear as sharply defined raised plaques, sometimes likened to a 'frozen doormat'. Later induration, ulceration and surrounding inflammation suggests the appearance of an invasive process (squamous cell carcinoma). Oral leukoplakia may be associated with a soreness or a burning sensation whereas vulval leukoplakia is usually pruritic.

Differential diagnosis

Oral leukoplakia should be distinguished from other oral leukokeratoses. These include oral lichen planus and certain familial and naevoid hyperplasias.

Vulval leukoplakia shows important differences from other vulval dermatoses and the key differential features are shown in *Table 18.7.*

Other vulval dermatoses sometime mistaken for vulval leukoplakia include 'white psoriasis', candidiasis, lichen planus, morphoea, Bowen's disease, Paget's disease and vitiligo.

Treatment

Once the diagnosis is confirmed histologically surgical excision or local destructive measures, e.g. cryotherapy, are advised. The removal of any irritant factor is important to prevent recurrence.

Table 18.7 Differential diagnosis of chronic vulval dermatoses

	Lichen simplex	Lichen sclerosus	Leukoplakia
Aetiology	Over 40, psychogenic	Childhood or 40–60 years	40–60 years
Pathogenesis	Frictional, itch–scratch cycle	Unknown ?superficial type of scleroderma	Unknown, occasionally follows lichen sclerosus or lichen simplex
Histopathology	Epidermal hyperplasia, rete-pegs clubbed or fused	Epidermal atrophy, upper dermis oedematous with homogenization	Intraepidermal neoplasia, dermal hyalinization
Signs	Red or white thickened mucosa, increased markings	White parchment wrinkling, occasional purpura, bullae, erosions, follicular plugs	Milky white thickening, cracks, fissures, no follicular plugging
Location	Vulva, pubis, groins	Vulva, perianal, natal cleft, perineum	Mucous membrane and mucocutaneous border only
	Labia minora: free	Labia minora: affected	Labia minora: affected
Skin elsewhere	Lichen simplex in 5 per cent of cases	Lichen sclerosus on trunk in 30 per cent of cases	Normal
Symptoms	Pruritus	Pruritus	Pruritus
Prognosis	Very rarely premalignant	Rarely premalignant (then via leukoplakia)	Invasive carcinoma sometimes develops
Treatment	Topical steroids*	Topical steroids*, cryotherapy, vulvectomy	Cryotherapy, vulvectomy

* Potent topical steroids are best avoided for prolonged use on mucous membranes.

Erythroplasia (*Plate 18.22*)

Red velvety patches appear on the oral or genital mucosa characterized by intraepidermal Bowenoid change. Erythroplasia is commoner
than leukoplakia on the oral mucosa.

Histopathology

The findings are identical with those found in Bowen's disease.

Clinical features

Erythroplasia presents as a slightly elevated and brightly erythematous plaque. The surface is velvety moist glistening or granular. It
may be found on the buccal mucosa, glans penis or vulval mucosa.
Although it always begins on a mucous membrane it may spread to
the skin by contiguity. Induration, verrucosity or ulceration are
indicative of invasive change.

Prognosis

The incidence of malignant change is greater than in Bowen's
disease or leukoplakia and the resulting squamous cell carcinoma is
more aggressive with a greater tendency to metastasize.

Differential diagnosis

From plasma cell balanitis, vulvitis and gingivitis, none of which are
premalignant. A fixed drug eruption or a patch of eroded psoriasis
can sometimes be mistaken for erythroplasia.

Treatment

Local excision, cryotherapy or topical 5-fluorouracil. Invasive lesions
must be treated as squamous cell carcinoma.

Summary and guidelines

The practitioner should by his training:

(1) recognize tumours that are malignant or potentially malignant;
(2) recognize premalignant dermatoses;
(3) be aware of the occupational hazards leading to skin cancer.

As a rule cutaneous neoplasms carry a good prognosis because early
diagnosis is possible and tumours are usually easily accessible to
surgery or radiotherapy. Mistakes in diagnosis and delays in
treatment do sometimes occur, not so much from lack of knowledge
or lack of suspicion on the part of the physician, but from
misinterpretation of the history and appearance of the lesion. Some
of the pitfalls are mentioned below. It should be remembered that the
general practitioner should be as well able to diagnose the common

skin tumours as the dermatologist. The specialist excels only because he is more circumspect, takes nothing for granted and realizes the necessity for early and adequate biopsy of any suspicious lesion. Some general guidelines may be formulated.

(1) Any skin tumour should be treated with suspicion. If in doubt refer as an urgent problem to an expert because early accurate diagnosis is of key importance.

(2) Do not be misled by the history. *The fact that a lesion has been present for many years does not exclude a highly malignant process.* A long-standing junctional naevus may only have become malignant in the last few weeks. *It is recent change which is significant.*

(3) Always remove any crust, inspect closely, palpate carefully and examine regional lymph nodes.

(4) Do not be misled by a lesion because it is small, causing no symptoms. Avoid a 'watch and wait' policy.

(5) Suspect any persistent papule, nodule, plaque or ulcer especially if bleeding or crusting has recently taken place.

(6) Any dark-grey, blue-black or black lesion is probably already malignant.

(7) Avoid 'blind' symptomatic treatment when the diagnosis is in doubt.

(8) Avoid cauterization or curettage—either excise or refer for expert opinion.

(9) Beware of the 'quick look' trap; 'while I'm here, doctor, I've got a spot on my leg', etc.

(10) Always provide the histopathologist with the clinical history and an adequate deep section of the lesion with some normal skin. Several sections may need to be studied.

19 Circulatory and allied disorders

R. J. Cairns
Terence Ryan

In this chapter disorders in which haemodynamic or vascular factors play a part in the symptomatology of the skin disorder are discussed under the following three major headings:

(1) circulatory disorders;
(2) urticaria and vasculitis;
(3) systemic autoimmune disease.

Circulatory disorders

Raynaud's phenomenon

A paroxysmal pallor of the digits provoked by cold is termed the Raynaud's phenomenon. The disorder is multicausal. In some instances excessive adrenergic discharge causes severe vasoconstriction; in others it is due to inherent sensitivity of the small arterioles to cold, changes in blood viscosity or to platelet emboli.

Two important subgroups exist:

(1) Raynaud's disease is by definition a primary disease without any demonstrable cause.
(2) Raynaud's syndrome is a secondary disease seen with many diverse causes. These include exposure to vibrating tools, neurological disease, cervical rib, cutaneous vasculitis, occlusive arterial disease, SLE, scleroderma, mixed connective tissue disease and circulating cold agglutinins, cryofibrinogen or cryoglobulins. Ergotism and heavy metal intoxication are rarer causes, whilst late onset Raynaud's phenomenon may appear with visceral malignancy. The primary disease is usually bilateral whereas the secondary Raynaud's syndrome is more frequently unilateral. Both variants are aggravated by beta blockers.

Clinical features

The characteristic attacks are precipitated by cold or emotional stress. Each paroxysm begins at the tip of one or more fingers with intense pallor which lasts several minutes and is followed by either cyanosis or the redness of reactive hyperaemia. An attack may end spontaneously or as a result of heating by placing the hands in warm water.

With severe disease the fingers may show progressive trophic changes. These appear as hardening of the skin with tapering (sclerodactyly) or superficial gangrenous ulceration. The feet may also be affected and less commonly the nose, cheeks, ears and chin.

Treatment

The vulnerable skin of the fingers should be protected from exposure to cold and minor trauma by appropriate gloves and the use of hand warmers. Likewise general chilling is best avoided because this may provoke reflex vasospasm of the extremities. Cigarette smoking should be discouraged. Priscol (Tolazoline) 25–30 mg thrice daily or Dibenyline (phenoxybenzamine) 10 mg thrice daily are valuable in mild cases. Reserpine 0.25 mg thrice daily or 10-methoxydeserpidinide 5 mg twice daily for two to three weeks are sometimes helpful. The prostacyclins promise to be most effective enhancers of blood flow but are at present not available.

Sympathectomy should be reserved for the few patients with severe disease and no remedial primary cause and in whom conservative management is unsuccessful.

Vascular reticulate dermatoses

There are several reticulate disorders with red-blue discoloration of the skin. All are due to capillary venular stasis in the superficial vascular tree furthest away from the cutaneous arterial supply. Such microstasis is found with disorders of microcirculation, hyperviscosity syndrome and luminal narrowing due to vasospasm or arteriosclerosis.

Clinical features

Three clinical types are recognized:

(1) Cutis marmorata—venular stasis occurring on skin exposed to cold and disappearing with warming.
(2) Primary livedo reticularis—an intensive red-blue mottling that persists despite warming of the skin.
(3) Secondary livido reticularis—a persistent mottling with evidence of vasculitis, microembolism or other associated disease.

Causes include immune complex disease, cryoproteins, bacterial endocarditis or other chronic infections of the blood stream, polycythaemia especially with thrombocytosis, or severe vasospasm as in phaeochromocytoma or from vasoconstrictor drugs.

Apart from involvement of the legs and feet, the thighs, lower abdomen, hands and arms may be affected in a few cases. Coldness, paraesthesia and numbness are frequent symptoms. In some instances purpura, atrophie blanche and ulceration accompany the eruption. Livedo reticularis should be distinguished from erythema ab igne. Livedoid vasculitis or cutaneous polyarteritis are particular forms of vasculitis showing similar distribution of the skin.

Aetiology

Causes include immune complex disease, cryoproteins, bacterial endocarditis or other chronic infections of the blood stream, polycythaemia especially with thrombocytosis, severe vasospasm as in phaechromocytoma, or vasoconstrictor drugs.

Treatment

In primary livedo reticularis protection from cold is the only treatment required. With ulceration or atrophie blanche on the legs lumbar sympathectomy should be considered in women.

With secondary livedo reticularis treatment is directed towards correcting the causative disorder.

Erythema ab igne *(Plate 19.1)*

Although not a primary vascular disease the pattern of this heat-induced disorder is determined by venular network. It is a reticulate dermatosis showing epidermal and dermal damage resulting from repeated subthreshold burn exposure to infrared radiation.

Aetiology

The development of the dermatosis is related to prolonged exposure to open fires or individual room heaters (gas or electric). The almost exclusive female sex incidence is due to the protective effect of clothing in men. Localization depends not only on the direction of radiation, but the contour of the skin, the thickness of the subcutis and the interposition of clothing. It is seen over the shins and pads of subcutaneous fat, sites where conduction of heat is poor; it is also seen in areas other than the shins and thighs where hot water bottles have been applied. It is common in hypothyroid subjects and is a valuable cutaneous sign of incipient hypothermia.

Clinical features

The skin changes of reticulate erythema, melanosis and hyperkeratosis are characteristic. The effects often clear in the summer months, but after several years' reappearance, involution is less complete, and keratosis and squamous cell carcinoma may develop within the heat damaged area.

Treatment

Hypothyroidism should be excluded. Clothing and covering creams prevent further exposure.

Chilblains

Perniosis and erythrocyanosis crurum are some of the other names which are applied to this syndrome.

Aetiology

The prime factors in the development of chilblains are individual susceptibility to cold and damp characterized by excessive vasospasm of arterioles on exposure to cold, and capillary and venular stasis. Local pressure from ill-fitting shoes or tight garments is also a factor. Post-capillary venular thrombosis occurs following microvenular stasis causing a venous capillary infarct.

Clinical features

Acute chilblains are the more common manifestation and are easily recognized when they appear on the fingers and toes. Other areas of predilection are the legs, feet, ears and, more rarely, the nose and cheeks. The affected sites burn and itch; they exhibit red or blue discoloration and are cold to the touch. Later these areas may become slightly swollen and feel infiltrated, or haemorrhagic blisters appear.

Micropapular chilblains are small infarcts usually affecting the fingers and toes.

Chronic chilblains arise from repeated exposure to cold in a susceptible person and appear as recurrent and chronic painful cutaneous lesions in the exposed area; they are violaceous, nodular, haemorrhagic or ulcerative; later scarring, fibrosis and atrophy of the skin and subcutaneous tissues occur.

The lower legs in girls are the sites most commonly affected; during the active phase the skin is cool to the touch, usually acrocyanotic and sometimes oedematous.

Differential diagnosis

The following conditions must be considered.

Erythema induratum: The nodules involve the calves rather than the lower part of the legs, ankles and feet, as in chronic chilblains. In general there is more nodularity and induration in erythema induratum and the ulcers are deeper. The lesions often persist in warmer weather.

Erythema nodosum: Exquisitely tender, violaceous and warm nodules affect the shins and extensor aspect of the arms. The patient may be pyrexial with polyarthralgia.

Nodular vasculitis: Red, painful nodules or inflammatory non-seasonal plaques occur on the calves of middle-aged women; chilblains occur in a younger age group.

Lupus erythematosus: When this involves the hands the lesions are more circumscribed than those of chilblains and occur between the joints and about the nail folds. There is no itching and although worse in winter the lesions often present in warm weather.

Cryoglobulinaemia: Purpura, cold urticaria and livedo reticularis may occur in a primary idiopathic form or secondary to diseases such as myeloma, leukaemia, and systemic autoimmune diseases.

Lupus pernio: A variant of sarcoidosis, affects the nose, ears and fingers.

Treatment

There is no specific prophylactic or circulatory drug treatment for chilblains. For the individual whose microcirculation reacts in this way to damp and cold, prophylaxis in the form of a warm environment and suitable clothing is of prime importance. Loose fitting warm gloves, sheepskin lined boots and the rejection of nylon stockings, tight cotton jeans and flimsy shoes in the cold weather are essential. It has been noted that office workers have a higher incidence than those in active occupations and that outdoor exposure does not seem to have any adverse effect. Some outdoor exercise is therefore indicated. Vasodilator drugs are disappointing.

Any local treatment must be directed towards easing the intense burning and itching sensation from which some patients suffer. Steroid creams or ointments are sometimes helpful if applied to the skin at the onset of symptoms.

Subjects prone to chilblains should avoid rapid warming of a chilled limb by means of hot bathing, hot water bottles or warming the extremity in front of the fire.

Sympathectomy may have to be considered in severe recurrent cases where there is much pain and risk of permanent disfigurement. These subjects, if they can afford it, would be well advised to take up permanent residence in a warm climate.

Venous ulceration (varicose ulcers)

The majority of ulcers of the leg seen in clinical practice have a vascular basis and venous ulcers form the commonest group, accounting for 95 per cent of all leg ulcers.

Most venous ulcers are seen in women over the age of 45 and result from damage to the valves of the deep venous system following phlebothrombosis. It follows that early diagnosis and treatment of deep vein thrombosis provides the key for preventing post-phlebitic sequelae of which ulceration of the lower leg is the most important.

Anatomy and physiology

A study of both the anatomy of the venous system and the normal mechanism of blood circulation in the lower limb is essential to understand the disorder of circulatory function that eventually leads to venous ulceration.

The veins of the lower limb consist of three related parts: the deep veins, the superficial veins and the veins connecting these two, called the perforating or communicating veins (*Figure 19.1*).

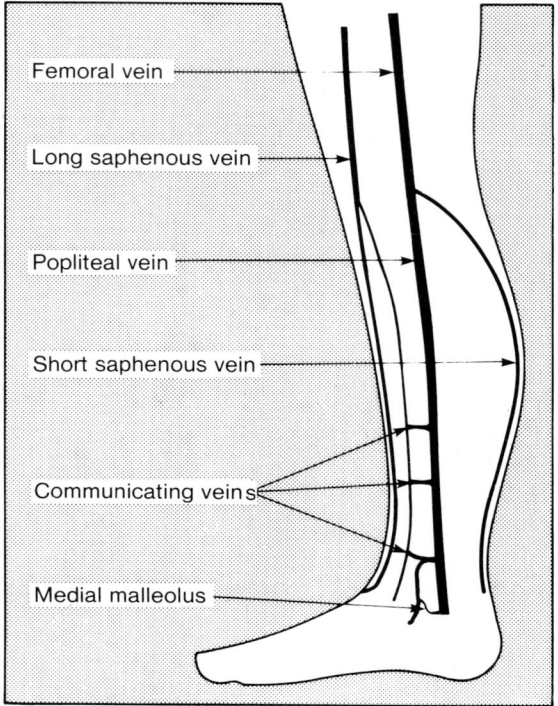

Figure 19.1 *Anatomy of superficial and deep veins in the leg*

In the healthy subject the perforating vessels are valved so that blood can normally only flow from the superficial to the deep veins and thence to the heart. Ninety per cent of the venous blood from the lower limb travels via the deep leg veins, the long and short saphenous veins and their branches taking only 10 per cent of the load.

The force driving the blood is derived from the so-called musculo-fascial pump of the calf. Contraction of the powerful muscles of the calf (gastrocnemius and soleus) within the inextensible fascial sheath exerts a pressure on the deep veins which when the valves are intact propels the blood upwards. With each step muscular contraction occurs. Thus the normal venous return depends on the combined efficiency of the calf pump and the deep venous valves.

In the ankle region the perforating veins are short, at right angles to the skin and guarded by a single valve. It is these venous channels that are the main drainage pathway from the skin of the ulcer-bearing area. On the medial side of the leg three perforating veins (Cockett's veins) are commonly found in line with the posterior border of the medial malleolus. The lower perforating vein is immediately behind the medial malleolus, the middle perforator four finger breadths above it, and the upper perforator four finger breadths above the middle one (*see Figure 19.1*). On the outer aspect of the ankle the position of the communicating veins is less constant. Other perforating veins are situated in the upper calf and thigh.

Causes of venous failure and ulceration

Many factors contribute to the failure of an effective venous return, thereby producing deep venous hypertension with secondary trophic changes. The important sequence of events and contributory factors are shown in *Figure 19.2*. It will be seen that venous ulcers are commonly post-thrombotic. Deep phlebothrombosis not infrequently follows pregnancy. Predisposing factors include obesity and occupational influences, particularly prolonged standing. Deep vein thrombosis is a hazard of bed rest; it is particularly liable to follow any abdominal operation and is prone to occur following a leg injury or in patients with a blood disorder such as polycythaemia. A massive thrombosis affecting the deep veins causes the 'white leg' syndrome or phlegmasia alba dolens, usually associated with pregnancy or parturition. However, such a definitive history of deep vein thrombosis in patients with venous ulceration is uncommon because phlebothrombosis is often symptomless.

After several weeks recanalization of the thrombus occurs and the valves in the deep veins are damaged. The resulting valvular

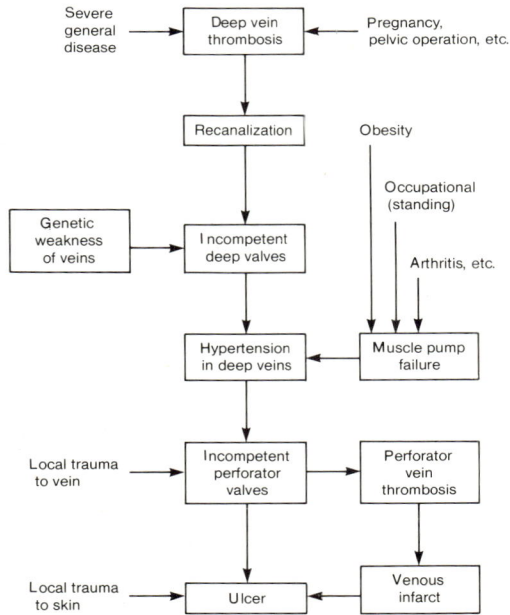

Figure 19.2 *Multiple factors leading to varicose ulcer*

incompetence is the prime cause of deep venous hypertension and the signs of this raised pressure first show in the perforating veins when the patient is upright and standing still. The result of continuous back pressure is either dilatation of the perforating veins and incompetence of the valve in each perforator (the ankle blow-out syndrome) or venous thrombosis of the perforating veins. The overlying skin suffers infarction, both the subcutaneous fat and dermis undergoing necrosis with resultant ulceration.

An important contributory cause to deep venous hypertension is weakness or failure of the musculofascial pump in the calf (*Figure 19.3*). Weakness may result from disuse atrophy of the muscles, neuromuscular or joint disease. Thus poliomyelitis, rheumatoid arthritis and osteoarthritis of the hip and knee are possible causes of muscle pump failure.

An occasional cause of venous hypertension is a congenital weakness of the muscular walls of the deep veins with incompetent valves. In such patients the symptoms of venous insufficiency appear in the absence of preceding deep vein thrombosis and a family history of similar disease is usual. Another, although uncommon cause of venous hypertension is a congenital arteriovenous fistula—a developmental abnormality in which arterial blood passes directly into the venous circulation. Such patients often show gross varicose veins and overgrowth of the affected leg. An acquired arteriovenous fistula is usually traumatic and the result of a penetrating wound which injures an artery and a nearby vein at the same time, so allowing arterial blood to pass directly into the vein.

Another occasional cause of damage to the deep valves and deep phlebothrombosis is the chemical insult from the injudicious use of sclerosing agents. Until a few years ago sclerosing agents were commonly used to ablate superficial varicose veins. This was

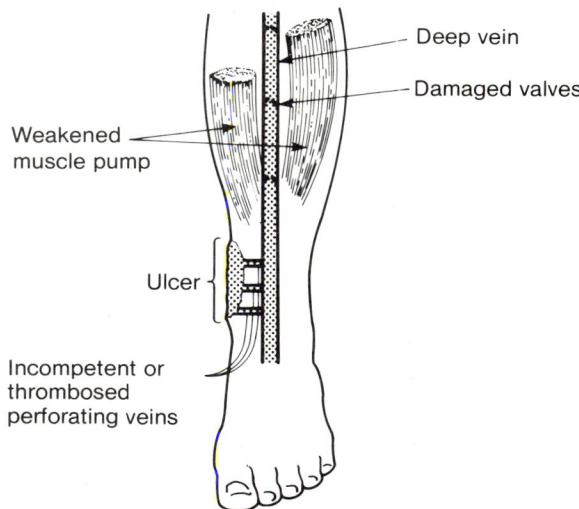

Figure 19.3 *Diagram of varicose ulcer mechanics*

performed by direct injection into superficial varicosities. However it is now known that the passage of such an irritant chemical through the perforating veins may cause damage to the deep valves.

Once a venous ulcer has appeared certain factors come into play which result in its perpetuation and even extension. Thus oedema is a potent cause of persistence although unrelated to its causation. Both venous oedema and ulceration are the result of deep venous hypertension. Infection of the ulcerated surface may lead to cellulitis and fibrosis of the surrounding tissues. Lymphoedema follows both immobility and failure of the calf muscle pump and is characteristic of Grade 5 venous failure (*see Table 19.1*). The dilated lymphatic channels commonly become infected and cellulitis leads to further lymphatic damage, lymph stasis and more oedema.

Clinical features

For convenience we shall designate degrees of venous failure Grades 1 to 5 (*see Table 19.1*). Grades 1, 2 and 3 are summarized in this table whereas Grades 4 and 5 are discussed in more detail.

Grade 4

This degree of venocapillary failure is the result of deep venous hypertension combined with moderate pump failure. The patient by this stage shows gross physical signs and suffers considerable disability. Such a degree of circulatory failure is reached perhaps only ten to 15 years after the first thrombotic episode. Superficial varicose veins are not conspicuous and, indeed, venous stars over the perforators are often obliterated by oedema. The oedema is marked and involves the toes, foot and malleolar hollows and extends for some distance up the calf. Phlebectasia and haemosiderosis may be seen, although commonly obscured by oedema. However, melanosis is sometimes marked. Secondary dermatitic changes—erythema, exudation, scaling and crusting are frequent. With mild dermatitis the changes include only redness and scaling; the area is pruritic. Marked eczematous dermatitis is often the result of inappropriate topical medication; the skin of the ankle region is easily irritated by primary irritants and particularly prone to develop an allergic contact dermatitis. Certain antibiotics, notably neomycin and soframycin, are particular offenders. As a result of primary dermatitis of the legs a distant sensitivity eruption may appear. Then redness and swelling of the face, eczematous eruptions on the arm flexures and thighs are commonly seen. Autosensitization eczema may even be the main presenting feature, the patient perhaps failing to mention that a leg ulcer is being treated with a proprietary or irritant preparation to which the skin is intolerant.

Venous ulceration is common with this degree of venous failure. The ulcer first appears as a localized crusted area overlying an incompetent perforating vein. Removal of the adherent crust reveals shallow ulceration. In some instances the ulcer appears at the site of

Table 19.1 Grades of veno-pump failure

Grade	1	2	3	4	5
Pathomechanism	Venous reflux	Gross leak Venous hypertension	Persistent venocapillary failure	Venocapillary failure	Venocapillary failure Lymphoedema Cellulitis Fibrosis
	Capillary leak rarely	Capillary leak usually			
	Pump intact	Pump usually intact	Slight pump failure	Moderate pump failure	Severe pump failure
Clinical features					
Venous findings	Tender perforators	Phlebectasia below malleolus	'Stars' over blown perforators	Not conspicuous	Venous ectasia submerged by oedema
Capillary haemosiderosis	Slight	'Peppering' variable	Marked near malleolus	Marked	'Submerged'
Purpura	Slight	Sometimes marked	Often marked	Marked	'Submerged'
White atrophy	Slight	Sometimes marked	Slight	Not evident	Not evident
Melanosis	Slight	Slight	Often marked	Gross	Inconstant
Oedema	None	None	Inframalleolar	Marked	Gross
Eczema	None	None	Absent or slight	Often	Usual
Ulcer	None	None	Rare	Frequent	Large
Treatment	Avoid trauma	Exercise	Exercise	Exercise	Control oedema
	Exercise	Crepe bandage for protection	Diuretics	Rehabilitation	Control infection then exercise and pressure bandage
	Special exercises for pregnancy, post operation		Pressure bandage	Diuretics	
				Pressure bandage	

injury near the ankle; a small abrasion or laceration fails to heal, and then extends and deepens producing an ulcer.

Treatment at this stage should be directed first to controlling the oedema of the leg by the use of diuretics; in very acute cases the dermatitic changes can be suppressed by prednisone 15 mg daily for five to six days. At the same time the patient should be encouraged to walk and exercise the leg, and within a few days when the oedema has subsided a medicated pressure bandage is applied. When associated disease is present which prevents effective functioning of the calf pump, e.g. rheumatoid or osteo-arthritis, it should be actively treated at an early stage.

Grade 5

This stage of venous impairment is associated with severe pump failure and lymphoedema is common. The patient, almost always an elderly woman, is severely disabled. A pathetic picture in her own home is presented by such an individual. She is often overweight, pale, undernourished, sitting close to a fire even on a warm day, and has gross oedema of the legs which she rests on a footstool. She has probably worn slippers and no shoes for many years, and sleeps all night in her chair. She never ventures out of the house and is surrounded by jars, tubes and cartons of ointment, all of which the district nurse has been applying with missionary zeal, to no benefit, for months or even years. The patient is apathetic and oedematous, and the foetor from infection with Gram-negative and anaerobic organisms pervades the atmosphere.

Venocapillary failure, muscle pump failure and lymphoedema are often complicated by cellulitis and fibrosis. Both legs are usually affected, oedema is gross, the skin is hyperkeratotic and, in some instances, coarsened with elephantiasic thickening. The ulceration is extensive and often deep, sometimes almost encircling the limb. Associated dermatitis is common.

The patient's attitude of apathy and resignation combined with general depression has led to prolonged immobility with further lymph stasis and leg stiffness. Pain and loss of sleep add to the distress. The gross oedema impairs healing of the ulcer and in these patients bacterial infection is commonly an important perpetuating factor. Both Gram-positive and particularly Gram-negative organisms delay healing by producing further oedema and fibrosis. Attacks of spreading cellulitis from either the ulcer area or from poor hygiene of the foot further damage lymphatic channels.

Treatment of this late stage is notoriously difficult because by now certain irreversible changes have occurred. The valves are irreparably damaged, the calf muscles have wasted, the ankle and knee joints are stiff and oedema and fibrosis of the muscles from vascular ischaemia prevent normal functioning of the limb. Any coexisting disease requires active and specific therapy. Anaemia, cardiac failure, arteriosclerosis and poor nutrition all require attention. Such patients usually require admission to hospital. The aim is to control both the oedema and infection, to remobilize the limb and to get the patient ambulant.

Differential diagnosis

The majority of ulcers of the lower limb are of venous origin. however, even when venous disorder is the prime basis of the disease, other diseases such as arteriosclerosis and diabetes may be present.

Purely arteriosclerotic ulcers differ from venous ulcers in their configuration and location. Arteriosclerotic ulcers are seen on the dorsum of the foot, the ankle or calf region. They are unrelated to perforating veins and are commonly polycyclic in outline. A characteristic feature is the presence of islands of normal tissue within the ulcerated area. Arteriolar ulcers are smaller, often multiple and painful. They commence as an erythematous disc, sometimes covered with a superficial bulla which abrades, leaving a shallow, painful ulcer. A common location is the lower part of the shin.

The history often points to the diagnosis of arterial insufficiency. Intermittent claudication suggests vascular ischaemia. Physical signs include absence of pulsation of the popliteal and dorsalis pedis arteries, and cyanosis or pallor of the toes. In some instances superficial gangrene of the digits is present.

Syphilitic ulceration has a vascular basis. Gummata with associated syphilitic endarteritis obliterans produces single or grouped nodules which ulcerate. These ulcers commonly occur on the upper part of the front of the shin.

In patients with poor peripheral circulation (acrocyanosis) chronic perniotic nodules appear in cold weather, usually on the lower third of the posterior aspect of the calf; they sometimes ulcerate.

Nodular vasculitis is a deep granulomatous disorder affecting the subcutaneous fat. The basis is vascular and ulceration sometimes occurs. A related disorder of tuberculous origin (Bazin's disease) more commonly ulcerates. The commonest location is at the back of the calf.

Large vessel vasculitis, as exemplified by polyarteritis nodosa, produces the classic triad of livedo racemosa, dermal nodules and ulcers. A common location is the front of the shin or the ankle region. A rare form of arteritis is Wegener's granuloma. Nasal, renal and pulmonary disease often overshadow the cutaneous lesions which are nodular and necrotic. Giant cell arteritis is a reported cause of leg ulceration.

A variety of systemic diseases may be present with ulcerative lesions on the lower limb. Gummata and Bazin's disease have already been mentioned. Pyoderma gangrenosum is a pustulonecrotic disorder characterized by large and rapidly spreading ulcerative areas. The ulcers may be circular or polycyclic in outline, surrounded by an infiltrative and pustular margin. They occur with both ulcerative colitis and rheumatoid arthritis. A similar ulcerative disorder is ecthyma gangrenosum which is based on septic infarction of the skin with *Pseudomonas pyocyaneus* in patients with septicaemia from this organism.

Certain blood disorders, particularly polycythaemia, spherocytic anaemia and sickle-cell anaemia may all produce leg ulceration.

Nodular panniculitis of the Weber–Christian type produces crops of nodules in the subcutaneous fat. Lesions occur at the front of the thighs and shins and in some instances liquefy, discharging fatty material (liquefying panniculitis).

Vegetating and granulomatous halogen eruptions produce infiltrated nodular and ulcerative tumours on any part of the body surface. Ulcerative bromoderma and ulcerative iododerma produce nodules and ulcers resembling neoplastic disease.

A rare cause of ulceration of the shin is underlying bone disease. For example osteomyelitis and Paget's disease may be associated with cutaneous ulceration.

Scleroderma and the rare Werner's syndrome which has scleroderma-like infiltration of the skin both show leg ulceration.

Neurotrophic ulceration due to the loss of cutaneous sensation combined with minor trauma of the skin occurs in tabes dorsalis, diabetes and other neurological disorders in which sensory loss is a feature. Neurotrophic ulcers are commonly found on the pressure bearing areas of the foot notably over the heads of metatarsals or the heel.

Certain infections produce ulceration with granuloma formation. Deep mycoses, such as actinomycoses, produce nodules and multiple sinuses or ulcers which discharge pus containing yellow granules. Tropical ulcers occur commonly on the legs and are frequently of diphtheritic origin. Ecthyma is an ulcerative form of impetigo which is seen in malnourished individuals. It is staphylococcal in origin and is common on the legs.

Certain tumours may first appear as an ulcerated lesion on the lower limb. Kaposi's sarcoma usually presents with multiple vascular nodules and oedema. Similarly Hodgkin's disease shows nodules and occasionally ulceration with polycyclic configuration. Malignant melanoma usually presents as a brown, grey or black flat lesion which extends, crusts and ulcerates.

Treatment

Venous ulceration is merely a symptom and invariably late result of deep venous insufficiency. The three guiding principles for treatment of venous leg ulcers are:

(1) The elimination of deep venous hypertension by continuous pressure bandaging applied with sufficient compression to counteract the abnormal venous pressure. The bandage should be applied from the base of the toes moulding to the contour of the ankle, up to the level of the tibial tuberosity so that the increased venous pressure over the whole of the leg is effectively neutralized. Pressure to the ulcerated area alone is ineffective.

Pressure bandaging should be used with caution in the presence of any ischaemic disorder of the lower limb.

(2) The maintenance and improvement of the pumping action of the calf muscles. The basis for this principle is that when a pressure bandage is worn there is an upward thrust with each contraction of the calf muscles even in the presence of incompetent valves. Active ambulation and regular heel raising exercises are of particular importance because many of these cases are elderly with stiffness of both the knee and ankle joints and disuse atrophy of the calf muscles. Many have literally forgotten how to walk and remedial exercises are of prime importance.

(3) The prevention and treatment of infection, eczema and lymphoedema. When stasis eczema is present the skin is prone to irritant or allergic dermatitis from topical medication, particularly under an occlusive dressing. The common offenders encountered causing an aggravation of stasis eczema are topical antibiotics. Greasy tulle gras preparations are best avoided. The control of infection in the ulcerated area is of secondary importance. Massive infection with Gram-negative organisms requires an effective topical antibiotic and cellulitis is best treated with systemic antibiotics. A povidone–iodine spray can be applied to the ulcer crater. The area surrounding the ulcer, particularly when it is eczematous, is effectively treated by the application of a bland absorbent paste such as Pasta Titanium Dioxide BPC. A medicated support bandage, Quinaband, Calaband or calamine impregnated cotton bandage is applied from the base of the toes to the tibial tuberosity. A pressure bandage such as ventilated diachylon, e.g. ventilated Lestreflex, is similarly applied completely covering the medicated bandage except when an ischaemic factor is present.

Early stages of venous insufficiency without ulceration or oedema require special forms of treatment and these are summarized in *Table 19.1*. Hospitalization is recommended only in certain cases of Grade 5 venous failure and for dealing with associated disease, e.g. anaemia, poor nutrition, cardiac failure.

Surgical reconstruction of the deep veins and their defective valves is at present impossible and surgical measures directed towards the ablation of associated superficial varicosities may further overload the deep system. Nevertheless, in certain cases surgery directed towards the removal or ablation of incompetent and useless perforating veins, particularly those near the ankle, may be curative.

The Cockett technique aims at tying the incompetent perforating veins above the ankle. Fegan devised a simple out-patient regime for localizing and injecting perforating veins. Following injection local pressure pads are applied, the legs bandaged and the patient kept ambulant.

When congenital arteriovenous fistula is responsible for deep venous hypertension and leg ulceration, it is sometimes possible to tie off the main communicating channels. Preliminary arteriography is necessary.

The general management of patients with leg ulcers is directed towards treating any associated disease. In obese patients weight reduction is of key importance. When present acute superficial thrombophlebitis responds well to butazolidine 100 mg thrice daily for six days; cellulitis requires a systemic antibiotic. With fibrosing panniculitis fibrinolytic therapy, e.g. stanozol (Stromba) 5 mg twice daily is required.

In Grades 4 and 5 venocapillary failure diuretics are valuable for controlling oedema before pressure bandaging. Hydrosaluric tablets 50 mg twice daily for four to five days is usually sufficient. When arterial insufficiency is present vasodilators probably help to improve local circulation.

Elderly patients are often anaemic, sideropenic and undernourished. Vitamin supplements and iron should be given.

In chronic leg ulcers excellent results have been claimed for preparing the ulcer for autografting with dressings of cultured human amnion. The vascular response fills the ulcer bed with granulation tissue. Autografts are applied after five days of amnion application.

Urticaria and vasculitis

Urticaria and vasculitis represent a response of small blood vessels to injury. The target tissue may be a component of the vessel wall such as an endothelial cell, a smooth muscle cell or an adjacent mast cell. Alternatively the target may be cells of the tissue supplied by the blood vessels, such as an epidermal cell in the case of an upper dermal capillary or fat cell supplied by subcutaneous vessels.

The time response depends on the severity of the injury as well as on the speed and efficiency of removal of the noxae and subsequent repair of the damaged tissue. Thus urticaria and vasculitis are often seen as the abnormal response to a relatively minor injury, a consequence of inadequate or of over-reaction by the tissues and sometimes perpetuated by an inadequate or exaggerated process of repair. An excessive white cell response or excessive fibrin deposition are examples of local responses which often contribute to vasculitis.

Small blood vessels have a limited repertoire of response including increased permeability, white cell diapedesis, bleeding, coagulation and thrombosis. Weals, purpura and gangrene are the most important clinical signs. Depending particularly on host factors controlling responses to injury some patients present with urticaria, others with purpura and others with widespread infarction. However, a mixed picture is common so that tender and persistent weals become purpuric and infarction occurs at sites of purpura. Oedema or necrosis of the perivascular and extravascular tissue accounts for vesicles, bullae or deep nodules.

The clinical picture depends on such factors as (1) intensity of the injury, (2) the time at which it is observed during the reponse and repair, and (3) the depth of the vascular lesions. Superficial vasculitis sometimes causes blisters or pustules whereas deep vasculitis produces large nodules.

Venules are the commonest vessels involved since they are always more vulnerable because of slow blood flow, leakiness and relative hypoxia, but arterial smooth muscle is quickly damaged by hypoxia.

Severe infarction occurs mainly as a result of ischaemia. Commonly necrosis of the wall of a medium sized dermal arteriole results when peripheral vessels supplied by it are continually congested or thrombosed or when the vessel itself is in vasospasm as in severe hypertension.

Urticaria (*Plate 19.2*) and vasculitis may be localized to one area of skin and such localization is associated with a more benign prognosis. A systemic and thereby severer disease is seen when more than one site or organ is affected. Severe anaphylaxis or widespread systemic vasculitis are examples of severe disease with multiple organ involvement.

Pathogenetic mechanisms producing vasculitis

(1) Circulating immune complexes are the most often incriminated. Viruses such as hepatitis B, bacteria such as the haemolytic streptococcus (Lancefield group A) or autoantibodies of rheumatoid arthritis are common antigens.
(2) Infective agents may directly damage blood vessels and with bacteraemia and micro-organisms sometimes provoke either widespread disseminated intravascular coagulation or focal vascular lesions.
(3) Drugs may directly injure a vessel but more often they alter the vascular response to minor injury. Drugs causing vasospasm, blocking fibrinolysis or enhancing permeability can be shown to encourage experimental vasculitis.
(4) Local repetitive injury. Some of the more bizarre patterns of vascular injury occur at sites of trauma where protective mechanisms in the tissues are exhausted. Thus angioedema may follow minor dental surgery or pyoderma gangrenosum follow venepuncture of the skin.

The Schwartzmann phenomenon is an example of a pathological process occurring when a further injury in the neighbourhood of a recently infected tissue results in an inflammatory coagulation of the affected vascular tree.

Plastic surgeons are familiar with ischaemic necrosis when manipulating skin that has suffered recent insults (the phenomenon of delay).

Urticaria and vasculitis are occasional manifestations of severe underlying disease such as infection, autoimmune disease or neoplasia. The antigens and noxious agents responsible for vascular damage include almost the whole range of living agents, drugs and also autoantibodies.

Factors influencing the tissue response

Impaired removal of antigen may be due to congenital or acquired defects in the immune system, such as decreased complement or impaired phagocytosis.

Exhaustion of the fibrinolytic system or enhancement of coagulation and thrombosis are common accompaniments of vasculitis.

Emotional, hormonal or drug effects are frequently recorded in association with urticaria and vasculitis.

Stasis, shock or cooling, contribute to the localization of haematogenous agents. Exhaustion of fibrinolysis and encouragement of coagulation as well as granuloma formation follows failure of recruitment of blood-borne opsonizing agents or factors essential for phagocytosis and intracellular destruction of bacteria.

The spectrum of vasculitis

During the past 150 years numerous names have been given to different patterns of vasculitis. There is so much overlap that the value of so much delineation is now doubtful. However, certain groupings of physical signs occur frequently enough to be labelled by a single name for the purpose of communication. Such names include Henoch–Schönlein purpura, necrotizing vasculitis, systemic hypersensitivity angiitis, polyarteritis nodosa, capillaritis, erythema multiforme, erythema nodosum, pityriasis lichenoides et varioliformis acuta, erythema elevatum diutinum and giant cell arteritis.

Histopathology

The microscopic changes range from evidence of slight oedema through various degrees of leucocytic infiltration to coagulation and thrombosis with necrosis. Minimal changes include swelling, distortion and separation of endothelial cells with intracellular and extracellular collections of fluid.

Leucocytoclasis is the term given to infiltration and destruction of neutrophils in the vessel wall and surrounding tissues. *Fibrinoid* is the exudation into the vessel wall of plasma proteins and coagulation products. There may be ischaemic necrosis of the smooth muscle contained in the walls of medium-sized blood vessels with evidence of disruption of the wall. Usually there is evidence of injury to the tissues supplied—spongiosis or necrosis of the epidermis or disruption of fat cells. Later pathology includes the activity of the mononuclear phagocytic system which may be filled with haemosiderin, lipids and fibrin and giant cell formation.

Immunofluorescent studies of early lesions provide circumstantial evidence of immune complex deposition.

Investigation

Whatever the type of urticaria or vasculitis the possibility of underlying systemic disease should be considered. While some forms of urticaria or vasculitis are recognized instantly as benign and requiring little investigation, most merit a search for the trigger as well as the underlying host factor that explains why the patient is reacting abnormally. Some patterns are associated more commonly with certain known triggers than others.

For example, streptococcal sore throat and Henoch–Schönlein purpura, herpes simplex and erythema multiforme, sarcoid and erythema nodosum; in a difficult case, whatever the morphology, a check list (*Table 19.2*) may be useful.

Table 19.2 Routine investigation should include a search for triggers of vasculitis as well as for constitutional defects

Infection:	Streptococcal sore throat
	Tuberculosis
	Leprosy, or any history of recent 'flu'-like illness, cystitis, sinusitis or vaccinations
Food and drugs:	Aspirin—headache pills, throat lozenges
	Purgatives
	Health foods
	Soft drinks—especially highly coloured and in large quantities
	Antibiotics
	Any medicine given for any specific illness
	Any recent intake of food or drugs to which the patient is known to be allergic
Constitutional:	Undue exposure to extremes of temperature in the environment, to bright sunlight or to cold winds
	Any known chronic illness such as: diabetes mellitus, blood disorders, rheumatoid arthritis or other autoimmune disease, chronic respiratory disease, disorders of the bowel or liver, or hypertension
	Malignant disease
	Recent surgery or pregnancy
	Any unusual degree of anxiety or an anxious personality
Local constitution:	Trauma, cold exposure, gravitational stasis, changes in vascular anatomy or in cellular infiltration

Urticaria and angioedema

Urticaria is caused by a transient exudation of fluid into the dermis. Angiodema is essentially the same but is more often used to describe deep swellings (*Plate 19.3*) which may be confined to a single site such

274

as the lip or throat. It represents the increased permeability of the earliest or acute phase of inflammation mediated by histamine, acetyl choline, and serotonin. However, there is overlap with more chronic inflammation as in vasculitis. Henoch–Schönlein purpura in children is often predominantly urticarial. It is probably helpful to regard weals that last 12 hours to three days and which are tender to the touch, as the equivalent of the earliest phase of vasculitis. The mediators involved include the kinins, plasmin, complement, coagulation factors and the products of white cells such as proteases and lymphokines.

The signs and symptoms of urticaria depend on the mediators of and the transience, size, and depth of the swelling as well as the extent of the skin involvement.

Some specific patterns of urticaria

Cholinergic urticaria

This is provoked by emotion, exercise or heat. Small 2 mm-sized weals which sting, last for up to 15 minutes and are surrounded by a prominent flush. Related to the blush reflex, such urticaria is common in the teenager or young adult. It can be helped by reassurance and the more tranquillizing of the antihistamines, e.g. hydroxyzine (Atarax) or anticholenergic drugs.

Physical urticaria

Dermographism (*Plate 19.4*) is an excessive triple response to friction or pressure occurring in about 5 per cent of the population. It is mediated mainly by histamine. Tender urticaria sometimes develops four or more hours after pressure is applied to the skin. In some patients it is part of a generalized ordinary urticaria, while in others it may represent the localization by pressure of immune complexes, or the exhaustion by ischaemia of local protease inhibitors. Cold urticaria is usually due to an abnormal sensitivity of the mast cell to cooling, but cryoglobulins and cryofibrinogens may be precipitated by cold. Patients who release large amounts of histamine in the cold should always be accompanied when swimming because of the risk of sudden death.

Solar urticaria immediately follows exposure to sunlight. Repeated exposure may result in tolerance but erythropoietic protoporphyria and systemic lupus erythematosus must be excluded.

Hereditary angiodema

A rare but extremely important condition because of the risk of severe laryngeal oedema. Absence of an inhibitor of the activated first component of complement is responsible for the syndrome. Danazol is the treatment of choice but epsilon aminocaproic acid or transfusions of fresh plasma seem to control some cases.

275

Acute urticaria

The aetiology is commonly iatrogenic, e.g. due to antisera such as antitetanic serum, or penicillin. Certain individuals develop acute urticaria as a manifestation of food sensitivity. The onset is sudden, with swelling and urticarial lesions which may last a few hours or several days. The lesions have a white, palpable central oedematous area with a variable halo of erythema. The size and shape varies widely and the individual lesions rarely persist over 48 hours. Joint swellings, abdominal pain and rarely oedema of the pharynx and larynx develop. The severest clinical type is anaphylactic shock.

Treatment

Oedema of the mouth, tongue, pharynx and larynx constitutes an acute medical emergency demanding adrenaline and airway maintenance. The following steps must be taken:

(1) adrenaline (1/1000) 0.5 ml injected slowly intramuscularly; not more than 0.5 ml should be given at first;
(2) intravenous infusion of 5% dextrose containing 100 mg of hydrocortisone; if no immediate response, 100 mg of hydrocortisone to be injected into the tubing;
(3) ephedrine 30 mg and chlorpheniramine (Piriton) 50 mg to be given by mouth. For less severe reaction adrenaline (1/1000) 0.2–0.5 ml to be given subcutaneously, with chlorpheniramide by mouth.

Chronic and recurrent urticaria

Chronic urticaria lasts from a few weeks to many years, usually with variable intervals of freedom. Severe itching is always present. Weals are scattered widely and the extent of the skin affected will often change from day to day.

The pathogenesis of urticaria is discussed above but the following check list may be helpful in the questioning and advice to patients.

Drugs—aspirin, penicillin, sera, codeine, morphine.
Foods—fish, eggs, tomatoes, milk, nuts, salicylates and benzoates, and colour agents (e.g. tartrazine).
Physical agents—heat, cold, pressure, light.
Psychogenic causes—frustration, guilt, repressed hostility, blushing and flushing.
Systemic disease—candidiasis.
Parasitic infestations—trichinosis, roundworms, tape-worms, onchocerciasis.
Systemic vasculitis—SLE, Still's disease.
Rare disorders—mast cell disease, erythroietic protoporphyria.
Inhalant allergens—pollen, dust, perfume, feathers etc.

Papular urticaria (lichen urticatus) (*See* Chapter 11)

Diagnosis of urticaria

Physical examination serves to distinguish between the different types of urticaria. It may also exclude other skin diseases with an urticarial component, e.g. dermatitis herpetiformis or allergic vasculitis, and a general examination may reveal the underlying primary cause.

The history is the most important diagnostic aid, though its value is greater in acute urticaria than in the chronic forms. However, in chronic urticaria a careful history may reveal a relationship to drug ingestion, trauma, cold or sunlight. A transient swelling can sometimes be induced in the physical urticarias by applying ice to the skin.

Skin testing in chronic urticaria is unrewarding; unfortunately positive skin tests often develop that are irrelevant and misleading.

Treatment of urticaria

(For the treatment of *acute urticaria see* p. 276)

The main objective in the treatment of allergic urticaria is to eliminate exposure to the offending allergen, and in symptomatic urticaria to treat the primary disease. When the eruption is persistent, socially embarrassing, or associated with gross swelling, hospital admission is occasionally required to control medication, diet and environmental factors. Treatment is often palliative and empirical, because many cases of urticaria are either non-allergic or the allergen remains undiscovered. The cause of chronic urticaria is determined in only about 20 per cent of cases.

Aspirin and indomethacin (salicylate benzoate) aggravate chronic urticaria; strict avoidance does not always lead to cure.

Elimination regimes may be useful in individual cases.

Antihistamines are often effective, though they may have to be administered in double or treble the normal therapeutic dosage. In those cases where antihistamines alone are ineffective, they may be used in combination with an H2 blocker, e.g. cimetidine (Tagamet). In some instances cyproheptadine (Periactin)—a histamine, acetylcholine, serotonin antagonist—is more effective than an antihistamine alone, and especially so in cold urticaria. When antihistamines are ineffective, mast cell stabilizers such as cromones or cromone-like drugs may be used; sodium cromoglycate (Nalcrom), doxantrazole and the newer ketotifen (Zaditen) may be worth a trial. Similarly alpha agonists—e.g. ephedrine 15 mg at 8 am and 12 noon—are sometimes helpful. When urticaria is a manifestation of immune complex disease (type III allergy) dapsone and steroids may be required to control the eruption. The elimination of trigger factors, i.e. aspirin, alcohol, etc. should be encouraged; the wearing of light, cool clothing should be advocated and when psychological factors are evident, sedatives and tranquillizers should be prescribed.

Topical therapy based on the applications of a cooling lotion such as menthol 0.25% in lin. calamine is often soothing. The use of topical antihistamines should be avoided because these agents are allergenic when applied to the skin and can produce contact eczema. It should be remembered that some antihistamines contain the azo-dye tartrazine which can cause urticaria in certain individuals. Cholinergic urticaria may respond to propantheline bromide (Pro-Banthine) or hyoscine bromide (Pamine).

Corticosteroids are only rarely justified, but urticaria that is very persistent and does not respond to antihistamines may do so to steroids.

Capillaritis

Capillaritis is often accompanied by purpura uncomplicated by urticaria or infarction in which the upper dermal vessels dilate, elongate and allow red cells to escape in small quantities. In the lower legs diapedesis of red cells is sometimes a consequence of venous hypertension, but more rarely a low-grade upper dermal injury from drugs or a contact dermatitis is responsible. The clinical picture is like a sprinkling of red pepper due to haemosiderosis derived from altered blood. Epidermal reaction ranges from a shiny smooth atrophy to exfoliation and scaling.

Causes of capillaritis

Khaki dermatitis: certain contact dermatoses, e.g. clothing.
Drugs: antibiotics, quinine, carbromal, barbiturates, quinidine, meprobamate.
Stasis eczema: pigmented dermatosis of the lower leg due to venous hypertension.
Symptomatic: part of systemic disease, e.g. SLE, cryoglobulinaemia, hyperglobulinaemia.
Living agents: viral exanthemata, e.g. measles.
Idiopathic: some transient itching purpuras.
Certain eponymic labels have been attached to several clinical entities that are based on capillaritis:
Gougerot-Blum disease: a purpuric lichenoid dermatosis.
Schamberg's disease: a progressive pigmented dermatosis in young men.
Majocci's disease: an annular telangiectatic eruption.

Histopathology

Acute cases show vasodilatation, diapedesis of red cells, perivascular infiltration and occasional intravascular thrombosis. Subacute and more chronic cases show capillary dilatation and proliferation, and chronic inflammatory cells predominantly in the dermal papillae, secondary pigmentation and haemosiderin or melanin is a late feature.

Clinical features

The eruption is widespread and symmetrical, affecting the lower limbs more often than the trunk and upper limbs. When drug sensitization is the cause, onset is sudden, although Carbromal eruption often spreads progressively until the drug is discontinued.

Henoch–Schönlein purpura *(Plate 19.5)*

A disorder commoner in children than adults, that most usually follows streptococcal tonsillitis.

Aetiology

The majority of cases are caused by sensitization initiated by haemolytic streptococcal infection. The primary infection—a sore throat, septic finger or patch of impetigo—is followed in ten to 14 days by the triad of cutaneous eruption, arthralgia and dysenteric symptoms. However, in the adult, many diverse infections, an autoimmune disease, drugs or neoplasm can be the trigger factor.

Histopathology

Leucocytoclastic angiitis, which gives the impression of numerous neutrophils in various stages of disintegration ensheathing the upper dermal vessels. This is accompanied by a variable degree of bleeding. Platelet aggregation and necrosis of the vessel and surrounding tissues.

Clinical features

Urticarial weals, purpura, erythematous discs, sometimes with central bullae and less commonly necrosis, ecchymoses and deep cutaneous swelling are found often following a sore throat. The symmetrical distribution and localization on the extensor surface of the limbs and the buttocks is characteristic. Arthralgia and gastrointestinal pain and haemorrhage may occur. Cropping and the polymorphic nature of the eruption is characteristic. Submucous intestinal haemorrhage may cause intussusception. A patient who has Henoch–Schönlein purpura is a candidate for acute rheumatism or acute nephritis and clinical and laboratory tests should be made to exclude coexistent cardiac or renal disease.

Prognosis

Complete recovery is usual unless severe renal involvement is present. A daily check of the urine is made for albumin and erythrocytes. A watch for hypertension, nitrogen retention and involvement of larger vessels (ischaemic necrosis or even disseminated intravascular coagulation) is important. Acute rheumatism or nephritis coexisting with this type of purpura carries the prognosis of rheumatic disease.

Differential diagnosis

Thrombocytopenic purpura: there is less polymorphism of lesion, usually purpura and ecchymoses only. Splenomegaly is usually present.

Treatment

Most patients require only an initial period of rest with an antibiotic when a bacterial cause is proven. Steroids or immunosuppressive drugs should be given in adequate doses only to diminish severe painful oedema and arthralgia, and are of doubtful value in the prevention of cardiac and renal complications. Treatment is continued for some weeks and tailed off cautiously.

Necrotizing vasculitis *(Plate 19.6)*

A polymorphic syndrome of erythematous discs, purpura and nodules. There are many similarities with both pityriasis lichenoides acuta and Henoch–Schönlein purpura. Instances are recorded in which the precipitating antigen has been drugs (penicillin, iodides), chemicals (weed killer) and bacterial infection.

Histology

The findings are those of a venulitis with leucocytoclasis, neutrophils, nuclear debris, fibrinoid vessel change often combined with ischaemic necrosis of the surrounding vessels and overlying tissue.

Clinical features

Three types of lesions constituting Gourgerot's triad are seen:

(1) Erythematous papules, 1–10 mm diameter resembling urticaria or erythema multiforme.
(2) Purpuric macules and papules, 1–5 mm in diameter.
(3) Dermal nodules, 2–7 mm in diameter.

Occasional additional lesions are bullae and necrotic ulcers. The course of the disease is often chronic, persisting over many years. In acute cases where cropping occurs, arthralgia and mild systemic symptoms may be present.

Diagnosis

Similar skin changes are seen from bacteraemia. Gonococcal and meningococcal infection may be difficult to exclude.

Treatment

Elimination of offending drugs, foci of infection or other causative agents. Corticosteroids may aggravate the condition. Severer forms with granulomatous changes in the upper respiratory tract or lung respond best to cyclophosphamide or azathioprine. Dapsone is sometimes effective.

Systemic hypersensitivity angiitis

A widespread acute severe vasculitis affecting both the viscera and the skin of adults.

Aetiology

Causative drugs include sulphonamides, barbiturates, pyrazolones, and rarely penicillin. The fulminating haemorrhagic and gangrenous lesions occasionally appearing in infectious fevers such as chickenpox are probably based on vasculitis of this type. When a drug aetiology is suspected the possibility of an underlying autoimmune disease should be considered.

Histopathology

There is intense fibrinoid change in the small vessels with an acute perivascular cellular infiltrate. Eosinophils often predominate. Sometimes extravascular granulomas are found (Churg–Strauss syndrome).

Clinical features

The cutaneous signs are often overshadowed by the systemic disorder and cover the whole range of changes seen in acute vasculitis. The commonest lesions are urticaria and erythema multiforme, although bullae, scald-like desquamation and necrosis may occur. A subacute variety with granuloma formation has been recorded. Mucosal and ocular lesions are not infrequent and systemic complications include renal failure, transient pulmonary infiltrations and myocarditis.

Treatment

Corticosteroids are life saving and must be given in large doses (prednisolone 60 mg daily) as soon as possible.

Polyarteritis nodosa

A systemic disorder based on multiple foci of vasculitis affecting medium sized subcutaneous and visceral vessels. The hallmark is segmental necrosis of the muscle or media of the vessel due to ischaemia or invasion of the wall. Most commonly it is part of a severe vasculitis affecting the whole of the arteriolar capillary venular tree. The impaired microcirculation allows immune complexes or other noxious agents to lodge in the vessel walls and the release of vasoactive mediators. Rarely the disease is confined to the skin.

Aetiology

In the majority of cases no cause is found but in a minority vascular lesions develop as part of a drug sensitivity reaction or immune complex disease as in other types of vasculitis. Hepatitis B is the antigen in certain cases.

Histopathology

The vascular changes are characteristic and diagnostic. Medium-sized muscular vessels show focal fibrinoid necrosis of the media. Vessel wall infiltration with leucocytes and eosinophils is followed by granuloma formation and fibrosis. Thrombosis and small aneurysms are common and ecchymoses or skin infarcts are encountered.

Clinical features

Thrombosis and rupture of arteries result in infarction and severe ecchymoses. Urticaria, purpura, erythema multiforme and erythema nodosum-like nodules are the associated lesions of other patterns of vasculitis.

Visceral involvement may be widespread and the patient febrile. Leucocytosis is usual. Systemic vasculitis may lead to a clinical presentation with bronchial asthma, pneumonitis or cardiac infarct and involvement of the nervous system with cerebral vascular attacks or peripheral neuritis.

Hypertension and renal failure are common associations and consequences. Other presentations include polyarthralgia, mesenteric thrombosis and myopathy. The onset may be insidious, with malaise, pyrexia and paraesthesia.

Diagnosis

Polyarteritis nodosa is a label often applied to patients who cannot otherwise be clearly categorized. The combination of cutaneous signs with multisystem involvement is essential for the diagnosis, e.g. multiple aneurysms in renal arteriogram or histological evidence in a muscle biopsy. Malignant hypertension, systemic autoimmune disease or vasculitis described above, as well as coagulation or platelet diseases, should first be excluded.

Treatment

When purely cutaneous, systemic steroids are rarely justified; dapsone may be helpful. In early systemic disease corticosteroids are beneficial and limit the inflammatory process, though when vasculitis and necrosis are advanced, healing occurs with fibrosis and this may cause ischaemic damage. Prednisolone 60 mg daily is required for effective control and when the acute stage is controlled low dosage cyclophosphamide should be introduced and the steroid dose reduced.

Temporal arteritis

This disorder is often part of a widespread disease—polymyalgia rheumatica. Localized arteritis of the temporal artery (giant-cell arteritis) causes ischaemic ulceration of the scalp. Other serious results include blindness and ulceration of the tongue. Corticosteroids are an effective treatment.

Disseminated intravascular coagulation

Occasionally, as a result of the same kind of microvascular injury as causes vasculitis, widespread coagulation results. The capillaries and venules are filled with fibrin and the skin has a slaty-blue discoloration and fails to blanche when gently pressed. Such patients are usually very ill and infection or neoplasia is the commonest cause of this condition. Essential findings are reduced platelets, urinary blood fibrin degradation products and prolonged prothrombin time. Heparin is the appropriate therapy.

Erythema multiforme (*Plate 19.7*)

The clinical varieties of this distinctive erythema with epidermal necrosis fall conveniently into two groups: (1) the minor form that is associated with little or no systemic upset; and (2) the major form (Stevens–Johnson syndrome), often with pulmonary, renal or intestinal complications and severe constitutional upset.

Minor type

Aetiology

It may result from vascular sensitization to a virus—e.g. vaccinia, orf, herpes simplex—bacteria or fungi. Drugs such as sulphonamides and barbiturates and rarely actinic sensitivity provoke an eruption of this type. In many instances no cause can be found although visceral malignancy in rare instances provides the antigenic stimulus.

Histopathology

The dermal vasculitis shows variable perivascular cellular infiltration and the epidermis is often disrupted over the centre of the lesion.

Clinical features

Erythematous discs often with characteristic central target-like lesions appear ten to 14 days after herpes simplex or primary vaccination. Frequently there is no preceding clinical infection. The more common sites involved are the dorsa of the hands and feet. The extensor aspects of the knees and elbows and the buccal mucosa and lips. When the eruption is a manifestation of drug sensitivity it may appear within a day or two of taking the offending drug, although sometimes the onset may be delayed for a week or two.

Prognosis

Recurrences although frequent and disabling are harmless. However, erythema multiforme appearing for the first time in a patient over 40 in the absence of drug or viral aetiology calls for a careful search for internal malignancy.

Treatment

Antihistamines often provide effective control of irritation and sometimes shorten an attack. Patients who develop erythema multiforme regularly ten to 14 days after herpes simplex should attempt to anticipate and abort the eruption with herpid, antihistamines and sometimes with steroids.

Major type (Stevens–Johnson syndrome) (*Plate 13.5*)

Aetiology

The causative organisms and drugs resemble those which provoke the minor type of eruption; in addition particular factors are long-acting sulphonamides, barbiturates and pyrazolones such as butazolidine. The reaction may occur anything from the second to the 24th day after starting therapy but the mean time is about the tenth day. The condition is sometimes caused by mycoplasma infection.

Histopathology

Fibrinoid vasculitis with extravasation of erythrocytes is seen in the dermis. Overlying epidermal spongiosis and necrosis with subepidermal bulla formation are frequently found. Sometimes intraepidermal bullae are present.

Clinical features

The onset is sudden. Initially the eruption, which is widespread, is morbilliform; soon discoid lesions, vesicles and bullae appear and there may be purpura. Occasionally large sheets of epidermis separate leaving an area resembling a scald. When this phenomenon is extensive it constitutes one form of Lyell's syndrome (toxic epidermal necrolysis). Severe constitutional symptoms and high fever are noted early together with conjunctivitis, erosive stomatitis and crusting of the lips. Genital involvement is common and damage to the genitourinary system may produce urethritis, vaginitis, albuminuria, haematuria, urinary retention and anuria. Pulmonary involvement with patchy pneumonitis is common. There is sometimes pharyngeal and intestinal involvement without skin lesions. Glomerulonephritis is recognized as part of the widespread vascular damage.

Prognosis

Before the advent of corticosteroids and antibiotics the mortality rate was high; even now the mortality is over 25 per cent. Death results from pneumonitis, widespread vasculitis, especially renal, or toxaemia following secondary infection. Recurrences of this type of erythema multiforme are not infrequent.

Differential diagnosis

Other oculo-mucocutaneous syndromes: Reiter's syndrome; urethritis; conjunctivitis; arthritis, balanitis, and vesiculo-keratotic lesions of the palms and soles (keratoderma blenorrhagica). Behcet's disease: aphthous, stomal and genital ulcers; severe ocular disease; erythema nodosum. Stevens–Johnson syndrome is sometimes mistaken for measles or other viral disease and patients are admitted to infectious fever hospitals.

Treatment

Severe cases pose a combined therapeutic and nursing problem. It is important that adequate doses of corticosteroids be administered as soon as possible. If the patient finds difficulty in swallowing, steroids or ACTH should be given as an intravenous drip. Antibiotic cover is required to prevent secondary infection and the dose of oral steroids slowly tailed off over two or three weeks. An average dosage schedule commences with 40 mg of prednisolone daily for the first week, decreasing stepwise over three weeks. The advice of an ophthalmologist may be required for the management of severe eye involvement.

Erythema nodosum (EN) *(Plate 19.8)*

A transient nodular eruption, often appearing in crops, affecting predominantly the front of the shins. Fever and polyarthralgia are commonly present. The nodules are tender, often exquisitely so, and with resolution show a sequence of colour seen in a bruise. EN is most frequently seen in children and young adults, particularly females.

Aetiology

The EN develops during the process of active sensitization and is initiated by diverse antigenic stimuli. It represents an Arthus-type reaction with accompanying immune complexes. The vascular damage involves venules in the lower dermis and the adjoining subcutis and has a probable immunological basis.

Table 19.3   Causes of erythema nodosum

Virus	Bacteria	Fungi	Drugs	Systemic diseases	Occasional causes
Lympho-granuloma venereum Ornithosis Cat-scratch fever	*Streptococcal infection *Tuberculosis Leprosy Syphilis	Systemic mycoses	Sulpha-thiazole Barbitur-ates Halogens Sulphones The 'pill'	*Sarcoidosis Ulcerative colitis Hodgkin's disease Bacteraemia Crohn's disease	Reactions to vaccines Behcet's syndrome Yersiniosis

* The three commonest causes in Great Britain.

In cases of primary tuberculosis erythema nodosum appears at about the time of Mantoux conversion, whereas with streptococcal infection it commonly appears seven to ten days after the height of the attack. Other bacterial causes of erythema nodosum include leprosy, syphilis and yersinia infection.

Viral infections are an uncommon cause; they include lympho-granuloma venereum, cat-scratch fever and ornithosis.

Fungal infections are another rare cause of this disorder. EN occurs with systemic mycoses and sometimes as a distant reaction from a patch of animal ringworm.

Certain drugs, notably sulphathiazole, barbiturates, iodides and sulphones are occasional causes. In a patient from an endemic area drug-provoked leprous erythema nodosum should be considered.

More commonly, systemic disease provokes erythema nodosum; it is seen with sarcoidosis, Hodgkin's disease and meningococcaemia. It is a rare reaction of vaccination.

The commonest causes in Great Britain are streptococcal sensitization, drug eruptions, sarcoidosis and tuberculosis. Often no definite cause is found—idiopathic erythema nodosum.

Histopathology

Marked perivascular infiltrates with neutrophils, lymphocytes and histiocytes surround the deeper dermal blood vessels; occasionally small granulomata are seen. Vascular changes are curiously inconspicuous. The subcutis shows septal panniculitis and often a perivenous septal infiltrate with neutrophils.

Clinical features

Tender erythematous nodules and plaques appear suddenly on the front of the shins; occasionally lesions are found on the front of the thighs and upper limbs. Nodules range from 1 to 10 cm in diameter, are pink or dusky red and exquisitely tender. With resolution a characteristic sequence of colours ranging through purple, green and yellow is seen. Cropping of new lesions may occur every few weeks. Individual nodules last one to five weeks. Polyarthralgia and nodular episcleritis may accompany erythema nodosum.

Diagnosis

The colour, extreme tenderness, appearance and location of the nodules are characteristic, and the presence of malaise and polyar-thralgia gives added confirmation of the diagnosis. A history of a recent sore throat and a rise in antistreptolysin titre is supportive evidence of streptococcal sensitization. Evidence in favour of a tuberculous basis includes recent Mantoux conversion, unilateral hilar lymphadenopathy and a history of contact with a tuberculous subject.

Sarcoidosis is likely with bilateral lymphadenopathy and increased gamma globulin. A coexisting iritis or facial palsy adds further weight to the diagnosis and a positive Kveim test is confirmatory.

A drug eruption should be suspected with a history of previous drug sensitivity.

Differential diagnosis

Bruises, bites and chilblains may cause diagnostic difficulties. Phlebitis may closely mimic erythema nodosum, but oedema is usually marked and the lesions are unilateral.

Bacteraemia causes multiple bacterial emboli in the skin; strepto-cocci, meningococci and gonococci may be responsible. Blood culture is usually positive. Intermittent fever and visceral manifestations are usual.

Nodules from more chronic vasculitis include nodular vasculitis with persistent nodules on the calf rather than the shin.

Bazin's disease presents with dusky nodules that are often ulcerative and associated with an occult or an overt tuberculous focus.

Polyarteritis nodosa may occur with mild systemic involvement and a triad of skin lesions: livedo racemosa, nodules and ulceration.

Certain nodular erythemas appear in the absence of a normal immunological response. These nodules appear with lepromatous leprosy which shows little inflammatory infiltration but many micro-organisms.

Sarcoid granulomas appear in leprosy, syphilis and certain deep fungal infections. Sarcoidosis shows persistent dusky nodules on the upper limbs, trunk, thighs and shins; apple jelly nodules may also be seen on diascopy. There is hypergammaglobulinaemia and the Kveim test is usually positive.

Panniculitis: An inflammation of subcutaneous fat, in which the nodules are deep and the skin surface often slightly depressed. The thighs as well as the shins are often affected. It is rarely due to pancreatic disease.

Erythema nodosum-like lesions with ulceration should lead to reassessment of the diagnosis and pyoderma gangrenosum, Bazin's disease or polyarteritis nodosa should be considered.

Treatment

This depends on the cause and every effort should be made to reach an aetiological diagnosis. With bacterial infection the appropriate antibiotic is administered. Antihistamines are of little value and steroids only rarely justified.

Pityriasis lichenoides et varioliformis acuta (Mucha–Habermann disease) (*Plate 22.1*)

An acute exanthem-like dermatosis with papulo-vesicles resembling chickenpox, haemorrhagic crusts and pitted scars. Rarer more infarctive forms both clinically and histologically resemble necrotizing vasculitis (*see above*).

Histopathology

The essential changes are capillaritis with overlying epidermal necrosis; some lesions may show lymphoma-like features (lymphomatoid papulosis).

Clinical features

Acute attacks begin with widespread eruption affecting the trunk and limbs. Vesicles, pustules and papulo-necrotic lesions with haemorrhagic crusts are characteristic. Erythemato-squamous papules are seen; they range up to 1 cm in diameter and show central clearing closely resembling the discoid lesions of pityriasis rosea. Close enquiry sometimes reveals that repeated attacks follow mild upper respiratory infection after an interval of seven to ten days. A minority of patients as well as characteristic lesions show purpura and aphthous ulcers in the mouth. A single attack usually lasts six to eight weeks and some patients have repeated attacks over a period of years.

Treatment

This is essentially symptomatic. However, dapsone or tetracycline is worth a trial.

Pityriasis lichenoides chronica

See Chapter 22.

Erythema elevatum diutinum (*Plate 19.9*)

An acute vasculitis which becomes chronic with healing by fibrosis.

Persistent dusky erythematous plaques are found on the knuckles, knees and elbows.

Granuloma annulare (GA) *(Plate 19.10)*

A fairly common and characteristic annular eruption with single or multiple patches usually seen on the extensor aspect of the limbs particularly the hands. It affects children more often than adults.

Aetiology

Many instances are unrelated to any preceding or associated disease. However, disseminated and symmetrical lesions sometimes follow an attack of tonsillitis or measles. Widespread atypical cases are at times found in association with diabetes and occasionally patches are apparently provoked by ultraviolet exposure or insect bites.

The pathomechanism is unknown although probably the dermal connective tissue is damaged as a result of an immune reaction.

Histopathology

The hallmark of granuloma annulare is a palisaded granuloma with central mucin and surrounding histiocytes seen in the mid-dermis. The changes are sometimes diffuse without well defined foci.

Clinical features

The earliest lesion is a papule, pale pink or skin coloured, that slowly enlarges without central clearing. The resultant ring is slightly elevated and the border sharply demarcated, with other lesions appearing as the ring slowly enlarges. Many patches cease to spread once a diameter of 2–3 cm is reached. Rare variants include lesions with central atrophy and necrosis and others with small papular lesions with no tendency to ring formation. Widespread papules and plaques are sometimes seen with diabetes mellitus.

Investigations

The ASO titre is often raised and with diabetes the glucose tolerance test is diagnostic.

Differential diagnosis

Although the annular pattern of GA may suggest ringworm, close inspection shows dermal not epidermal lesions without the vesicles or scales seen in tinea circinata.

Necrobiosis lipoidica, with or without diabetes, may closely simulate GA particularly when the eruption is present on typical GA sites. However, lipoid necrobiosis usually has a yellow tinge and marked central atrophy. Particular diagnostic difficulties arise when the two conditions coexist.

Erythema elevatum diutinum—another dermal connective tissue disorder with vasculitis—shows plaques rather than rings but again the similarity to GA is sometimes striking.

Tuberculoid leprosy produces similar lesions to GA although hypopigmentation and anaesthesia provide valuable diagnostic clues.

Treatment

Because spontaneous resolution may occur at any time it is difficult to assess the effects of treatment. However, any trauma such as taking a biopsy often initiates involution. The same effect is produced by freezing with ethyl chloride or 'Freon', applying carbon dioxide snow or liquid nitrogen. Intralesional injections of triamcinolone hexacetonide are sometimes useful.

Systemic autoimmune disease

Systemic lupus erythematosus (SLE) (*Plate 19.11*)

A complex systemic disorder characterized by multisystem involvement resulting from vascular damage and fibrinoid connective tissue changes.

Aetiology

The basis of the disorder is autoimmune whereby groups of antibody-producing cells change and produce circulating antibodies against the patient's own double stranded DNA; these antibodies become fixed and damage both vascular and connective tissue. Often a history of drug reaction precedes the onset of the illness, sulphonamides, butazolidin and penicillin being most frequently involved. Other drugs such as hydrallazine and procainamide alter DNA and produce a syndrome closely resembling SLE and the symptoms usually resolve when the offending drug is stopped.

Genetic factors are sometimes relevant since familial cases are recorded. Females are predominantly affected. Some idiopathic cases are perhaps provoked by ultraviolet exposure. DNA becomes antigenic in SLE-like disease due to congenital complement deficiency.

Histopathology

In the skin and viscera three coexisting changes are found: fibrinoid vasculitis affecting capillaries and arterioles; fibrinoid collagen change in the perivascular and extravascular tissue, and dermal infiltration with lymphocytes and occasional neutrophils.

The epidermis overlying these combined changes shows liquefaction of the basal layer, pigmentary incontinence and epidermal atrophy.

Clinical features

The onset is often insidious with general malaise, pyrexia, anaemia and arthralgia. Other presentations simulate acute rheumatism, thrombocytopenic purpura, hepatitis and pneumonia. Rarely a non-itching urticaria is the initial first finding. Splenomegaly and generalized lymph node enlargement are usual.

In mild cases the cutaneous changes are non-specific, perhaps with only a persistent blush over the cheeks and 'V' of the neck. The paronychial folds often show telangiectasia. The more definitive cutaneous lesions, many of which are based on vasculitis, include purpura, erythema multiforme, dermal and hypodermal nodules and haemorrhagic infarcts. Rarely Raynaud's attacks, digital gangrene, bullae and ulceration are seen.

The visceral manifestations may relate to any of the body systems and include pneumonia, pleurisy and pleural effusion, pericarditis, endocarditis, myocarditis, epilepsy, psychosis, neuropathy, cerebral vascular disease, nephritis, nephrosis, anaemia, leucopenia and thrombocytopenia.

Diagnosis

In mild cases examination reveals moderate fever, mild anaemia, leucopenia and a raised ESR. Albumin and erythrocytes are frequently found in the urine. The antinuclear factor test is usually strongly positive and LE cells may be demonstrated. Antibodies to double stranded DNA are demonstrable. Complement is low in active disease. Immunofluorescent studies show deposition of IgG on the basement membrane both on affected and unaffected covered skin.

Treatment

Corticosteroids have proved life-saving in many cases; when given early they probably prevent irreversible organ damage. They reduce the discomfort of the acute inflammatory phase of the disease such as fever and arthritis. In mild cases antimalarials may be effective in controlling the symptoms. Immunosuppressive drugs, notably azathioprine, are valuable when corticosteroids are contraindicated and are required with progressive renal deterioration. They are useful in combination with steroids since in the long term they allow a much smaller dose to be given.

Exposure to sunlight should be avoided; in severe cases it may be necessary to nurse the patient in a darkened room. Unnecessary medication should be avoided, especially reactive drugs such as pyrazolones or sulphonamides in view of their liability to exacerbate the disease.

Chronic discoid lupus erythematosus (DLE) *(Plate 19.12)*

A patchy and persistent erythemato-squamous eruption with characteristic follicular plugging, telangiectasia and atrophy.

291

Aetiology

Although the cause is uncertain autoimmune mechanisms and genetic factors are relevant. DLE is commoner in women than men and occurs usually between the age of 25 and 40. Sometimes the eruption follows trauma or exposure to bright sunlight. It is the same disease as SLE but may be regarded as the benign end of the spectrum—a shift towards SLE is unusual and is seen in 1–5 per cent of cases.

Histopathology

The epidermis shows diffuse hyperkeratosis which extends into dilated hair follicles. There is epidermal atrophy in some areas and acanthosis in others, whilst the basal layers shows liquefaction degeneration. The dermis shows areas of focal collagen degeneration and dense collections of lymphocytes around blood vessels and appendages.

Clinical features

The face and scalp (*Plate 19.13*) are the sites of predilection. The nose, cheeks and malar areas are commonly affected and the classic 'butterfly' distribution is rarely seen. Sometimes the fingers show discoid lesions and nail fold telangiectases, and these are often associated with poor peripheral circulation (chilblain type LE). Individual lesions range from a few millimetres to 2 cm in diameter. They are red and scaly, often with follicular plugging. Removal of a thickened adherent scale reveals characteristic 'carpet tacking'; small spiny projections previously impacted in dilated hair follicles. With lower power-lens atrophy and telangiectasis are clearly visible.

The discoid lesions of LE spread peripherally with satellite lesions which fuse to produce a large irregular area of redness, scaling and atrophy.

Discoid patches on the scalp produce an irreversible scarred alopecia.

Investigations

IgG can be demonstrated in the epidermal basement membrane in the lesional skin only. Antinuclear antibodies are sometimes present.

Prognosis

Spontaneous resolution is unusual. Exacerbations sometimes appear after exposure to intense sunlight.

Treatment

Avoidance of excessive ultraviolet exposure is important. Modern treatment has greatly improved the prognosis in what was formerly a chronic disfiguring disease. However, even with current therapy, relapses are frequent. Accurate application of a potent steroid such as clobetasol propionate (Dermovate) to the lesions is helpful. Good results are sometimes achieved with triamcinolone hexacetonide intralesional injections. Systemically administered antimalarials often produce rapid resolution, but they may cause corneal opacities and retinopathy. The antimalarials given are mepacrine (quinacrine) 100 mg daily, or chloroquine (Avloclor), hydroxychloroquine (Plaquenil) and amodiaquine (Camoquin) 200 mg twice daily. These drugs are first given for four to six weeks when the patient is reassessed, with particular attention to any visual symptoms. Because of the danger of corneal or retinal damage with antimalarial therapy a monthly slit-lamp examination and visual field check is advisable.

Opaque covering creams (Covermark, Ardena, etc.) are useful as sun-screening and masking agents. Male patients prefer benzophenone (Uvistat) which is a sun-screen without any masking effects.

Dermatomyositis

A rare combined disorder of skin and muscle with a distinctive eruption and progressive weakness of the limb girdle muscles.

Aetiology

It is regarded as having an autoimmune basis. In some instances there are overlapping features with SLE and scleroderma. The disease occurs at any age although about 25 per cent of cases appear first in childhood. In adults 30–40 per cent of cases are seen with associated visceral malignancy.

Clinical features

Skin lesions may precede, accompany or follow the myositis. Insidious muscular weakness is often the first symptom although an eruption is frequently present when the patient first seeks advice. The early skin changes include telangiectasia with a cyanotic erythema of the upper eyelids and knuckle regions. With more acute onset the eruption may mimic an acute contact dermatitis or a photosensitivity eruption; indeed light exposure may provoke dermatomyositis. Heliotrope coloration of the eyelids is characteristic; erythema of the forehead, butterfly area of the face and light exposed triangle of the neck is commonly seen and telangiectasia and scaling are sometimes found over the deltoid region. The changes in the hands and fingers are diagnostic: scaly telangiectatic erythema over the knuckles and extensor tendons (purple parchment patches or Gottron spots) (*Plate 19.14*) combined with nail fold telangiectasis. In more chronic cases the skin changes may be poikilodermatous or sclerodermatous and widespread muscular and cutaneous calcification is sometimes encountered.

Investigations

Muscle biopsy, muscle enzyme studies are useful and reflect the activity of the myopathy. Serum aldolase is a more sensitive indicator of muscle damage than the creatine phosphokinase; electromyographic studies may be diagnostic. The urinary excretion of creatine is increased. The antinuclear, LE cell and Latex tests may be positive.

Treatment

In an adult a careful search for a malignant tumour is mandatory. Corticosteroids are effective in controlling the symptoms and prednisolone 60 mg daily is usually an effective initial dose. As soon as a response occurs as judged by serum enzyme levels the dose should be reduced gradually.

Scleroderma

The term scleroderma literally means 'hard skin'. Among the diseases encountered with scleroderma are localized plaques, guttate or linear lesions confined to the skin and a widespread process involving much of the skin with associated visceral involvement. Widespread scleroderma causes severe disturbance of cutaneous and visceral function.

From clinical, histological and immunological data some forms of the disease appear to have an autoimmune basis. It is a late feature of graft versus host disease following marrow transplant.

Classification of the sclerodermas

Cutaneous

Localized: morphoea, lichen sclerosus of genitalia.
Linear: 'coup de sabre', limb type with soft tissue and bone atrophy.
Widespread: generalized morphoea, subcutaneous morphoea (eosinophilic fasciitis), lichen sclerosus et atrophicus.

Systemic

Acute diffuse scleroderma with overlapping features of dermatomyositis, SLE.
Sjögren's syndrome.
Calcinosis, sclerodactyly, Raynaud's disease and telangiectasis (CSRT syndrome).
Progressive systemic sclerosis.

Sclerodermoid syndromes

Sclerodema.	Werner's syndrome.
Paraproteinaemias.	Phaeochromocytoma.
Porphyria variegata.	Carcinoid.
Phenylketonuria.	Vinyl chloride disease.
Mucopolysaccharidosis.	Graft versus host disease.

Morphoea (*Plate 19.15*)

A localized scleroderma which shows round or oval irregular plaques. These are smooth, indurated, yellow-white in colour with a lilac halo. Later the patches become atrophic and ivory-white and after some time involute completely. The subcutis and underlying muscle may be affected.

A more diffuse type with widespread cutaneous involvement is sometimes encountered and rarely linear forms are recognized. A subcutaneous variant with eosinophilia sometimes appears after vigorous exercise (eosinophilic fasciitis).

Systemic scleroderma (*Plates 19.16* and *19.17*)

Telangiectasia of the face and hands is a usual feature. Calcification in the subcutaneous tissues sometimes occurs.

Acrosclerosis is the commonest form of systemic scleroderma and is usually seen in women. It is rarely progressive. Raynaud's phenomenon and sclerosis of the fingers and face are characteristic. Skin involvement of the trunk and limbs is only rarely seen. Visceral involvement is uncommon although failure of oesophageal peristalsis is a major diagnostic sign of the disease. Paralysis of the gastro-oesophageal sphincter with gastric influx, oesophagitis and stricture are found as late complications.

Acute diffuse scleroderma commonly begins on the face and trunk and is seen in both sexes. Raynaud's phenomenon is often absent but may be severe; the onset and course of the disease are rapid and progressive with simultaneous involvement of the skin and internal organs. The lungs, heart, kidneys and liver as well as the gastrointestinal tract are affected. Progressive organ fibrosis and organ failure, especially of the kidneys, are the cause of death. The ESR is raised and rheumatoid and antinuclear antibodies are usually found.

Treatment

Although no specific therapy for scleroderma exists certain drugs can provide relief symptoms. Vasoactive drugs are used to control Raynaud's phenomenon. These include phenoxybenzamine, tolazolidine, and nicotinic acid. Anti-inflammatory agents include salicylates, potassium aminobenzoate, antimalarials and corticosteroids. Physiotherapy may help to keep the patient mobile and to prevent contractures.

Lichen sclerosus et atrophicus (*Plate 19.18*)

This most commonly affects the vulva and perianal skin, occasionally the glans penis and foreskin. Many authorities regard this condition as a variant of localized scleroderma affecting the superficial dermis.

Lichen sclerosus is characterized by regular or polygonal flat-topped white papules which usually coalesce to form plaques; in the later stage of the disease keratotic plugging and delling may be noticed. The upper trunk, neck, vulval and anal areas are the usual sites of predilection; itching at the latter site can be severe. Local steroid ointments are helpful especially in the male.

Mixed connective tissue syndromes

Some patients have a wide range of symptoms and signs that defy a more precise diagnosis than connective tissue disease. In most of the patients the overlap is marked in the initial stages; later a more definite pattern towards rheumatoid arthritis, systemic lupus erythematosus, dermatomyositis, scleroderma or polyarteritis nodosa gradually emerges.

Mixed connective tissue disease (Sharp's syndrome) applies to a smaller group of patients who retain features of more than one connective tissue disease; myositis and Raynaud's syndrome occur in about 75 per cent. Skin changes are not a prominent feature, but there may be diffuse hair loss or telangiectasia. The low incidence of renal disease is accompanied by a benign course and a good response to small doses of corticosteroids. The presence of antibodies to extractable nuclear antigen (ENA) is characteristic; ANF is speckled and there is a normal complement level.

A similar clinical disorder is provoked by exposure to vinyl chloride.

20 Psychological factors in skin disease

Patrick Hall-Smith

It is generally agreed that about 30 per cent of all patients seen for any cause have disorders initiated by psychic and emotional factors and that another 30 per cent suffer from organic disease with a large functional overlay.

The question as to why one patient should react to emotional stress by a set pattern of cutaneous changes while another patient subject to identical stress produces a different pattern, or no skin change at all, may be partially explained by the theory of constitutional predisposition or organ inferiority, which in man is genetically determined.

There is still some divergence of opinion among dermatologists as to which conditions may be rightly classed as psychodermatoses; the following conditions (modified from Lewis and Cormia) would be accepted by most authorities:

Dermatoses always psychological in origin:

(1) dermatitis artefacta:
(2) neurotic excoriations;
(3) trichotillomania;
(4) parasitophobia.

Dermatoses combining psychogenic and other aetiological factors:

(1) lichen simplex chronicus;
(2) pruritus;
(3) urticaria;
(4) hyperhidrosis;
(5) pompholyx of hands and feet;
(6) discoid eczema;
(7) acne excoriée;
(8) acne necrotica.

Dermatoses which may be aggravated by psychogenic factors:

(1) atopic dermatitis;
(2) alopecia areata;
(3) rosacea;
(4) contact and sensitization dermatoses;
(5) seborrhoeic dermatitis, otitis externa and pyococcal dermatoses;
(6) psoriasis;
(7) anogenital pruritus;
(8) lichen planus;
(9) herpes simplex.

Dermatitis artefacta (*Plates 20.1* and *20.2*)

The patient consciously produces the artefacts but denies responsibility for them. This denial distinguishes the disorder from neurotic excoriations. The bizarre or geometrically shaped lesions produced by an instrument are seen on parts of the body easily reached by the hand, depending on whether the patient is right or left handed. The distinct pattern of the lesions distinguishes the condition from other dermatoses. A liquid, either acid or caustic, may produce a linear streak as a drop runs downward on the skin surface.

In a follow-up of a large series of such cases, nearly a third were still disabled psychologically and unfit for work 12 years after the onset.

Neurotic excoriations (*Plate 20.3*)

This is the result of compulsive picking and scratching by the patient. The lesions are produced by the fingernails and usually occur on the arms and legs, face or upper back. The excoriations are usually covered with a haemorrhagic scabbed crust surrounded by an erythematous border; later a scar with hyperpigmentation may remain.

Trichotillomania (*Figure 14.3,* p. 159)

Patients are often children who have an uncontrollable desire to pull out their hair. Irregular-shaped bald patches may be found on the scalp with associated broken-off and twisted hairs.

Parasitophobia (delusions of parasitosis)

The subjects are often elderly patients who complain of itching or a crawling sensation (formication) beneath the skin and insist that they are infested with some parasite. They scratch and gouge at their skin and try to substantiate their claim that they are infested by producing matchboxes containing epithelial debris which they regard as the causative parasite. Their delusion is such that no amount of explanation will shake it.

Lichen simplex chronicus (neurodermite) *(Plate 20.4)*

The condition is characterized by circumscribed lichenified plaques on the nape of the neck, the inner surface of the thighs, extensor surface of the forearms or just below the elbows and knees, though almost any part of the body surface may manifest such a patch. Involvement of the nape of the neck (often termed suboccipital dermatitis) nearly always occurs in women; it is rarely seen in men. Another form, again seen in women, is confined to the upper eyelids, which may be thickened and reddened as a result of rubbing.

Treatment

Steroid ointments or creams are the most effective local treatments. As a short-term measure one of the more potent local steroids such as Betnovate, Propaderm, or Dermovate are indicated. Tar pastes under a firm dressing, or complete occlusion of the site if it should be on arm or leg, with a medicated bandage such as Tarband or Viscopaste is indicated. Intradermal injection of triamcinolone is also effective on circumscribed patches. Superficial x-ray therapy may also have a place in selected cases.

Pruritus

Psychogenic pruritus can be divided into generalized or localized forms, including pruritus ani, pruritus vulvae and pruritus of the scalp.

It is emphasized that before commencing treatment for any apparent functional pruritus, whether generalized or local, it is essential to exclude all possible organic causes. Nothing is more damaging to the reputation of any physician than to miss glycosuria, a faint icterus, vulval moniliasis or threadworms.

The treatment of a functional case is not a simple matter of one short interview with a sympathetic psychiatrist; insight alone is not tantamount to cure. Skin conditions such as psoriasis, atopic eczema or urticaria must be managed in general as physical illnesses. Of the three conditions urticaria is most commonly regarded as psychosomatic in origin; in fact it is almost totally unresponsive to psychiatric treatment, despite the claims which have been made. The role of psychological factors in these conditions has been much overemphasized, partly as a result of their unknown aetiology, and partly because the patient often describes them as 'nervous' rashes. What psychiatric symptoms do occur are almost always secondary, either to the irritation, the disfigurement, or the patient–doctor relationship. The use of a mild tranquillizer, and particularly a hypnotic, so that scratching during sleep is minimized; discussion and explanation are helpful in management. Whitlock, in a review of papers dealing with the use of psychotropic drugs in dermatology, states that it is improbable that psychotropic drugs as such will have much direct influence on skin symptoms unless they have pharmacological actions separate from their anxiolytic or antidepressant properties.

The manner in which the doctor handles the patient with a skin eruption is important in determining patient–doctor attitudes. The hostility which psychiatrists so often see as a determining factor underlying psychosomatic skin eruptions is almost certainly secondary to the patient's encounters with the medical milieu. The doctor should be familiar with what nakedness, skin blemishes, and the different areas of the body which are affected might mean to the individual. Physical contact—the handling of the eruption by the doctor—is a method of rapidly establishing rapport by showing the patient that the doctor is not revulsed by, or afraid of, the disease. Most experienced and sympathetic dermatologists recognize that disfiguring skin diseases such as nodulocystic acne and widespread florid psoriasis cause loss of confidence in the patient and handicap social intercourse. Psychologically unstable subjects with such an additional burden may express their frustration and lack of response to treatment in antisocial behaviour. Effective dermatological treatment, in some cases, resolves these behavioural problems.

21 Inherited cutaneous disorders

F. M. Pope

Inherited ichthyoses

These are a very heterogeneous group and autosomal dominant (*Figure 21.1*), recessive and sex-linked recessive forms were first clearly separated by R. S. Wells. Anatomical differences are slight and variations of epidermal thickness and the presence or absence of a granular layer distinguish the small scaled autosomal dominant from the large browny scaled sex-linked recessive type. Dramatic epidermal ballooning and hydropic degeneration is characteristic of the rare autosomal dominant bullous erythrodermic pattern. Severe autosomal recessive patterns include the lethal harlequin fetus (*Figure 21.2*) and the collodion baby which produces severe adult disease. Rare combinations with mental deficiency, retinitis pigmentosa, hypogonadism, peripheral neuropathy are included in Refsum syndrome and Sjogren–Larsen syndrome. The latter has been associated with a phytanic acid alpha hydroxylase abnormality and the latter less impressively with variable aminoaciduria. Recently patients with sex-linked recessive ichthyosis have been shown to be steroid sulphatase deficient. Amongst other things, this causes inefficient conversion of dihydroepiandrosterol to oestriol with resulting poor cervical ripening and prolonged or delayed labour. There is thus a strong family history of post-mature boy babies. The ichthyosis is unlikely to be the direct result of steroid imbalance and may mean that sulphatase deficiency directly affects the production of other proteins such as keratin, membrane constituents or phospholipid. Inherited abnormalities of these various proteins and lipids are likely and should eventually allow more detailed classification of these varied disorders (*Table 21.1*).

Treatment

This is generally unsatisfactory and symptomatic; 10% urea in a water-miscible base (Calmurid or Aquadrate), salicylic acid in ung. emulsificans and various bath oils and emulsifying ointments are the mainstay of treatment. Generally retinoic acid is not indicated, but

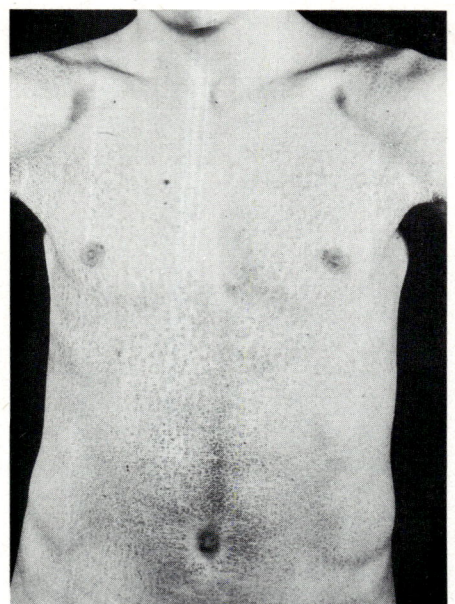

Figure 21.1 *Typical large flaky scaling of inherited sex-linked ichthyosis*

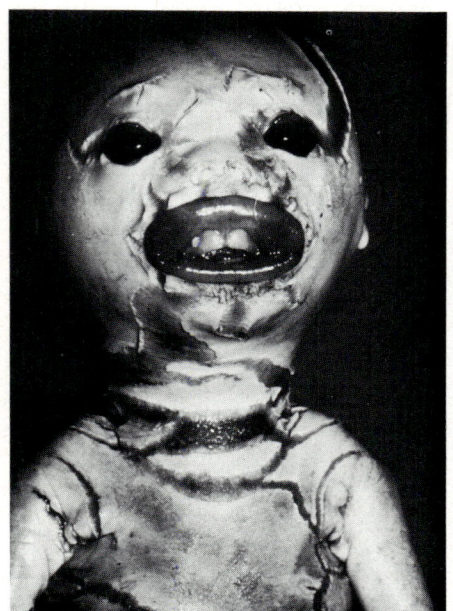

Figure 21.2 *Fetus with the lethal type autosomal recessive ichthyosis. Note widespread fissuring of flexures*

Table 21.1   Classification of the various inherited ichthyoses

	Dominant	Sex-linked	Erythrodermic Recessive Non-bullous	Erythrodermic Recessive lamellar	Dominant bullous
Frequency	1/300	1/500	?	?	3/1 000 000
Site	Face, flexures free	Scalp, face, neck, flexures affected	General-ized	General-ized	General-ized
Onset	Before 3 months	After 3 months	at birth		at birth
Scales	Small fine	Large dark			
Histology	Diminished granular layer	Prominent granular layer	Epidermal thickening		Hydropic degenera-tion Desmoso-mal defect

systemic steroids can be life saving in the severe congenital erythodermas. Better treatment will undoubtedly follow improved molecular understanding of these various diseases. The use of systemic retinoids in this group of disorders has produced good results but requires further evaluation.

Pachyonychia congenita

This is an autosomal dominant abnormality of hard keratin in which there is marked hyperconvexity and thickening of hand and toe nails. Sometimes there is hyperkeratosis of the palms and soles and, less frequently, pitting of these areas.

Hair abnormalities

Hair keratin is a hard, sulphur-rich protein. Numerous biochemical abnormalities are known in sheep and probably several await identification in man. A useful clinical division separates those with and without hair fragility.

With hair fragility

These include monilethrix, trichorrhexis invaginata (bamboo hair), trichorrhexis nodosa and Menkes syndrome.

(1) Monilethrix—this is a simple autosomal dominant trait in which the hair is lobulated. Brittle nails, keratosis pilaris, juvenile cataracts and dental abnormalities also occur.
(2) Bamboo hair (trichorrhexis invaginata)—bamboo hair, ichthyosis and atopic eczema combine to form Netherton's syndrome. No specific keratin abnormality has been identified.
(3) Trichlorrhexis nodosa—there are two forms of the disorder. The commoner is an isolated hair shaft anomaly in which tooth and nail changes are occasionally associated. Much more rarely the nodular hair is accompanied by mental retardation and arginosuccinuria. Here arginosuccinuric acid is not cleaved to arginine and fumaric acid. Since arginine comprises 10 per cent of hair keratin, faulty keratin and hair formation results.
(4) Pili torti—here the hair looks like an overtwisted wire. There are several varieties.
(5) With copper deficiency (Menkes syndrome)—this is a sex-linked recessive syndrome and affected boys show the combination of twisted kinked hair, seborrhoeic eczema, failure to thrive, mental retardation with neurological signs, obstructed tortuous arteries and hypothermia. Danks in 1971 realized the analogy between copper deficient swine (which have similar arterial problems) and sheep which produce abnormally twisted wool—useless commercially. He was then able to show that affected humans are low in copper and absorb it very poorly. Copper is an essential co-enzyme for lysyl oxidase (which crosslinks collagen and elastin and could produce arterial problems). It is important for keratin crosslinks and also cytochrome oxidase which could produce hypothermia and a tendency to infection (because of inadequate neutrophilic phagocytons and autodigestion). Female heterozygons for the gene have minor degrees of pili torti but do not have arterial problems. Copper replacement therefore has not been successful.

Hair shaft anomalies without fragility

(1) Pili annulati—alternate light and dark bands are due to air-filled cavities within the hair. A pseudo pili annulati occurs in which there are alternating light and dark bands but no cavities.
(2) Woolly hair—there are autosomal dominant, recessive and patchy naevoid types.

Ectodermal dysplasias

Epidermal and dental abnormalities are associated in two groups of disorders, one of which has defective sweat glands and the other does not. The former is a sex-linked recessive and the latter autosomal dominant.

Anhidrotic ectodermal dysplasia

There are sex-linked recessive and autosomal dominant types. Carrier females of the sex-linked type have mildly impaired sweating and minor dental abnormalities in contrast to the thin skin, absent or rudimentary sweat glands, sparse hair, wrinkled skin, large ears and conical sparse teeth (*Figure 21.3*) which affect their sons. The carrier women have two distinct populations of sweat glands (normal and rudimentary) scattered at random over their body surfaces. This is a classic example of lyonization of the X chromosome. This is a phenomenon by which one of the two X chromosomes carried in each female cell is inactivated (at random) within each cell. This prevents the imposition of an abnormal genetic load (from the genes in each X chromosome) which females would otherwise carry. A good example in cats is the ginger gene which in X-linked males with only one X chromosome (and without the option of inactivation) carry the ginger gene whereas their mothers are invariably tortoiseshell (due to random inactivation of the ginger X and non-ginger X respectively. Similar considerations apply to other human X-linked disorders of course.

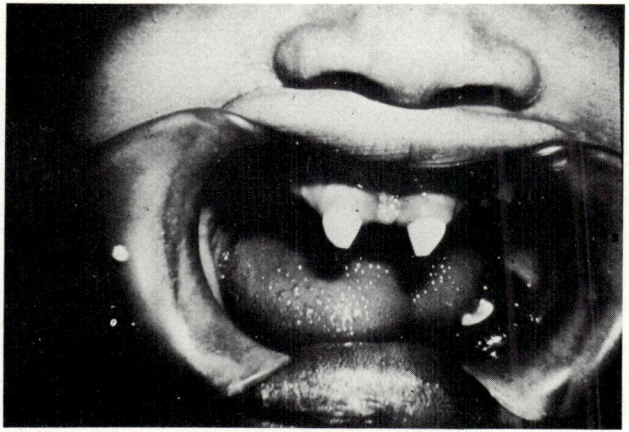

Figure 21.3   *Teeth of anhidrotic ectodermal dysplasia*

Hidrotic ectodermal dysplasia

Thin brittle hair and normal sweating is associated with a nail dystrophy, keratoderma palmaris and plantaris and normal teeth. Inheritance is autosomal dominant.

Epidermal abnormalities

Darier's disease and Hailey–Hailey disease or benign familial pemphigus are two of the commoner inherited epidermal diseases.

Both are inherited as autosomal dominant and cell contact and adhesion are impaired and result in a superficial blistering.

Darier's disease

This is an autosomal dominant with low fertility but a high mutation rate. Characteristically widespread crusted papules abound in the flexures, trunk, flanks, face, forehead, ears and especially the scalp (*Plate 21.1*). The distribution closely resembles seborrhoeic eczema. A peculiar longitudinal ridging and nail thickening also occurs.

Histopathology (*Figure 3.2,* p. 25)

The epidermis shows poor internal adhesion with frequent individual darkly stained cells (corps ronds). Electron microscopy suggests that tonofilaments and desmosomes which normally anchor cell to cell and basement membrane to basal cell are considerably stretched. Treatment is generally unsatisfactory, although topical vitamin A (Retin A) and systemic retinoids are sometimes helpful.

Benign familial pemphigus (Hailey–Hailey syndrome) (*see Chapter 13*)

Inherited abnormalities associated with cancer

Several inherited cutaneous syndromes herald later cancerous tumours. In most of them, the actual connection between the cancer and the particular skin disease is obscure.

Gardner's syndrome (colonic polyposis type III)

Gardner first noted the association between certain multiple epidermoid cysts and large intestinal polyps and later cancer of the colon. Multiple sebaceous cysts, bony osteomas, fibromas and fibrosarcomas are all well documented. Colonic polyps are present as early as the second decade and invariably become malignant. The other manifestations are variable but colonic cancer always complicates the colonic polyps.

Palmoplantar hyperkeratosis (tylosis)
(*Plate 21.2* and *Figure 21.4*)

Hyperkeratosis of the palms and soles is a common autosomal dominant trait which is extremely heterogeneous clinically. Howell-Evans and colleagues have described two unique families from

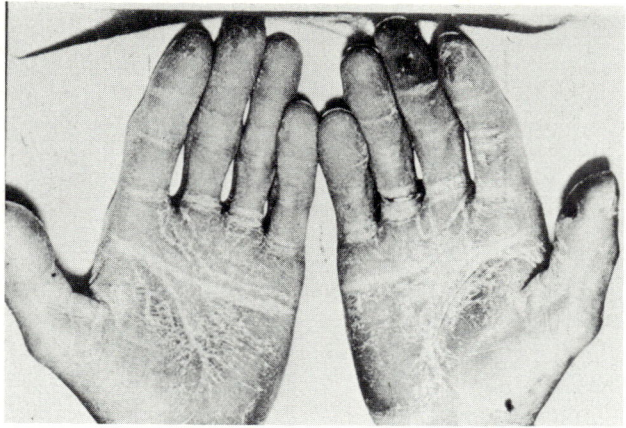

Figure 21.4   *Hyperkeratosis palmaris (inherited tylosis)*

Liverpool in which tylosis was invariably a marker of later oesophageal cancer. Similar sporadic cases have been described around the world but none has been as convincing and consistently associated with oesophageal cancer as the Liverpool families. The latter are probably one large family and unique. There is no definite explanation of the connection between the palmoplantar thickening and the oeseophageal cancer. Although it is quoted as an example of pleiotropism, which is the variable effect of a single mutated gene at different anatomical sites, no mechanism is yet identified.

Another possibility is that the cancer promoting gene is closely associated with, but separated from, the skin thickening gene. Although skin and lower oesophagus are both lined by stratified squamous epithelium, the occurrence of cancer in one and not the other is puzzling.

Bloom's syndrome

This is an autosomal recessive disorder in which a facial butterfly erythema is associated with cutaneous atrophy and light sensitivity. Chromosome breakages increase susceptibility to ultraviolet induced fibroblast damage and leukaemia is significantly more common in these patients. Heterozygotes have an increased frequency of more common internal cancers than the general population.

Xeroderma pigmentosum *(Figure 21.5)*

Xeroderma pigmentosum is a heterogeneous group of similar diseases in which an abnormal cellular susceptibility to ultraviolet light produces irreversibly damaged skin with atrophy, freckling and telangiectasia. There is a particular predisposition to all cutaneous cancers including basal and squamous carcinomas and malignant

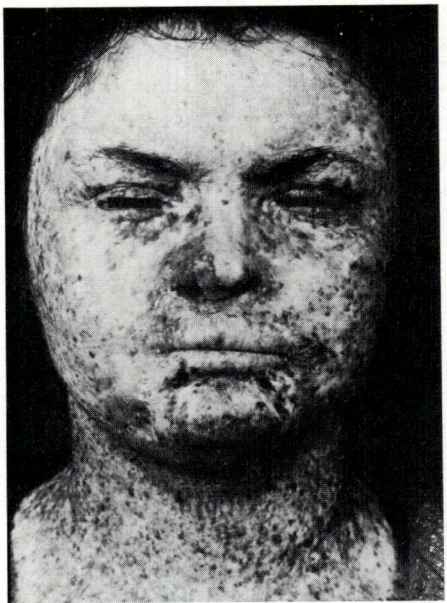

Figure 21.5   *Generalized hyperpigmentation and atrophy of a typical patient with xeroderma pigmentosum. There is an extending cutaneous cancer of the right nasolabial margin*

melanomas. Tumours can occur in patients as young as three years old. Cleaver demonstrated in 1968 that cultured skin fibroblasts from such patients lack the ability to repair DNA damaged by ultraviolet light. Xeroderma pigmentosum differs from the normal only in this repair capacity, as normal and abnormal cells are equally badly damaged. The disease is heterogeneous and five types are currently recognized, each with different abnormalities. Complementation experiments do not always correct the abnormality. Such experiments utilize medium from one set of growing fibroblasts to grow another set. Enzyme mutations along a metabolic pathway can produce whole families of fundamentally similar diseases. Then the *in vitro* addition of medium A (deficient in enzyme X but containing all others) to fibroblasts B (deficient in Y) or B to A will correct an inherited disease and produce normal end products. Good examples are the Hunter and Hurler syndromes in both of which mucopolysaccharides accumulate for different enzymic reasons. The addition of either serum to either fibroblast line corrects this abnormality in culture. Certain forms of xeroderma pigmentosum fibroblasts show such cross correction implying that ultraviolet induced DNA repair has several mechanisms. The failure of cross correction on the other hand can have a number of explanations. These include specific enzymic variations (iso-enzymes) complicated multiple mutations along metabolic pathways, or more fundamental errors such as gene deletions (DNA missing) or mRNA abnormalities. In any event both autosomal recessive and sex-linked recessive forms of xeroderma pigmentosum have been identified and each of these groups are heterogeneous. Xeroderma pigmentosum is a good example of how modern molecular biological techniques can completely unravel certain disease mechanisms. The implications of such research may also have far reaching relevance to other more common cancers.

Peutz–Jegher syndrome (*Figure 21.6*)

This autosomal dominant trait shows a typical perioral freckling, associated with variable gastrointestinal pigmentation, sometimes more widespread cutaneous pigmentation and intestinal polyposis. The polyps are actually found throughout the upper small intestine but are most frequently duodenal. *In situ* malignancy is common and metastatic cancers have been described in stomach, duodenum and other parts of the small intestine. The oral mucous membrane, lips, face, hands, palms and soles may all show the characteristic pigmented macules. Abdominal pain, haematemesis and melaena occur. Finger clubbing and ovarian granulosa cell tumours have been described. The penetrance is variable and the mechanism of disease unknown. One possibility may be an overproduction of a small intestinal polypeptide which allows the stimulation of pigmentation and duodenal polyp formation.

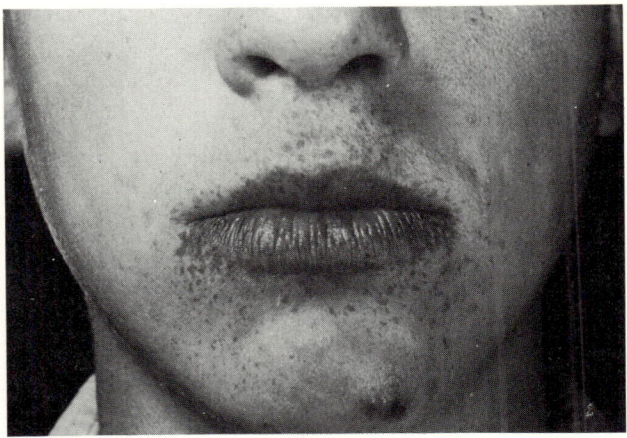

Figure 21.6 *Typical circumoral and labial distribution of the pigmented macules of the Peutz–Jegher syndrome*

Pigmentary abnormalities

There are two broad groups of abnormalities, those with increased and those with decreased pigmentation.

Diminished pigmentation

Melanin is derived from tyrosine by a number of intermediate precursors; the final rate limiting step being controlled by tyrosinase. Albinism is a clinically and genetically isolated disorder in which melanin production is blocked along the pathway. Tyrosinase negative and positive types can be separated by hair root culture. Tyrosinase positive types form melanin in the presence of tyrosinase whereas the negative ones do not. The enzyme abnormality lies at different points along the melanin pathway. Albino Negroes are normally tyrosinase positive and albino Caucasians are generally tyrosinase negative. Autosomal recessive inheritance is the rule although there are autosomal dominant and localized sex-linked recessive types. Albinism can be generalized (skin, hair, eyes, central nervous system) or localized—ocular albinism in which the skin and hair are normal.

Autosomal recessive albinism (*see Chapter 15*)

Albino skin contains amelanotic melanocytes with premelanosome-like granules. Trevor-Roper described a family in which two albinos had normal children, the implication being that there are several alleles for albinism. Nance described a possible third variant in an Amish family in which classic albinism was present at birth but later the child developed fair hair and some skin pigmentation. He found an unusual phaeomelanin in the urine. Albinoidism is a separate genetic entity in which skin pigmentation is reduced (pale skin and fair hair) together with ocular albinism, nystagmus and myopia. The albinism gene also impairs the muscular coordination of the eyes with resulting nystagmus. The nerve nuclei which control such movements are badly connected possibly because melanin has a neurotransmitter function which influences the pattern of connecting neurones on certain central locations.

Ocular albinism spares the skin but translucent irises, retinal depigmentation, photophobia and nystagmus recur. There is autosomal recessive and sex-linked inheritance and Fitzpatrick has described an autosomal dominant form. The impaired pigmentation of the common autosomal recessive generalized albinism allows easy ultraviolet light damage to skin and predisposes to various cancers including squamous cell and malignant melanomas.

Waardenburg syndrome

This is an autosomal dominant in which a localized depigmentation of the scalp hair (as a white forelock), leucoderma, white eyelashes and heterochromia iridis are associated with cochlear degeneration and deafness. Sometimes there is premature greying of the hair and the fundus may be albinotic or partially depigmented. The disorder is especially common in South Australia. All white-haired, blue eyed cats are similarly affected and there is experimental evidence that deafness is initiated shortly after birth because of an excessive endolymphatic production. Hirschsprung's disease has been described in association with humans.

Defects with increased pigmentation

Café au lait patches

Café au lait patches with axillary freckles are characteristic of neurofibromatosis. Giant dopa positive melanosomes are common but not diagnostic.

Albright syndrome

This affects girls who have precocious puberty, polyostotic cystic fibrous bony dysplasia and a distinctive unilateral naevoid hyperpigmentation (sometimes in the distribution of the fifth cranial nerve), but more commonly in a root pattern on the trunk. There can be a generalized increased melanin pigmentation too. Hyperparathyroidism and gigantism are sometimes associated. Very similar cutaneous changes can occur without the bony and endocrine abnormalities and can also affect males.

Leopard syndrome (cardiomyopathic lentiginosis) (*Figure 21.7*)

Walther first described the association of familial multiple lentigines and electrocardiographic changes. Gordon described clear autosomal dominance and coined the acronym leopard (lentigines, ECG changes, ocular hypertelorism pulmonary stenosis, atrophic gonads, retardation and deafness) to describe the essential features. Unfortunately pulmonary stenosis, gonadal atrophy, deafness and retardation are by no means consistent but the term leopard in its own right is a good one. The cardiovascular features include pulmonary stenosis and various heart murmurs and Moynahan first drew attention to endocardial and myocardial fibroelastosis. Polani and Moynahan later described left-sided obstructive cardiomyopathy in addition to their earlier observations, but none of their patients were deaf. Such clinical variation implies genetic variability.

Basement membrane abnormalities

Epidermal basement membrane is a biochemically complex but structurally amorphous membrane which has a large collagenous and significant glycoprotein content. The collagen is unique to basement membrane but there may be variability of basement membrane type. There is circumstantial evidence that skin is antigenically different from lung and renal basement membranes. Goodpasture's syndrome, in which severe lung damage and acute

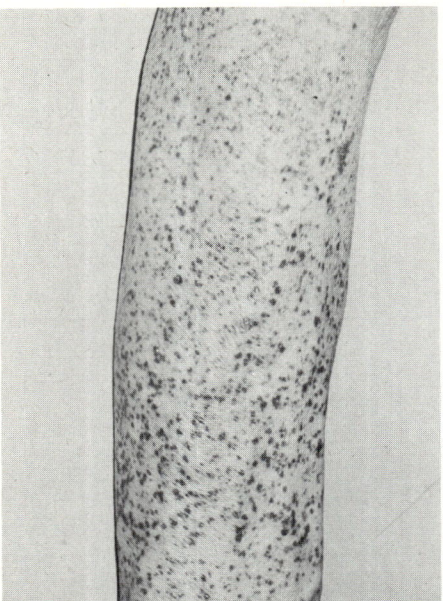

Figure 21.7 *Leopard syndrome showing unusual macular lentigines distributed over forearms*

glomerulonephritis are associated with antibasement membrane antibodies, is quite distinct from pemphigoid in which similar antibodies attack only the skin and occasionally the upper gastrointestinal tract. Two groups of inherited abnormality in which basement membrane may be at fault include the nail-patella syndrome and the various types of epidermolysis bullosa.

Nail-patella syndrome

The combination of small, distorted nails, absent or hypoplastic patellae, iliac horns and abnormalities of pronation and supination of the elbows comprises this autosomal dominant syndrome. There may be two forms; with and without renal disease. The latter is a basement membrane change sometimes associated with glomerulonephritis and sometimes with a less obvious nephrosis. Collagen fibrils have been demonstrated in the basement membranes of the mesangium. Normally basement membrane is amorphous and does not contain fibres. There is a distinct genetic linkage with the ABO blood group locus which is closely situated in the same chromosome.

Epidermolysis bullosa (*Figures 13.1* and *13.2*, pp. 142 and 143)

Blistering from minimal friction characterizes this syndrome which represents a group of disorders with different clinical and genetic characteristics. Rook recognizes three autosomal dominant and two autosomal recessives, whereas McKusick lists as many as eight autosomal dominant and five autosomal recessive patterns. Such heterogeneity may indicate considerable biochemical variability and it is possible in some of them that basement membrane collagens are at fault. Other possibilities include an abnormality in anchoring fibril proteins, which may be collagenous or perhaps more related to keratin proteins. Abnormalities in collagenase activity have also been postulated to explain some types of epidermolysis. The autosomal dominant forms are relatively trivial and include the moderately troublesome dystrophic type with scarring and the mild simplex and Cockayne patterns. In some cases at least collagenous abnormalities are likely and in particular the lethal recessive variety is reminiscent of the fatal disorder of sheep and cattle—dermatosparaxis.

(For clinical variants of epidermolysis bullosa *see Chapter 13.*)

Dermal abnormalities

Dermal mucopolysaccharides, collagen and elastin comprise the vast majority of the dermis. Nerves, muscle, sweat glands, blood vessels and sebaceous glands form most of the remainder. Blood vessels also contain considerable amounts of collagen as does perineurium.

Various inherited abnormalities of these structures and substances are described below.

Inherited abnormalities of collagen

Recently abnormalities of collagen chemistry have been shown to cause specific types of disease. Thus fragile skin, easily ruptured blood vessels, pleural rupture, brittle bones and tendon rupture may all be caused by such inherited mutations in collagen pattern. Collagen is a high molecular weight triple helical protein weighing 470 000 daltons. Three intertwined crosslinked helical chains produce its characteristic chemical stability and structural characteristics. Five collagen types are now recognized and types I, III and V are widely distributed in the dermis, and type IV forms the collagenous component of basement membrane.

Many cutaneous syndromes undoubtedly have underlying collagenous abnormalities. The Ehlers–Danlos syndrome (EDS) is probably the best known of them. Four of the eight or so varieties of EDS have had specific biochemical abnormalities demonstrated. These are types IV, V, VI and VII. Osteogenesis imperfecta is proving equally complicated and five or more biochemical lesions are now recognized.

Ehlers–Danlos syndrome (*Figure 21.8*)

Type I—gravis (no biochemical defects identified) is the classic form of the syndrome and is the original type described by Ehlers and

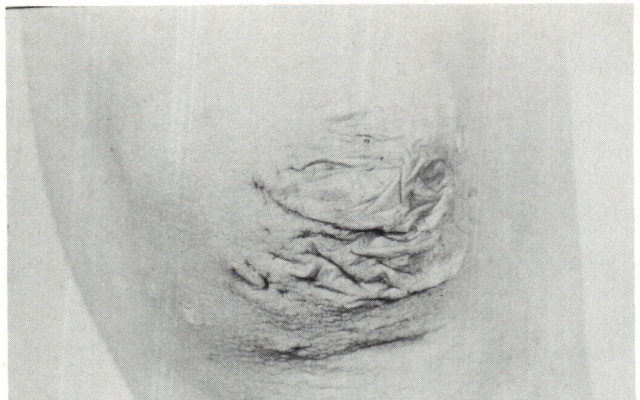

Figure 21.8 *Ehlers–Danlos syndrome (cutis hyper-elastica) showing typical papyraceous scars*

Danlos. Extremely hyperextensible skin and joints, wide papyraceous scars, joint hyperextensibility and fibrous nodules are characteristic. Like the less severe EDS type II (mitis) and the common EDS III in which hyperextensible joints are inherited as autosomal dominants, the fundamental biochemical causes are unknown. Occasionally mitral valve prolapse and rarely aortic rupture complicate EDS I and II, and EDS III is complicated by painful joints and premature osteoarthrosis (presumably from excessive wear and tear).

EDS types IV, V, VI and VII—the essential clinical and biochemical features are summarized in *Table 21.2*. They are proving increasingly complicated and several subgroups of each are now recognized.

Table 21.2 Chemical abnormalities in Ehlers–Danlos syndrome

Type	Inheritance	Clinical features	Biochemistry
EDS IV (ecchymotic acrogeria)	(1) Autosomal recessive	Pinched nose Owl eyes Premature ageing Arterial rupture	Type III collagen deficiency
	(2) Autosomal dominant	Normal face Thin skin	Type III collagen deficiency
EDS V	Sex-linked recessive	Non specific	(1) Lysyl oxidase deficiency (2) Normal enzyme levels
EDS VI	Autosomal recessive	Scoliosis Retinal detachment Aortic rupture	(1) Hydroxylysine deficiency (2) Normal hydroxylysine
EDS VII	Autosomal dominant	Short stature Extreme joint laxity	Procollagen N extension peptide mutation

Elastosis perforans serpinginosa (Lutz–Miescher syndrome)
(*Figure 21.9*)

This is a collection of hyperkeratotic papules often with a raised edge and clearing centre reminiscent of a cutaneous fungal infection. Histology shows the characteristic elastic tissue infiltration and extrusion through the epidermis. Clinical lesions occur anywhere, most typically over the neck. A number of inherited diseases of connective tissue have been described in association with the disorder. These include pseudoxanthoma elasticum (PXE), Ehlers–Danlos syndrome, acrogeria of Gottron or EDS type IV, osteogenesis imperfecta, arterial and cerebral aneurysms, copper deficiency, capillary angiomas, cystinosis and renal stones and a syndrome of multiple orthopaedic defects with gynaecomastia. Possible mechanisms include collagen abnormalities allowing an abnormal relative increase of elastin (EDS, acrogeria, Marfan syndrome, aneurysms, osteogenesis imperfecta) an actual alteration of elastic fibres (PXE) and unexplained—mongolism and cystinosis. In any event the occurrence of elastosis perforans requires a careful search for the underlying diseases mentioned above.

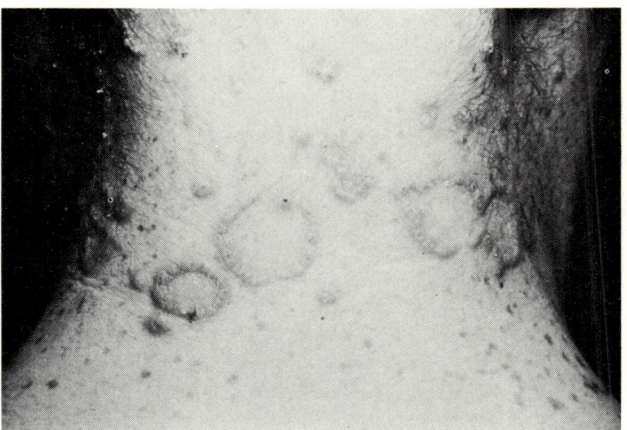

Figure 21.9 *Typically raised circinate crateriform lesions of Mieschers elastoma*

Mucopolysaccharide abnormalities

Mucopolysaccharides are complex polymers of acetylated or sulphated polysaccharide chains attached to a central protein core. The normal balance between production and destruction is grossly altered if the degradative lysosomal enzymes are diminished. Under these circumstances, heparin and dermatan sulphate accumulate. A whole group of clinical defects characterized by thickened skin, hypertrichosis, coarsened broadened features, kyphoscoliosis, joint tightening, hepatosplenomegaly, mental retardation and corneal clouding are the result. Except for the Hunter syndrome which is a sex-linked recessive, inheritance is autosomal recessive.

Inherited abnormalities of elastin

Elastin is a high molecular weight fibrous protein widespread in skin, blood vessels, lungs, intestine and tendons and is rich in glycine, proline, lysine and valine. Histologically there are micro-fibrillar and globular forms. The biochemistry is not sufficiently well understood to allow the logical biochemical separation of various diseases, as is the case with collagen. Both cultured fibroblasts and muscle cells (especially of blood vessels) can synthesize the protein. Various degradative enzymes (elastases) are capable of digestion and are liberated from the pancreas, but are also present in granulocytes. There are certain well known abnormalities of elastin formation and degradation which are relevant to dermatology.

Abnormalities of the elastic fibre

Pseudoxanthoma elasticum (PXE) (*Figure 21.10*) is an inherited abnormality in which elastic fibres are abnormally fragmented. The typical skin changes are in areas which are often stretched such as

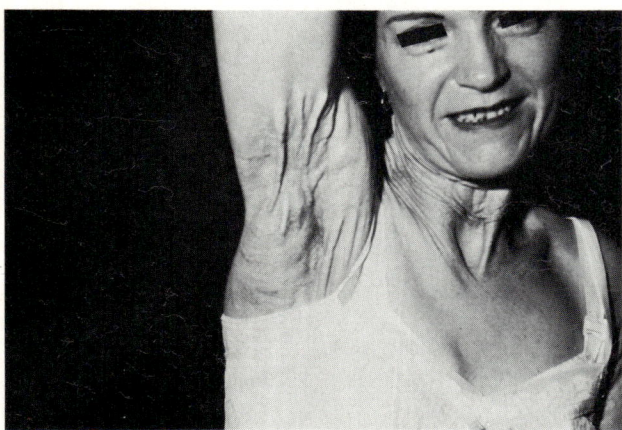

Figure 21.10   *Typical PXE of neck and axillae*

the neck, elbows, groins and popliteal fossae. The abnormality is presumably generalized within the skin and also elsewhere in the body. Similar changes affect arteries producing impalpable radial pulses, extensive calcification, premature coronary artery disease and gastrointestinal bleeding. Splitting of Bruch's membrane, a subretinal layer of elastic fibres, forms the classic angioid streaks through which the more deeply coloured choroid is contrasted with the retina (*Figure 21.11*). Microhaemorrhages and scarring in association with the streaks cause macular scarring and typical

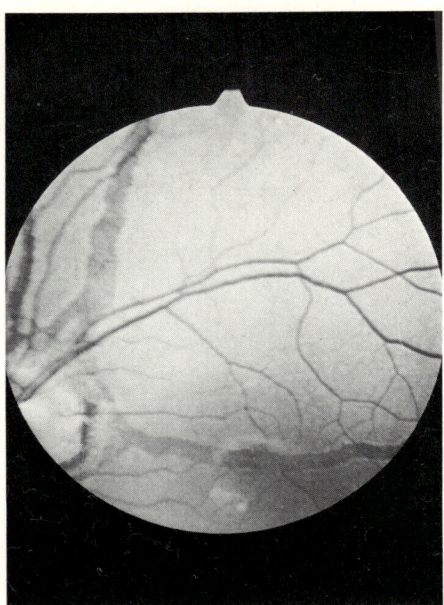

Figure 21.11 *Retinal photograph showing angioid streaking from the optic disc at 1 and 3 o'clock. There is early macular degeneration*

central scotomas. Occasionally, the lungs are affected, either by emphysema or even more rarely by an extensive 'snow storm' micronodulation (due to calcification). The syndrome is genetically and clinically heterogeneous and there are at least two autosomal dominant and two autosomal recessive forms. The rare juvenile Paget's disease with PXE may be an entirely different variety as may the occasional patient with severe kyphoscoliosis and high myopia with PXE. Of the four recognized types, type I autosomal dominant and recessive are the most severe, whereas type II dominant has many features reminiscent of an inherited collagen defect (with loose jointedness, pectus excavatus, varicose veins, blue sclerae and hernias). Specific biochemical defects await identification. Calcification is probably secondary to the underlying elastic degeneration although some workers suggest a primary abnormality.

Abnormalities with excessive elastic loss

A number of inherited traits are characterized by elastin deficiency. Autosomal recessive and dominant diseases with abnormally sparse elastic fibres—the congenital cutis laxas—are described. The skin hangs in redundant folds looking much too big for the patient (beagle syndrome). Laryngeal (deep husky voice), lung (emphysema), gastrointestinal (megacolon diverticulae), renal tract (hydroureter and bladder diverticulae) occur with lack of elastic material. Rare lethal

317

autosomal recessive forms with pulmonary hypertension and emphysema occur. No specific biochemical abnormalities have been described. A specific elastase which is inhibited by α2 macroglobulin and α1 antitrypsin are well known, but no such inhibitor abnormalities have been described in congenital cutis laxa. Other possibilities include an abnormal substrate (elastic fibre), an abnormally active elastase or an inefficient enzyme–inhibitor complex. Other cases of loose skin which may be confused with cutis laxa include recessive type II PXE and some types of Ehlers–Danlos syndrome. Unlike classic cutis laxa the elastic fibres are normal, degenerated or increased.

Blood vessel abnormalities

Inherited capillary and venous angiomas are common and probably have heterogeneous causes. Haemangiomata are among the commonest disorders of this type encountered in infancy (*see* Chapter 18).

Familial telangiectasia (Osler–Weber–Rendu syndrome) (*Plate 21.3*)

This is an autosomal dominant with variable penetrance. Widespread non-pulsatile pinhead-sized telangiectases are scattered over hands, limbs, palate, nasopharynx, tongue and gastrointestinal tract. Sometimes there are larger nodular lesions over the face and forehead and capillary haemangiomas can be the presenting feature in childhood. Nose bleeds are common, as is gastrointestinal bleeding with chronic anaemia in the elderly. Pulmonary arteriovenous fistulae, aortic and central nervous aneurysms and cirrhosis of the liver have all been recorded. Possibly they indicate a generalized abnormality of blood vessel formation or composition. The syndrome is clinically variable. A family is recorded with recurrent haemoptyses transmitted as an autosomal dominant trait in three generations. Bronchoscopy has failed to show a source of bleeding, but all affected persons have bronchial and sublingual telangiectasia but normal skin. Another common variant is widespread linear facial telangiectases with numerous cutaneous angiomas and capillary telangiectases, nose bleeds and gastrointestinal bleeding without buccal telangiectasia. (The cause of the OWR syndrome is obscure. The widespread nature of the lesions suggests a blood vessel composition abnormality.) One possibility that merits careful study is that an inherited abnormality of collagen is the cause.

Ataxia telangiectasia (Louis–Bar syndrome)

This is an autosomal recessive disorder in which conjunctival facial and peripheral telangiectases are associated with cerebellar ataxia and various immunological abnormalities. These include IgA and IgE deficiency, lymphocytopenia and thymic atrophy with T cell lymphomas. Cellular degeneration with Purkinje cell damage, cell degeneration, nystagmus and slurred speech are the rule. The telangiectasia usually precede the neurological signs. There is a predisposition to cancer in homozygotes and heterozygotes. DNA repair to ionizing radiation is faulty.

Angiokeratoma corporis diffusum (Anderson–Fabry disease)

This remarkable sex-linked recessive disease is caused by a specific ceramide galactosidase deficiency. Ceramide and neutral glycolipid then accumulate in skin, blood vessel, kidneys, gut, peripheral and central nervous system. Cultured skin fibroblasts or lymphocytes can be used to demonstrate and confirm the enzyme abnormality and the enzyme can be measured in plucked scalp hair roots. The disease is analogous to other glycolipid accumulations such as Tay–Sachs disease. The rash which appears before puberty consists of dark red telangiectases which do not blanch on pressure. Scrotal, abdominal and thigh lesions are characteristic, but the distribution can be much less widespread. Paraesthesiae, impaired sweating, headaches, and muscular pains are typical and are caused by lipid deposits in those areas. Spun urine typically shows albumin, red cells and lipid bodies and renal biopsy shows a PAS positive glycolipid in the glomerular vessels. Skin biopsy also shows PAS positive vessels and electron microscopy shows the characteristic concentric lamellations of glycolipid. Slit lamp examination may show corneal clouding. Progressive renal failure or an infiltrative cardiomyopathy is the usual end result.

Although renal transplantation has been claimed to induce more normal enzyme levels in recipients the effect is usually temporary.

Other inherited abnormalities affecting fibrous tissue

Neurofibromatosis (Von Recklinghausen's disease) (*Figure 21.12*)

This is a common autosomal dominant with variable penetrance. Cutaneous changes include multiple café au lait patches and cutaneous nodules of neurilemmal origin. At least five patches over 1 cm in diameter must be present, and axillary freckling can occur either alone or in combination with fibrous nodules. (The latter are entirely collagenous.) More commonly the patient is covered with nodules. Although the pigmented patches contain melanocytes with giant melanosomes, these are not invariable and can be indistiguishable from the patches of Albright's syndrome. The clinical signs are extremely variable within families because of the effect of modifying genes.

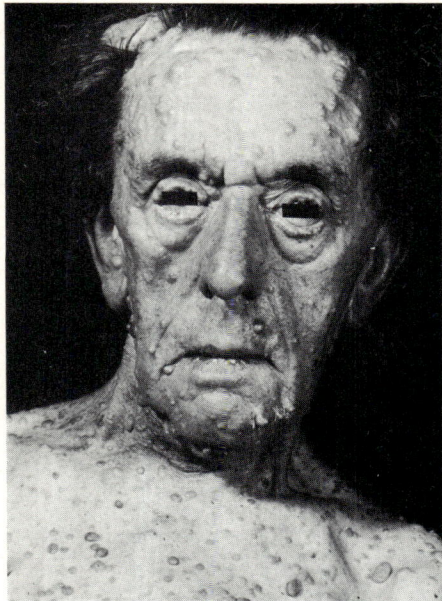

Figure 21.12 *Multiple neurofibromatosis showing the typical subcutaneous nodules and papillomas*

Complications

Neurofibromas can be widespread throughout the central nervous system and are especially common in the cranial nerves. Auditory neuromas, trigeminal neuralgia and ophthalmoplegia, cervical and root neurofibromas and meningiomas are frequent. Phaeochromocytomas, cardiac tumours, scoliosis, osteoporosis, bony cysts and pathological fractures have all been described. Plexiform neuromas can be cosmetically disfiguring especially around the face.

Heterogeneity of the syndrome

Loose jointedness, hyperextensible skin and blue sclerae are common in some families and probably imply an inherited defect of connective tissue. Several patients with coincident Ehlers–Danlos syndrome are reported. Although many families with neurofibromatosis do not show these features, it is likely that the group with connective tissue abnormalities have an underlying inherited collagen abnormality which also causes the neurofibromatosis. The neural sheath is rich in type III collagen and cultured perineural cells can produce collagenous material in culture. More recently central and peripheral forms of neurofibromatosis have been described. The peripheral form is the classic type in which extensive cutaneous nodules occur, whereas the central type has mainly central nervous lesions. Nerve growth factor elevations have been described in both.

Angiofibromas (tuberose sclerosis, adenoma sebaceum) (*Plate 21.4*)

Tuberose sclerosis (epiloia) is an autosomal dominant disorder in which a facial butterfly angiofibromatous rash is associated with systemic fibrous nodules, mental retardation and epilepsy. Originally considered sebaceous hypertrophy, the facial rash is really a vascular fibrous proliferation. Other cutaneous associations include periungual fibromas, shagreen patches which are thickened, dermal fibrosis, and ovoid ash-leaf like patches of depigmentation. Fibrous nodules also affect the gums, palate, tongue and larynx.

Abnormal neutrophil function

Neutrophils are chemotactically attracted to sites of bacterial infection and ingest (phagocytose) and then digest the invaders. Chemotactic factors are liberated not only by the invading organisms but also by the various complement derivatives of the host. For example, C3a, C5a and C5, 6, 7 complexes induce oxygen consumption from H_2O_2 production. NADPH oxidase is necessary for proper neutrophil function and myeloperoxidase reacts with H_2O_2 to allow bacterial killing. Abnormalities in any of these steps can produce defective polymorph function and cause specific syndromes usually with cutaneous changes.

Chronic granulomatous diseases

This is a clinically and genetically heterogeneous group of diseases in which there are recurrent staphylococcal infections of the skin, lymph nodes, lung, liver and bone. Multiple abscesses filled with lipid-rich macrophages are common. Poorly phagocytozed organisms include *S. aureus, E. coli, Pseudomonas, Candida* and *Aspergillus*.

Immunoglobulin levels are diffusely raised and T and B cell functions are unimpaired. Although chemotaxis and phagocytosis are normal, bacterial killing is deficient. Hydrogen peroxide is not generated by staphylococci, but is generated by other organisms and presumably several intermediate steps in the generation of peroxide can be blocked.

A reasonable screening test for neutrophil function is the nitroblue tetrazolium test which expresses function in terms of the efficiency of conversion of the blue test dye to a black product. Recently, a deficiency in cytochrome C, an essential cofactor for superoxide production, has been shown in carriers and affected patients. Sex-linked and autosomal recessive inheritance occurs. Treatment includes the prompt use of the relevant antibodies.

Myeloperoxidase deficiency

Normal human polymorphs contain peroxidase positive granules which contain the enzyme myeloperoxidase. Some patients with severe adult onset systemic candidiasis have deficient myeloperoxidase activity. Inheritance is autosomal recessive.

Chediak–Higashi syndrome

This is a rare autosomal recessive disease in which eosinophilic peroxidase positive granules are contained in myeloblasts and promyelocytes. The blood and bone marrow are depleted in mature neutrophils and the patients die before ten years of age of overwhelming infection and malignant lymphomas. Inheritance is autosomal recessive and the clinical features include oculocutaneous albinism, photophobia and nystagmus, repeated staphylococcal infections, lymphadenopathy and lymphoreticular proliferation, hepatosplenomegaly and hypogammaglobulinaemia. Both melanocytes and neutrophils have large granules and a possible explanation of such diverse abnormalities is that microtubule formation is defective. McKusick classifies the disease as Albinism type III, types I and II being the allelic forms of classic albinism mentioned earlier. Similar abnormalities to the Chediak–Higashi syndrome also occur in mouse, cattle, mink and killer whales. Neutrophil chemotaxis and bacterial killing are impaired. Whether the handling of other infective agents such as cancer-forming viruses can also cause the malignant lymphomas in these patients is speculative.

Inherited abnormalities of complement

Complement is a complex serum protein family recognized by Bordet in 1895 as essential for certain antigen–antibody reactions. It is contained within serum as an inert form but can be activated by either the classic or alternative pathways. Such activation produces a cascade of complement components each acting in sequence as an enzyme to produce the next. Increasing numbers of complement deficiency states are becoming recognized. Most of them have not been associated with particular diseases and it is overaction of the system by a deficiency of $C\bar{1}$ inhibitor (allowing the complement cascade to overproduce) that is the best known of these abnormalities. This produces hereditary angioneurotic oedema. The complement pathway is activated by two distinct (not interrelated) ways. Firstly C3 is converted to C3b via the antigen-antibody activation of C1r and C1q—the classic pathway, and secondly by the alternative pathway, mediated by factors such as endotoxin and lipopolysaccharide. In either case the result of C3 conversion (or fixation) is to allow it to bind with neutrophils, red cells and lymphocytes and so initiate various immunological reactions by these cells. The produc-

322

tion of C3 cleavage by the classic pathway involves the action of C1q, C1r, C1s, C4, C2 which finally generate the enzyme complex for the conversion of C3 to C3b. Subsequently C5 is cleaved to C5b and complexes involving C6, 7, 8 and 9 come into play. These latter allow the classic complement levels to appear in cell membranes (producing cell lysis and death by immune mechanisms).

Hereditary angioedema

Hereditary angioedema (HAO) is an autosomal dominant deficiency of C1 esterase inhibitor protein. This normally inhibits activated C1s, one of the three constituents of the first component of complement and also inhibits the enzyme activity of Hageman factor, kallekrein and Factor Xl. It allows plasmin and C1 to react with C2 and release extremely vasoactive mediators. C2 and C4 are overconsumed and there is a strongly associated tendency to immune complex formation with resulting glomerulonephritis. This deficiency is inherited as an autosomal dominant and normally the active inhibitor levels are 50 per cent of normal, but fall during attacks to almost zero. In this instance the gene is deleted but another form of the disorder with immunologically detectable but presumably inactive inhibitor occurs; presumably due to an amino acid substitution or frame shift mutation. The clinical onset can be at any time from childhood to early adult life. Cutaneous changes include local subcutaneous oedema with or without urticaria. Unfortunately, subepithelial laryngeal oedema is especially dangerous and can cause rapid death. Abdominal swellings with recurrent abdominal pain and intestinal obstruction often occur, and sometimes because of the unrecognized cause laparotomy and even resection is undertaken. What activates the C1 esterase is unknown but the vasoactive C2 can be produced at several points in the pathway. Proteinase inhibitors can help attacks and epsilon aminocaproic acid and tranexamic acid are both useful. Danazol, an anabolic virilizing androgenic steroid stimulates C1 esterase inhibitor synthesis (presumably, the normal gene product) within weeks, C4 consumption stops and levels increase to normal. Excitingly in those individuals with immunologically inactive deficiency, it is the normal C1 esterase inhibitor that is selectively stimulated (rather than its abnormal mutated allele).

Other complement deficiencies

There is no clear pattern by which the various complement component deficiencies can be correlated with the particular disease states with which they have been associated. These are tabulated below (after Lachman, 1976).

    C1q—hypogammaglobulinaemia,
    C1r⎫
        ⎬SLE,
    C1s⎭

C2—vasculitis, SLE, Henoch–Schönlein purpura,
C3—immune deficiency,
C4—atypical SLE,
C5—SLE,
C6—meningococcal and gonococcal septicaemia,
C7—scleroderma, Raynaud's, CRST syndrome,
C8—gonococcal sepsis.

Thus C1r, C4, C2 and C̄1 inhibitors have all been associated with immune complex diseases. One possible explanation is that deficiency of these factors does not allow efficient use of the classic pathway so that infective (viral?) agents cannot be properly dealt with, persisting and causing the disease. Alternatively the deficiency is coincidental and unrelated to the diseases themselves. C6 and 8 deficiency have each been linked with overwhelming gonococcal infections and may possibly be connected with direct immune responses to these organisms. Abnormal activation of the alternative complement pathway producing low serum complement levels, and C3 deposition in glomeruli occurs in inherited partial lipodystrophy. Complement abnormalities precede the nephritis and are possibly the direct cause of it. Serum from these patients contains an abnormal complement activating factor (C3 nephritic factor).

Miscellaneous dermatoses, including disorders of the sweat glands

R. J. Cairns
Patrick Hall-Smith

The poikilodermas

Poikiloderma is a complex polymorphic skin change resulting from a wide variety of causes. The lesions include telangiectatic reticulate erythema, punctate haemorrhages, atrophy—sometimes with a cigarette paper-like pleating—patchy pigmentation and depigmentation; miliary lichenoid scaly papules constitute an inconstant feature. A good example of this change is x-ray atrophy.

Poikiloderma is important because of the association with systemic disease and the possibility of malignant change occurring within the abnormal skin.

The causes of the *poikiloderma syndrome* fall under four major headings:

(1) Autoimmune disease

Dermatomyositis either in the acute stage or when subsiding may present with the cutaneous lesions of poikiloderma. The face, hands and front of the chest are particularly affected. Likewise, systemic lupus erythematosus and less commonly scleroderma may show skin changes of poikiloderma. It is important to consider the possibility of an underlying visceral neoplasm in cases of dermatomyositis first appearing in adult life; the older the patient the more likely the association with internal malignancy.

(2) Lymphomatous change

Poikiloderma often with marked lichenoid papules and sometimes with plaques of parapsoriasis constitutes a common precursor of cutaneous lymphoma. The coexistence of infiltrated plaques and localized areas of poikiloderma suggests that the transformation into cutaneous lymphoma, particularly mycosis fungoides (*Plate 17.4*), has already occurred. Strictly localized poikiloderma may remain unchanged for 20 to 30 years before manifesting frank signs of lymphoma.

(3) Congenital gene determined poikiloderma

The *Rothmund–Thomson* syndrome begins with poikiloderma on the cheeks, hands and buttocks. The cutaneous changes fade in time leaving atrophy. Malignant change to intraepidermal epithelioma or frank squamous cell carcinoma is frequently seen. *Xeroderma pigmentosum* shows all the changes of poikiloderma and light is the activating factor which provokes malignant change in these individuals, based on an enzyme defect responsible for skin repair after ultraviolet damage.

(4) Exogenous factors

Prolonged exposure to sunlight, x-ray, and skin damage from chronic photosensitization, particularly from tar and mineral oils, result in poikilodermatous changes. Like the congenital group, patients with exogenous poikiloderma may develop epitheliomatous changes within the skin-damaged areas.

Parapsoriasis

Several dermatoses of different aetiology and natural history were grouped by earlier generations of dermatologists as parapsoriasis because of the resemblance to psoriasis and a complex terminology thus evolved. The terms, some eponymic, are included in parenthesis:

(1) Pityriasis lichenoides (*Plate 22.1*)

The acute variety (Mucha–Habermann disease, Chapter 19) is probably based on allergic vasculitis affecting the dermal arterioles with subsequent infarction. Haemorrhagic papules appear in crops, become crusted and leave pitted varioliform scars; there may be some systemic upset. Less frequent lesions include vesicles, papules and nodules, all of which form part of the Ruiter syndrome of allergic cutaneous vasculitis. Rarely visceral lesions are encountered.

The chronic variety shows multiple scaly lesions which occur profusely on the trunk and limbs (pityriasis lichenoides of Juliusberg). The face, hands and feet are spared. The lesions come and go, with no tendency for confluence, and are covered with a characteristic micaceous scale which on removal as a thin flake leaves a slightly depressed surface without the characteristic punctate bleeding of psoriasis. This chronic guttate eruption persists for many years without the development of a lymphoma.

(2) Lymphomatous parapsoriasis

This group comprises several pre-lymphomatous dermatoses in which the appearance of a definite lymphoma occurs after a variable period of years. Fairly distinctive entities are recognized:

(a) Guttate type

The lesions are small, up to 1 cm across, and somewhat resemble pityriasis lichenoides chronica. However, the patches are fixed, do not vary in intensity and are covered with rather adherent scales which are thick and not mica-like in appearance.

(b) Plaque type (*Plate 17.6*)

This is the well-known *parapsoriasis en plaques*. It is the commonest clinical picture, areas ranging in size from 1–10 cm, simulating both psoriasis and discoid eczema. Patches are well defined in the initial stage but later may become confluent, although they can remain unchanged for many years. Itching is a feature. The face and hands are not usually affected. The lesions are radioresistant, but respond to ultraviolet light. Infiltration suggests transformation into cutaneous lymphoma; other features suggestive of malignant change include atrophic poikilodermatous areas, involvement of the face and systemic upset.

(c) Parapsoriasis lichenoides

Miliary lichenoid lesions predominate, with pigmentary changes making it difficult to distinguish the condition from poikiloderma; such changes are a precursor of skin lymphoma.

Mucous membrane disorders

The buccal mucosa and tongue may be affected in skin disease; mucosal changes are indeed diagnostic of certain disorders. Thus a fine white lace-like pattern admixed with white puncta is diagnostic of buccal lichen planus (*Plate 22.2*). Pemphigus vulgaris will show eroded bullae on the buccal mucosa as a first sign. Other bullous disorders include mucous membrane pemphigoid (cicatrical pemphigoid) and epidermolysis bullosa.

The mucosal lesions of secondary syphilis (snail-track ulcers) are of diagnostic importance. Haemorrhagic crusting of the lips and buccal erosions combined with conjunctivitis constitute an integral part of the Stevens–Johnson syndrome (*Plate 13.5*). Koplik's spots of measles are well-known. Changes of malnutrition and the white adherent deposit of oral candidiasis are frequently seen; the white adherent thickening of leukoplakia is also familiar, with the inner cheeks, tongue and lips being affected; likewise the vulval mucosa may show white thickening characteristic of this premalignant dermatosis.

Geographic tongue is a transient disorder with patchy loss of the lingual epithelium leading to red map-like areas which are static or occasionally migrate across the dorsa of the tongue (*Figure 22.1*). It probably represents a reactive pattern of the tongue to several different disorders. The condition has been associated with Reiter's disease and psoriasis, with features of atopy commoner in affected patients than in non-affected individuals.

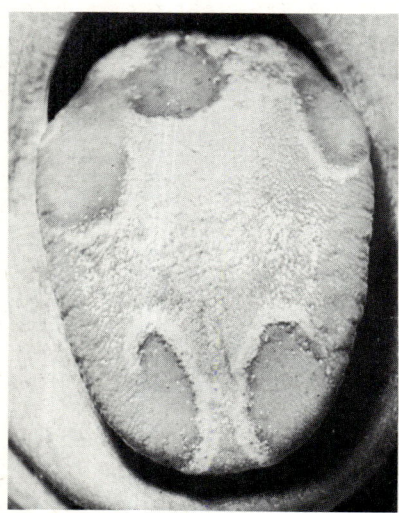

Figure 22.1   Geographic tongue

Hyperhidrosis

Hyperhidrosis is excessive sweating, which may be localized or generalized.

Localized hyperhidrosis

This occurs in the palms, on the soles, axillae, groins and perineum. It may be emotional, though familial predisposition and sometimes neurological disease may be causative. This last may produce asymmetrical hyperhidrosis.

Generalized hyperhidrosis

This is usually the result of environmental warmth and humidity. Infections and endocrine disorders, e.g. thyrotoxicosis, the menopause and obesity may all cause an increase in temperature affecting the heat centre in the hypothalamus. This is thermoregulatory sweating.

Gustatory hyperhidrosis

Some sweating of the forehead, upper lip, nose and perioral area after eating spicy and highly seasoned foods can be regarded as normal. Marked hyperhidrosis at these sites can occur after disease or trauma to the autonomic nervous system. Von Frey's syndrome occurs after damage or disease to the parotid gland affecting the auriculo-temporal nerve.

Treatment

Topical 20% aluminium chloride hexahydrate solution in ethanol (Anhydrol Forte) is effective in most cases of axillary, palmar and plantar hyperhidrosis. The areas to be treated should be completely dry and should not be washed immediately prior to application; nor should the preparation be applied to broken or eczematized skin. The solution is best applied before going to bed on two successive nights, followed by a rest period of two nights, and the cycle then repeated. The patient should be able to assess the response and increase or decrease usage accordingly. Transient irritation or redness is controlled by hydrocortisone cream 1%. In a few severe cases of axillary hyperhidrosis unresponsive to aluminium chloride hexahydrate solution, the Hurley–Shelley operation can be undertaken. This entails the excision of an ellipse of central axillary skin containing the sweat gland-bearing area. Likewise uncontrolled palmar hyperhidrosis may require cervical sympathectomy. Drugs such as propantheline bromide (Probanthine) are disappointing. Plantar hyperhidrosis may also be treated with 20–40% formalin, though watch should be kept for sensitization.

Aluminium chloride hexahydrate solution 20% may also be used in gustatory hyperhidrosis, though surgical intervention may be necessary in some cases.

Hypohidrosis

Hypohidrosis—sometimes termed anhidrosis—means greatly diminished or absence of sweating. Kay and Maibach list the following conditions associated with anhidrosis:

(1) congenital ectodermal defect;
(2) quinacrine (atabrine) anhidrosis;
(3) metal poisoning;
(4) miliaria profunda—thermogenic anhidrosis or following exposure to radiant heat;
(5) CNS or spinal cord injury;
(6) Sjörgren's syndrome;
(7) metabolic, endocrine and systemic disease such as orthostatic hypotension (limited to legs), diabetic neuropathy and multiple myeloma.

Hypohidrosis may also occur in psoriasis.

Miliaria is the result of plugging or rupture of the sweat ducts. In infants it may be a physiological phenomenon. It can occur at any age. It is divided into three types depending on the level of obstruction of the sweat duct:

(1) Miliaria crystallina (sudamina), due to superficial plugging, causing a clear vesicle with minimal inflammation.
(2) Miliaria rubra (prickly heat) in which punctate erythematous papules cause severe itching.
(3) Miliaria profunda (mamillaria)—occasionally seen in the tropics and manifested by 1–3 mm papules affecting the trunk and limbs. Discomfort is minimal.

Treatment

The patient should be placed in a cool environment. Air conditioning is the ideal if available. Wool fat BP (anhydrous lanolin) may unblock occluded pores. Aqueous cream BP may also prove helpful. Alcohol 95% is worth a trial.

Fox Fordyce disease

This is a rare condition occurring mostly in women between puberty and the menopause. It manifests itself by skin-coloured or pigmented follicular papules most commonly occurring in the axillae, though the breasts, umbilicus, pubic and vulval areas may also be involved. The ages of onset, resolution and the fact that it may disappear during pregnancy point to an endocrine causation.

Treatment

Topical corticosteroids, the contraceptive pill and surgical excision of the affected site have all been used with varying degrees of success and failure.

23 Drug eruptions

Ashley Levantine

With the ever-increasing number of available drugs, adverse reactions are becoming more frequent. Cutaneous reactions are the commonest complications of drug therapy, but there may also be visceral reactions. Most drugs have been reported as causing a reaction, but the high risk group includes antibiotics (particularly penicillin), sulphonamides and barbiturates.

The incidence of drug eruptions is very difficult to assess. Not all eruptions are reported, and often cutaneous changes of other origin are falsely attributed to drugs. Self-medication and unknown ingestion of drugs, such as quinine in bitter lemon, increase the risk of adverse reactions.

Drugs seldom reach the patient as 100 per cent pure chemicals; in addition to the active ingredients there is a vehicle and there are various coatings, flavouring and colouring agents.

Classification and mechanism of drug reactions

The mechanisms of most drug reactions are unknown. Reactions are often attributed to drug sensitivity on insufficient evidence.

Overdosage

Reaction is directly related to the total amount of drug in the body. Usually the symptoms of overdosage are an exaggeration of the pharmacological action of the drug. Overdosage may be absolute, due to deliberate over-ingestion or over-prescribing, or relative, due to an underlying abnormality in the patient. Thus different rates of absorption, metabolism and excretion may influence the possibilities of a reaction. The action of drugs metabolized by the liver may be enhanced and prolonged in liver disease. Diminished renal function, such as occurs in the elderly and in renal disease, may similarly result in overdosage.

Intolerance

Intolerance occurs when there is a low threshold to the normal pharmacological action of a drug. Thus an abnormally small dose produces the characteristic effects of the drug. Excretion defects may predispose an individual to drug intolerance.

Idiosyncrasy

Idiosyncrasy is an uncharacteristic response to a drug which is not due to an immunological mechanism.

Both intolerance and idiosyncrasy may result from pharmaco-genetic mechanisms.

Pharmacogenetics

Very few drugs are eliminated from the body unchanged. They may be metabolized by oxidation, reduction, hydrolysis or conjugation. The various enzymes involved are subject to variations on an hereditary basis, so that there may be differences in the way in which individuals metabolize drugs. Slow acetylation, for example, is inherited as an autosomal recessive trait. Slow acetylators accumulate high levels of isoniazid on normal doses of the drug and may develop signs of toxicity, such as peripheral neuropathy. Patients with glucose-6-phosphate dehydrogenase deficiency may develop acute haemolysis when exposed to certain drugs.

Acute toxicity

Acute toxicity may result from overdosage, or an abnormally fast or great absorption of the drug. Certain drugs have predictable toxic effects due to their pharmacological nature. In spite of its widespread use and high incidence of allergic reactions, penicillin has a surprisingly low incidence of toxicity.

Chronic toxicity

Chronic toxicity results from the chronic accumulation of drugs and their metabolites. This may be a simple deposition of the drug in the phagocytic cells of the skin and mucous membranes. Argyria is due to deposition of silver and may result from absorption after the prolonged application of silver salts to the mucous membranes. Chronic arsenical accumulation produces a wide variety of adverse reactions, notably keratoses (*Figure 23.1*), cutaneous and internal malignancies, and the classic 'rain-drop' pigmentation.

Secondary effects

Secondary effects are indirect effects mainly due to the disturbance caused by the drug in homeostatic and other control mechanisms. Candidiasis of the anogenital region and oral mucous membranes after the administration of broad spectrum antibiotics is a common example. This phenomenon is probably due to the suppression of natural competitors, thus allowing *Candida albicans* to multiply at an increased rate. Corticosteroids and immunosuppressive drugs may also favour the multiplication of candida.

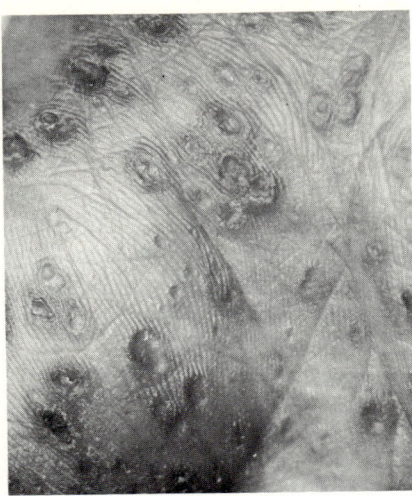

Figure 23.1 *Palmar arsenical keratosis*

Exacerbation of existing or latent disease

Certain drugs may activate existing or latent systemic disease. Administration of barbiturates or oral contraceptives may worsen acute intermittent porphyria, or precipitate attacks in subjects with latent porphyria. A Jarisch–Herxheimer reaction may be provoked if a patient with early syphilis is treated with penicillin. Psoriatic patients are often sensitive to antimalarial drugs, which may provoke a widespread pustular eruption with exfoliation.

Hypersensitivity

Hypersensitivity reactions develop from an allergic sensitization to a drug. This results from previous exposure to that drug or to a chemically related substance. Some of these reactions result in tissue damage.

The size of the molecule has considerable influence on the ability of a drug to induce antibody response. Most drugs, due to the small size of their molecule, are incomplete antigens. They, or their degradation products, must therefore act as haptens by combining usually covalently, with a larger molecule before they can become immunogenic. The role of this carrier molecule is assumed to be played by autologous proteins. The modified protein which results from this combination is treated as a foreign protein or antigen, and therefore antibody formation occurs.

Research into drug allergy has been concentrated mainly on penicillin, and the haptenic determinants of most other drugs have not been determined. The penicillins contain a number of haptenic determinants with high sensitizing potential. The major haptenic determinant in penicillin allergy is the penicilloyl group. Penicillin also contains several other antigens, collectively referred to as the

333

minor determinants. These include penicillin breakdown products and protein impurities.

Tissue damaging reactions from hypersensitivity to drugs are classified into four types:

(1) *Type I* reactions correspond to immediate type hypersensitivity. The main antibody involved is IgE. Patients with type I skin reactions to penicillin have markedly raised serum IgE levels. Clinically, type I skin reactions are manifest as acute anaphylaxis and urticaria.

(2) *Type II* reactions are cytotoxic and are brought about by antibody reacting with antigens on the surface of cells and fixing complement. Acute haemolytic anaemia and allergic thrombocytopenic purpura are due to this mechanism. The antibodies in this type of reaction are IgG and IgM.

(3) *Type III* reactions are the result of deposition of antigen–antibody complexes within the blood vessels or in the extravascular compartments of the capillary bed. The symptoms and signs depend on the organs that are involved. The kidneys and skin are the most commonly affected. The classic cutaneous manifestation of the type III reaction is the Arthus reaction. The lesions show vasculitis and haemorrhagic necrosis. Serum sickness is a systemic allergic reaction produced by circulating immune complexes. It is characterized by fever, rash, arthritis, lymphadenopathy, nephritis and oedema. Urticarial and maculopapular eruptions are particularly common. Many cases of drug sensitivity, in particular penicillin and sulphonamides, are examples of this type of reaction. Symptoms develop after a latent period of about six days or more, according to the time of maximal complement formation.

(4) *Type IV* reactions are those of delayed type hypersensitivity. This is cell mediated immunity; the initial sensitization takes ten to 14 days and the reaction then develops 24–48 hours after subsequent exposure to the allergen. Clinically delayed type hypersensitivity is most commonly manifest as contact eczema, and most exanthematous eruptions are thought to be due to this type of hypersensitivity.

Hypersensitivity to drugs is influenced by dosage and duration of administration. However, minute doses may elicit severe, even fatal, reactions in a sensitized subject. Allergic reactions to drugs seem to be less common in children, and this may be due to less previous exposure or to a less vigorous antibody response. Hypersensitivity does not appear to be greatly influenced by the route of administration of the drug.

Cross-sensitization occurs when allergic symptoms induced by one compound are subsequently produced in the same patient by one or more related substances. A knowledge of cross-sensitization is important, for the inadvertent substitution of secondary allergen may result in a severe reaction.

Clinical features

The clinical manifestations of drug eruptions are so varied that it is seldom possible to incriminate any one drug. Occasionally the eruption is pathognomonic. Carbromal, for example, produces small, irregular patches of punctate purpura (*Plate 23.1*), followed by brownish-red haemosiderin pigmentation and branny scaling. Identical eruptions may be seen from completely unrelated drugs, and different types of eruption may be seen with any one drug. Fever, lymphadenopathy and mucosal involvement may occur. Other tissues or organs may also be affected, leading to blood dyscrasias, hepatitis and nephritis.

In this chapter several of the more important cutaneous drug reactions are described. However, even the most comprehensive of reviews can provide no more than a rough guide to the diagnosis of drug eruptions.

Exanthematic eruptions

Exanthematic eruptions are the most frequent cutaneous reactions to drugs, and can vary greatly in their clinical features. The rash may simulate scarlatina or measles, or it may consist of a profuse eruption of small papules bearing no resemblance to an infective exanthem. Rarely does the type of eruption clearly indicate a particular offending drug.

The drugs that most commonly cause exanthematic eruptions are:

penicillin and related antibiotics,
sulphonamides,
phenylbutazone,
gold,
para-aminosalicylic acid,
allopurinol.

Less common causative agents include: isoniazid, barbiturates, phenothiazines and atropine,

Urticaria

Urticaria is probably the second most common cutaneous reaction to drugs. Drug-induced urticaria may be allergic or non-allergic.

Allergic urticaria may result from an immediate type of allergy and sometimes accompanies a severe anaphylactic reaction. Urticaria is particularly common in the serum-sickness syndrome.

Non-allergic urticaria results from drugs such as aspirin and morphine, which act as histamine liberators. Patients suffering from chronic idiopathic urticaria are often made worse by aspirin, which is capable of inducing both allergic and non-allergic urticaria.

Penicillin present in milk and dairy products may cause chronic urticaria. Drug and diet challenge tests have recently been formulated for investigating urticaria. The test substances include tartrazine, sodium benzoate, penicillin, acetylsalicylic acid and yeast extract.

The drugs that most commonly produce urticaria are:

penicillin,
salicylates,
sulphonamides,
codeine.

Purpura

Purpura induced by drugs may be thrombocytopenic or non-thrombocytopenic. Several drugs may produce both types, and allergic or toxic mechanisms may be involved with either type.

Thrombocytopenic purpura

Drugs causing thrombocytopenic purpura include a wide range, notably:

sedormid, which has been the subject of much research,
quinine,
aspirin,
para-aminosalicylic acid,
chlorothiazide and hydrochlorothiazide,
sulphonamides, and
cytostatics.

In *allergic thrombocytopenic purpura* the drug acts as a hapten, combining with the platelets and rendering them autoantigenic. When antibody is formed, the platelets combined with the drug react with it. The platelets agglutinate and, in the presence of complement, undergo lysis. *In vitro* tests for the investigation of drug-induced platelet lysis include the platelet agglutination test and the inhibition of clot retraction. Any drug which has a toxic effect on the bone marrow can cause thrombocytopenic purpura. Often other blood elements are affected similarly. Cytostatic drugs produce this type of reaction.

Non-thrombocytopenic purpura

A large number of drugs are capable of causing capillary damage, with or without any change in platelets. Sometimes the purpura is accompanied by obvious inflammatory lesions. Drugs which may produce capillary damage include:

carbromal,
acetylsalicylic acid,
sulphonamides,
barbiturates,
gold salts,
phenylbutazone,
quinine,
quinidine, and
meprobamate.

Carbromal produces a distinctive clinical picture. Rarely patch testing with a solution of carbromal induces local purpura.

Corticosteroid purpura

Corticosteroid purpura is due to the lack of support of the blood vessels associated with changes in the surrounding connective tissues. It occurs mainly on the forearms, hands and legs, following minor trauma, though occasionally it occurs spontaneously. The lesions vary considerably in size and shape and are usually symptomless. They show little in the way of inflammatory reactions.

Tartrazine and other food additives may also cause purpura, while the disease for which a drug has been given may be the cause of the eruption.

Eczematous eruptions

An eczematous eruption may develop in a patient already sensitized by external exposure to a particular drug or a chemically related substance. The eruption usually starts shortly after administration of the drug, and it may involve the sites affected by the original contact eczema. Continued administration may lead to a generalized eruption.

The more important causes of eczematous drug eruptions are:

penicillin,
sulphonamides,
neomycin,
phenothiazines,
antihistamines,
chlorothiazide and hydrochlorothiazide,
tolbutamide and chlorpropamide,
idodine, and
quinine.

Cross sensitivity may also result in eczematous eruptions. The para-amino group is a common sensitizer found in a large number of chemicals used externally, and in such drugs as local anaesthetics, sulphonamides, tolbutamide, and thiazide diuretics. Patch testing with the offending drug will often give a positive result.

Exfoliative dermatitis

Exfoliative dermatitis is one of the most serious cutaneous reactions to drugs. It may follow exanthematic eruptions or it may develop spontaneously. It usually starts weeks or even longer after commencing the drug, with a diffuse erythema spreading over the whole body, followed by exfoliation. In a severe reaction, generalized lymphadenopathy may occur. An eczematous eruption in patients previously sensitized by contact may also become generalized.

The drugs which most frequently cause exfoliative dermatitis are:

phenylbutazone and oxyphenbutazone,
gold salts,
organic arsenicals,
para-aminosalicylic acid,
hydantoin derivatives,
isoniazid, and
streptomycin.

Fixed drug eruptions occur at the same site or sites each time the offending drug is administered. The lesion is sharply demarcated, (*Figure 23.2*), circular or oval in shape, and occurs within hours of taking the drug. At first the colour is dusky red, later becoming violaceous or brown. The affected area may be oedematous and sometimes a large bulla develops. The lesion may be solitary at first, but with repeated attacks new lesions usually appear. The lesions occur most frequently on the trunk and proximal limbs, but the glans penis is a common site. Local or systemic symptoms are mild or absent. The eruption lasts for two or three days and healing takes place with pigmentation, which increases with subsequent attacks.

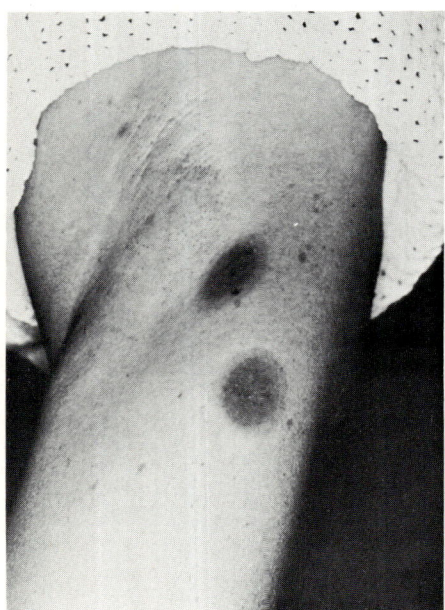

Figure 23.2   *Fixed drug eruption*

Many drugs have been reported to produce a fixed eruption, the most frequently incriminated being:

phenolphthalein, which is present in a large number of proprietary
    laxatives,
barbiturates,
oxyphenbutazone,

phenazone,
sulphonamides,
dapsone,
tetracyclines, and
chlordiazepoxide.

Colouring agents in foods, toothpastes and drug capsules may cause the eruption. Cross reactions to related and totally different types of drugs have been found. Readministration of the drug would provide a dependable test, but this cannot be recommended as a routine, for extensive bullous reactions sometimes occur. Occasionally patch testing on a quiescent area will give a positive result.

Lichenoid eruptions

Many drugs may produce an eruption which is indistinguishable from or very similar to lichen planus. The mechanism for its production is unknown. Often the histological picture is identical, though in some instances there is a moderate degree of parakeratosis or an admixture of eosinophils in the cellular infiltrate, neither of which is encountered in lichen planus. Lichenoid eruptions may mimic exactly the idiopathic condition, or they may show atypical features, such as marked scaling, eczematization, hypertrophic lesions and a tendency to a more intense residual pigmentation. Mucous membranes may be involved but are frequently spared. If hair loss occurs it may be severe and permanent.

The commonest drugs to cause lichenoid eruptions are:

quinine,
mepacrine,
chloroquine,
quinidine,
hydrochlorthiazide,
chlorothiazide,
gold, and
para-aminosalicylic acid.

Discontinuation of the drug usually leads to clinical improvement.

Bullous eruptions

Almost any eruption, when sufficiently severe, may produce vesicles and bullae. However, certain drugs may characteristically produce tense, thick-walled bullae, often few in number. This is particularly so with barbiturates, iodine and bromide reactions, and sulphonamides. Phenolphthalein tends to produce a fixed bullous eruption, and nalidixic acid a bullous photoreaction (*Plate 23.2*).

Drug-induced coma may be followed by bullae which occur at sites of pressure or trauma. This phenomenon is well recognized after barbiturate coma but it also occurs with several other drugs.

In severe erythema multiforme the centre of the target lesion may become bullous. In addition, bullae, usually haemorrhagic, appear on the mucosal surfaces.

Toxic epidermal necrolysis (Lyell's syndrome) (*Plates 23.3* and *23.4*)

This is a more serious condition. The illness is preceded by fever and toxaemia. Extensive areas of erythema resembling scalds develop into large flaccid bullae. Large areas of epidermis peel off, leaving an exudative, raw surface.

The drugs that cause toxic epidermal necrolysis are much the same as those that cause erythema multiforme. The drugs most commonly implicated in either condition are:

phenylbutazone,
sulphonamides,
sulphonyl-ureas,
barbiturates,
hydantoins, and
penicillin.

Drug-induced and staphylococcal-induced toxic epidermal necrolysis may sometimes be differentiated on histological grounds. In staphylococcal-induced cases epidermal cleavage will be seen in the granular layer of the epidermis, while in drug-induced cases there is a subepidermal split.

Acneiform eruptions

Certain drugs may aggravate existing acne or induce an acneiform eruption. Lesions are papulopustular but comedones are usually absent.

ACTH and corticosteroids induce acneiform eruptions after puberty. The papules are most numerous on the forehead and chin. Hyperplasia of sebaceous glands on the neck may give rise to so-called 'stippled skin'.

Tuberculostatic drugs such as isoniazid, ethionamide and ethambutol give rise to an eruption very similar to corticosteroid acne. This may spread to the whole trunk and buttocks.

Halogens may provoke an eruption similar in distribution to acne vulgaris. This usually occurs after prolonged administration and is acute in onset, with an active inflammatory reaction.

Anti-epileptic drugs such as phenobarbitone, hydantoins and trimethadione may induce an acneiform eruption or aggravate existing acne vulgaris. These drugs are thought to increase surface lipids, and a central mechanism is postulated.

Alopecia

Many drugs cause partial or complete loss of hair. The mode of action is uncertain, though it is known that antimitotic agents interfere with hair growth in the anagen or proliferative phase. Alopecia due to antimitotic agents begins shortly after administration but may not be noted for several weeks. The effect is dose dependent. When treatment is stopped the hair resumes its growth.

Hair loss due to antithyroid drugs is mainly localized to the scalp. These drugs include iodine, thiouracil and carbimazole. Loss of hair may occur due to hypothyroidism resulting from over-treatment. However, most patients with hair loss from antithyroid drugs are euthyroid.

All the anticoagulants are capable of inducing hair loss. With normal therapeutic doses this does not amount to obvious alopecia in most patients, unless higher doses are given. The scalp hair is mainly affected, though eyebrows, axillary and pubic regions may also be involved. There is usually a latent period of two to three months before diffuse alopecia begins.

Drug-induced changes in pigmentation

Drugs commonly produce increased pigmentation in the skin and its appendages, though they may also cause diminished pigmentation. Several different mechanisms are involved. Heavy metals are deposited diffusely in the dermis, bringing about a change in colour as a result of optical changes in the refraction and scattering of incident light. Some elements, such as arsenic, cause colour changes by altering melanin deposition. Other drugs, such as dapsone, produce changes by combining with haemoglobin to form methaemoglobin.

The commonest drugs causing pigmentary changes are:

metals: arsenic, silver, gold, bismuth, mercury,
antimalarials,
hydantoin derivatives,
cytostatic agents,
hormones: oral contraceptives, ACTH,
phenothiazines.

Inorganic arsenic was used in the past for many conditions, including psoriasis. It is still found in some 'tonics'. Occupational exposure occurs and water supplies may be contaminated. Prolonged ingestion of inorganic arsenic may result in a diffuse macular pigmentation, most pronounced on the trunk, where it may produce the well-known 'rain-drop' appearance. Argyria results from the deposition of silver in the dermis and in the mucous membranes. The continued application of silver salts to mucous membranes may result in sufficient being absorbed to produce side effects. The changes are first seen in the mouth as a diffuse slate-grey pigmentation of the gingiva and oral mucosa. The skin assumes a bluish-grey colour with accentuation on exposed areas. Prolonged administration of gold may result in a permanent, diffuse, blue-grey pigmentation on exposed areas.

Changes in skin pigmentation occur in about 25 per cent of patients receiving any of the antimalarials for periods of more than three or four months. When high doses of mepacrine are used in the prophylaxis of malaria, a generalized intense yellow discoloration of the skin occurs. Localized blue-black pigmentation may affect the pretibial areas, the face, hard palate and subungal regions, and may be produced by any of the antimalarials. All patients receiving antimalarials who develop pigmentation should undergo ophthalmological examination to exclude corneal deposits and retinal damage. Bleaching of the hair may occur after two to three months of chloroquine therapy. Only blonde, light brown and red-haired people are affected, and it is reversible on withdrawing the drug.

At least 10 per cent of patients receiving hydantoin derivatives develop pigmentation of the face resembling chloasma. Contributory factors include solar radiation and the individual ability of the skin to produce pigment.

Busulphan may produce a diffuse brown pigmentation of the face, forearms, chest and abdomen, particularly in patients with a dark complexion. Occasionally Addison's disease is simulated. Cyclophosphamide may produce melanosis of the finger and toe nails.

Oral contraceptives may produce chloasma, particularly in women who have developed such pigmentation in pregnancy. The incidence of chloasma increases with the length of time that the oral contraceptive is taken. Men taking oestrogens for prostatic carcinoma may develop nipple pigmentation. The mechanism of 'pill' chloasma is uncertain, but both oestrogen and progesterone are necessary to produce it. In contrast to the chloasma of pregnancy, that resulting from oral contraceptives fades slowly on cessation of the drug and is sometimes permanent. ACTH may produce pigmentation of an Addisonian pattern.

The prolonged use of chlorpromazine in large doses may produce progressive pigmentation, beginning with a tan or golden-brown colour in the summer months, mainly on exposed areas, followed by a slate-grey or bluish and later purplish appearance. When the drug is withdrawn, the pigmentation fades slowly, if at all. The related drug phenothiazine may also cause pigmentation.

Drug-induced photosensitivity

Photosensitivity is an abnormal reaction of the skin to light. The term includes phototoxicity, and nearly all drugs producing photoallergic reactions are also phototoxic.

Phototoxic reactions are dose dependent, both for the drug and sunlight, and the appearance is that of an intense sunburn reaction. It may occur on first exposure to the drug. A high incidence of phototoxic reactions is associated with demethylchlortetracycline. Occasionally a photo-onycholysis develops.

Photoallergic reactions, in common with other allergies, have a delay from first exposure to onset of the reaction. Flare-ups may occur at unexposed sites. After discontinuation of the drug the reaction tends to regress slowly. The majority of photoallergic reactions are due to external agents, which may be met in cosmetics and soaps.

The drugs that most commonly cause photosensitive reactions are:

tetracyclines,
phenothiazines,
chlorothiazide and hydrochlorothiazide, (*Plate 23.5*)
nalidixic acid (*Plate 23.2*),
sulphonamides and sulphonyl ureas.

Vascular reactions

Erythema nodosum

Erythema nodosum is most commonly caused by tuberculosis, streptococcal infection or sarcoidosis. Drug-induced erythema nodosum is rare and should only be suspected when all other possible causes have been excluded. Few drugs, except sulphonamides, have sufficient claim to be incriminated.

Polyarteritis nodosa

Although polyarteritis nodosa and other arteritic lesions appear to have followed the administration of a large number of drugs, there is no real proof of this; expected remission seldom follows withdrawal of the suspected drug.

Drug-induced systemic lupus erythematosus (SLE)

Syndromes indistinguishable from SLE have been reported following the administration of a large number of drugs, the commonest of which are:

hydrallazine,
isoniazid
phenytoin,
procainamide.

The cause of drug-induced SLE is unknown, but some patients have a genetic predisposition. In the majority of cases it is indistinguishable from spontaneously occurring SLE, though fever and renal involvement may be less common. Laboratory findings show LE cells, antinuclear and antinucleoprotein antibodies. Leucopenia and thrombocytopenia occur infrequently, and occasionally false positive serological tests for syphilis are found.

The disease is usually reversible on stopping the offending drug, although some cases of hydrallazine-induced SLE have had rather prolonged courses.

Selected drugs with more specific reactions

Ampicillin

Two main groups of rashes occur in the course of ampicillin therapy.

Firstly, a hypersensitivity rash, which is urticarial and similar to the rash associated with true penicillin hypersensitivity, may appear soon after the onset of treatment, or may be delayed for as long as three weeks. Anaphylactic reactions to ampicillin have only rarely been reported.

Secondly, and much more commonly, a rash specific to ampicillin may occur. Patients affected in this way need not necessarily be regarded as sensitive to other penicillins, which they may tolerate subsequently without ill effect. The typical ampicillin rash may appear on the first day of treatment, but is usually seen after five to 14 days. It is often first noticed after the ampicillin has been stopped, and it may continue to spread and become florid. The rash usually starts on the extensor aspects of the limbs, particularly on the bony prominences of the elbows and knees, spreading symmetrically to most parts of the body. It may be morbilliform or maculopapular before becoming confluent. Dull red at first, it may become haemorrhagic in severe cases, taking a week or more to subside before desquamating and staining. The mucous membranes may be involved. Itching is not a major symptom.

The cause of ampicillin rash is not known. Nearly all patients with infectious mononucleosis given ampicillin will show the rash (*Plate 23.6*), and a higher incidence has been reported in patients with cytomegalo virus mononucleosis and lymphatic leukaemia.

Practolol

Practolol is a selective beta-adrenoceptor blocking agent. It was withdrawn from general use because of severe side effects, including a characteristic rash, eye changes, impairment of hearing, sclerosing peritonitis, and an SLE syndrome.

The rash is often psoriasiform in character, most marked over the bony prominences, with guttate lesions on the trunk and erythematous macules with marginated scaling and gyrate patterns. There is hyperkeratosis of the palms, fingers and soles. Itching particularly affects the palms and soles. The rash develops slowly over several months and clears gradually on stopping the drug.

Diagnosis

Polypharmacy is very common, so that once a drug reaction has developed it is essential to enquire about all drugs that a patient is receiving. A detailed history should include the date on which each drug was first administered in relation to the onset of the eruption, whether the patient has taken the same or related drugs before, and if so, whether he has suffered a reaction. Often a patient may deny taking any drugs at all. Drugs popularly regarded as harmless, such as those bought without prescription, are often forgotten or not regarded as drugs. The history should include details of any chemical exposure at home or at work, and particulars of diet.

The timing of a drug reaction depends to a large extent on the mechanism, e.g. an anaphylactic reaction occurs within minutes of re-exposure to the drug. A reaction may not develop until after the drug has been stopped. Symptoms of serum sickness appear seven to ten days after the effective sensitizing dose. Long-acting depot preparations will modify the timing and duration of reaction. The effects of inorganic arsenic may not become apparent for many years.

In vivo tests

Discontinuation of the drug

Whenever a drug reaction is suspected, all therapy should, if possible be stopped. When a drug is essential for the patient, the commonest offenders should be withdrawn first. Disappearance of the reaction may be misleading; it may have been a naturally occurring self-limiting event unrelated to the drug. Slow excretion or depot preparations may cause prolonged reactions. Inadvertent substitution of the drug with one which is chemically related will result in the rash becoming progressive. Cross sensitization to chemicals in food and drink may complicate the situation. Penicillin may be present in sufficient quantity in milk and its products to sustain a hypersensitivity reaction.

Readministration

When a reaction has cleared, a test dose may reliably incriminate a drug. Fatal reactions to minimal amounts of a drug such as penicillin have been recorded. Readministration may be justified if a patient is dependent on a drug for which no chemically unrelated alternative is available, but all methods to combat an anaphylactic reaction should be at hand. Readministration will not always reproduce a drug reaction; hypersensitivity may disappear, or the test dose may be too small.

Skin tests

Skin tests are generally of limited value in the diagnosis of drug eruptions. A positive intradermal, scratch or prick test may merely indicate cutaneous hypersensitivity to the drug. A patient giving a positive skin test to the drug may tolerate its administration by other routes, while negative skin tests are often recorded in patients who have subsequently experienced systemic reactions. In view of the risk of severe, or even fatal reactions, intradermal testing should not be carried out in patients with a history of anaphylactic hypersensitivity. The use of skin tests is further limited by lack of knowledge of the actual allergen.

Intradermal tests

Knowledge of the antigenic determinants of penicillin has led to the development of skin tests of increasing reliability. Penicilloyl-polylysine, which is a conjugated form of the penicilloyl group, has been found to be most suitable for skin testing. The antigenic specificities of the skin-sensitizing antibodies in patients with immediate type reaction may not be due only to the penicilloyl group, and the minor antigenic determinants should also be tested. In practice, penicilloyl-polylysine is usually tested first; if negative, benzylpenicillin is tried. To avoid dangerous reactions it is safer to perform prick tests first, and if these are negative the agents are injected intradermally. Interpretation of the results may be difficult; though current intradermal tests for penicillin sensitivity show promising results, they are far from being routine procedure.

Passive transfer tests

Passive transfer tests involve the injection of reaginic serum into the skin of a normal subject. Reaginic antibody has a high affinity for human skin. Subsequent challenge of skin by drug antigen in skin injected with specifically sensitized serum produces a weal and flare reaction. This test, which forms the basis of the Prausnitz–Kustner reaction, is limited by the risk of developing serum hepatitis.

Patch tests

Patch tests are of limited value in the diagnosis of drug hypersensitivity, though they are useful in the diagnosis of allergic contact eczema. They may reveal the sensitizer, and establish the range of cross sensitivity in patients with an eczematous eruption provoked by drugs to which they have been previously sensitized by epidermal contact. Application of a drug to the skin involves a much greater risk of sensitization than if the drug is given systemically. This is particularly so with highly sensitizing drugs such as penicillin and chlorpromazine.

In vitro tests

Owing to the potential dangers of skin testing, extensive research has been done on laboratory tests, most of which concern drug hypersensitivity, with particular reference to penicillin.

Blood and tissue drug levels

Quantitative toxicological studies are of use in the diagnosis of overdose, but are not helpful in hypersensitivity tests, as the blood and tissue levels of a drug are not usually in the toxic range.

General investigations

A full blood count should be performed to exclude any blood dyscrasia. Eosinophilia may suggest that an eruption is due to a drug, but it is a non-specific and inconsistent finding.

Histopathology

In most drug eruptions the histological changes are non-specific and will only be indicative of the clinical features, e.g. urticaria and erythema multiforme. Bromides and iodides may cause pseudoepitheliomatous hyperplasia. In lichenified eruptions the changes may closely resemble those of idiopathic lichen planus, though the cellular infiltrate tends to be pleomorphic and less dense.

Detection of reaginic antibodies (IgE)

In vitro tests for measuring reaginic antibodies present practical difficulties and often conflicting results. Most of the methods are costly, requiring laboratory animals and sophisticated techniques, and they are therefore not suitable for use in every hospital.

Treatment of drug eruptions

Once diagnosed, the majority of mild drug eruptions subside rapidly when the drug is stopped. The decision whether or not to continue a drug suspected of causing a reaction will depend on availability of chemically unrelated drugs with similar pharmacological properties.

The natural duration of hypersensitivity varies from a few days to several years, so that apparently successful hyposensitization is difficult to evaluate. The procedure of hyposensitization usually consists of the administration, at short intervals, of initially minute but gradually increasing doses. In view of the risks involved, hyposensitization should only be carried out if the offending drug is essential for the patient's life or health. Adequate precautions should be taken to deal with anaphylactic reactions.

Large doses of antihistamines may be needed to control urticaria. A severe reaction may necessitate the use of systemic corticosteroids. Smaller doses of antihistamines may relieve itching in other types of drug eruptions, but do little to alter the course and duration. When choosing a drug for treatment of a reaction it is important that this drug is not chemically related to the offending agent. For example, an antihistamine of phenothiazine structure must not be prescribed to patients with a reaction induced by chlorpromazine.

The individual reactions described above are treated with both topical and systemic therapy, depending on their severity.

24 The photodermatoses

W. Frain-Bell

The action of light is important in the assessment and treatment of a number of conditions, some of which will involve systems additional to that of the skin. Growth in childhood, certain body rhythms and normal endocrine function are all dependent to some extent on regular exposure to daylight. Adequate amounts of ultraviolet radiation (UVR) are necessary for the production of vitamin D in the skin and thus for normal bone metabolism. There are risks therefore in any situation which leads to a change in environmental light. Such a change occurs when racially pigmented individuals move to a part of the world where the amounts of UVR are less than that to which they are accustomed, as in the case of the UK immigrant from the Indian subcontinent; inadequate amounts of vitamin D may then be produced in such a skin. A similar problem will arise in the housebound or institutionalized elderly, and in those whose occupation require long periods away from daylight. It may be also that the choice of artificial lighting should be based to a greater extent on the mix of wavelengths of the solar spectrum rather than simply that which is best for reading and working. The presence of the ozone layer in the upper atmosphere prevents damaging short wavelength UVR reaching the earth. It is also therefore important to control the amounts of propellent gases derived from aerosol sprays, from the exhaust gases of high flying aircraft, and from those produced by agricultural fertilizers, all of which may diminish this protective layer. It is surprising that although light is necessary for the preservation of life, cellular DNA should be so easily damaged by UVR. It is fortunate however that human skin cells have built-in methods of repair which quickly reverse this ultraviolet induced damage. These repair mechanisms are dependent on the presence of enzymes and when these are deficient those cells which are not killed outright by UVR develop mutagenic changes which in time will lead to malignant growths. Such an outcome is seen in xeroderma pigmentosum where, as a result of an inherited defect of enzyme activity involved in the mechanism of repair, skin malignancy develops in early life. The main protective mechanism in the human skin against the undesirable effects of UVR is the production of melanin pigmentation and the thickening of the epidermis. Melanin has the ability to absorb and scatter UVR and by its presence throughout the epidermal cell layer it helps to protect the actively growing basal layer of cells and the deeper structures. Following exposure to light, an immediate pigmentation develops as a result of oxidation of bleached melanin and this is due mainly to the longer wavelengths of ultraviolet light (UV-A) and to some extent to visible light (*Figure 24.1*). A later developing delayed pigmentation which appears some days after exposure, and which is mainly due to the shorter ultraviolet wavelengths (UV-B), results from the formation of new melanin and plays the major role, along with thickening of the epidermis, in protecting the skin from subsequent exposure to UVR. Any impairment in the production of this protective melanin pigmentation will lead to premature ageing and premalignant and malignant changes in the skin. The absence of melanin pigmentation, for example in albinism, is particularly serious, and also, but to a less extent, in the red haired fair complexioned Celt especially if the latter moves away from the northern hemisphere. The ease and availability of world-wide travel and increasing leisure and affluence means that the skin of the white Caucasian races will have to adapt to increasing ultraviolet exposure. For the foreseeable future however light-induced damage of the skin will remain a problem. It must also be appreciated that as life becomes more sophisticated there is exposure to an increasing number of substances which, on reaching the skin by direct contact or by ingestion, have the ability to absorb wavelengths from various parts of the solar spectrum, as a result of which some individuals become 'photosensitive'. For reasons which are poorly understood, the subsequent ability to react abnormally to light may persist for months and even years after apparent contact with the responsible photoactive substance has ceased.

Clinical features

The diagnosis of photosensitivity

The possibility that the skin is reacting to light should be suspected if there is a history of an eruption which, following exposure to the sun, appears on the uncovered skin only and varies in severity with the amount of exposure. An example of this would be normal sunburn erythema. A similar history and distribution of the skin reaction can occur also in those who, for a variety of reasons, are abnormally light sensitive. However, the history of abnormal light sensitivity may be less clear-cut (*see Table 24.1*) and particularly if the responsible wavelengths are present at times of the year outside the sunshine season, i.e. where the action spectrum of the eruption is broad and involves both the ultraviolet and visible light (*Figure 24.1*). In the normal subject sunburn occurs at the season of the year when there is likely to be exposure to increased amounts of short wavelength ultraviolet (UV-B), i.e. on bright sunny days with clear blue skies. In the abnormally light sensitive individual the eruption will be

Table 24.1   Some reasons why a clinical diagnosis of
photosensitivity may be missed

---

(1) *The eruption is usually but not always confined to the sunshine months.*
The subject may be sensitive to a broad spectrum of light which is
present throughout the year, and also therefore to irradiation from
indoor lighting of Tungsten or fluorescent type.
In light sensitivity dermatitis the reaction of the skin may be due to
factors additional to the photosensitivity and thus the response may be
present in some subjects both during and outside the sunshine season.

(2) *The eruption is usually but not always confined to the exposed skin.*
The skin covered by clothing may react to light passing through thin
fabrics.
The covered skin may be affected as part of the spread from the primary
eruption on exposed sites, a feature which is common to various
dermatoses whether light induced or not.
For reasons which are obscure, certain exposed areas fail to react, e.g.
the skin of the face in some female subjects with polymorphic light
eruption.

(3) *The subject denies any relationship between the eruption and exposure
to the sun.*
A reaction of the skin to light is usually denied in those subjects with a
broad action spectrum (i.e. ultraviolet and visible light) and in those
with aetiological factors additional to the photosensitivity.
Also, blistering and fragility of the skin in hepatic porphyria is rarely
linked by the patient to the exposure to light, whereas in
erythropoietic protoporphyria the complaint is often of severe
discomfort following exposure of the skin to sunlight.

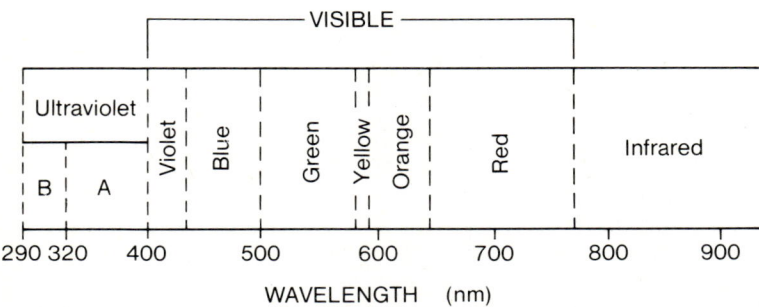

Figure 24.1   *Wavelengths—ultraviolet and visible light*

confined to this same sunshine season if in fact the action spectrum
is mainly in the UV-B and/or UV-A wavebands. If however visible
light wavelengths are involved then the skin reaction may persist all
the year round with or without apparent seasonal aggravation. Such
an affected individual will often discount any relationship between
the skin condition and exposure to light. Also, the eruption in the
abnormal light sensitive person may not always be confined to

uncovered skin and can appear on the covered areas since some fabrics will allow penetration of the responsible wavelengths. The eruption can also appear on covered sites due to factors other than the photosensitivity (*see* p. 354).

The morphological changes resulting from an abnormal reaction to light are of some diagnostic assistance, but since the skin is limited in its patterns of reaction these changes are not in themselves diagnostic, similar ones occurring in other dermatoses where light sensitivity is absent. However, certain of these skin changes are to be found more often in some of the photodermatoses than in others, and a recognition of these along with an appropriate history and distribution can be helpful in arriving at a correct diagnosis.

Photodermatoses

Photodermatoses is the term used to cover reactions of the skin in which an abnormal response to light plays some part. The term '*photosensitivity*' is used to indicate that the skin will react to light in a way that differs from normal. This term can therefore be applied to an individual who sunburns more easily on account of a fair complexion, or to one whose skin reacts because of the presence of a photoactive substance as in a light induced drug eruption or to those with idiopathic long-term photosensitivity, an example of which is polymorphic light eruption. The involvement of immunological pathways allows for the use of the term '*photoallergy*' in the same way as contact allergic dermatitis is used where a dermatitis response is due to a specific contact allergen. The term '*phototoxic*' reaction is used to indicate a reaction of the skin to light in the presence of a photoactive substance, the reaction depending on non-immunological mechanisms.

This phototoxic reaction is analogous to that occurring in contact irritant dermatitis where immunological mechanisms are also not involved. *Photocontact dermatitis* is used to describe a reaction of the skin following external contact with a substance which then combines with appropriate wavelengths of the solar spectrum to produce a reaction which may be of either photoallergic or phototoxic type. A *light induced drug eruption* describes a reaction where the presence in the skin of a therapeutically administered substance leads to a photosensitivity response.

Table 24.2 lists the various photodermatoses. Polymorphic light eruption is the commonest cutaneous photosensitivity reaction seen in the female and photosensitivity dermatitis commonest in the male. The reaction of the skin to light in the presence of a photoactive substance may occur from external contact with this substance (photocontact dermatitis), or following ingestion (light induced drug eruption), or from accumulations in the skin of excessive amounts of a metabolic product as in porphyria. Of the *non-light sensitive dermatoses* in which light plays some part, lupus erythematosus is probably the one which merits most consideration, otherwise this

Table 24.2   The photodermatoses

Polymorphic light eruption
Actinic prurigo
Solar urticaria
Hydroa vacciniforme

Photosensitivity dermatitis
Actinic reticuloid

Due to a photoactive substance
Photocontact dermatitis
Light induced drug eruption
Metabolic disease—porphyria

Effect of light on other dermatoses
Lupus erythematosus
Dermatomyositis
Eczema
Psoriasis
Lichen planus
Lymphocytoma

Darier's disease
Pemphigus
Acne aestivale
Juvenile spring eruption
Lymphocytic infiltration of lessner
Pellagra

Rare developmental abnormalities
Bloom's syndrome
Rothmund Thomson syndrome
Cockayne's syndrome
Hartnup's disease
Phenylketonuria
Xeroderma pigmentosum

group is relatively less important. The syndromes based on inherited *developmental abnormalities* affecting usually a number of body systems, are important despite their rarity in that a study of the cutaneous photosensitivity has led in some to a better understanding of the basic abnormal processes involved. This has been particularly so in xeroderma pigmentosum.

Polymorphic light eruption

This commonly affects females of any age, not infrequently starting in childhood and often lasting for many years. There tends to be a familial factor and a possible association with atopy. It consists of an erythematous reaction which at the start is usually that of numerous small irritating papules which in many instances become confluent forming variable oedematous erythema in which there may be an urticarial element. The sites affected are those of uncovered skin such as back of the hands, arms and legs, the neck, particularly the anterior 'V'; the face and other exposed sites may sometimes be spared and the reason for this is as yet to be satisfactorily explained.

The skin of covered sites can react similarly as a result of the penetration of thin fabrics by the responsible wavelengths. It is usual for the eruption to occur at any time during the sunshine months in direct relationship to the amount of exposure. In some individuals however the tendency of the skin to react becomes less as the summer season progresses and some form of unexplained 'desensitization' or tolerance appears to occur in this instance (*see* p 363). Occasionally the eruption will disappear for a period of years if there is a continuous exposure to increased amounts of sunshine. In some subjects in addition to the erythematous response more persistent lesions develop in the form of variable sized papules and nodules and lichenified plaques. To this has been applied the term '*actinic prurigo*' (*Plate 24.1*). Views differ as to whether actinic prurigo should be separated from polymorphic light eruption or not. The term 'actinic prurigo' is thus used to indicate cutaneous photosensitivity in which changes seen in the skin are more those of a pruriginous lichenified reaction, often with solar cheilitis, with a tendency to affect covered as well as exposed skin, although clinical photosensitivity is rarely in doubt. It usually is first seen in childhood going on into adult life with a tendency to clear up in the late teens or early twenties. A familial factor may again be present, and particularly so in countries such as South America. It would seem reasonable in view of the lack of knowledge of the mechanisms involved in polymorphic light eruption to accept actinic prurigo as a separate 'clinical entity'. However, it should be remembered that in children the reaction of exposed skin to light can not infrequently contain small prurigo papules, vesicles, eczema, and even sometimes superficial pitted scarring, features which are rarely, if ever, seen in adults with polymorphic light eruption/actinic prurigo.

In both polymorphic light eruption and in actinic prurigo the responsible wavelengths are to be found in the short wavelength ultraviolet (UV-B) with sometimes a spread into the long wavelength UV (UV-A) and even into the visible light in a minority of subjects. It is not uncommon however to find a normal action spectrum for erythema on phototesting and this may be due to the technique of monochromator irradiation (*see* p. 361) failing to simulate the natural conditions of exposure to the solar spectrum. Lastly there is *hydroa vacciniforme* which on clinical grounds once again would appear to be an abnormal response of the skin to light in which the photosensitivity cannot be confirmed by the standard phototesting technique. In this reaction there is a vesiculo-bullous response affecting most often the skin of the face and back of hands leading on to a stage of heavy crusting and finally vacciniform scarring (*Plate 24.2*).

An urticarial weal is a not uncommon component of a photosensitivity reaction of the skin, particularly, but not exclusively, of the polymorphic light eruption type. When it occurs in this condition the immediate urticarial weal is soon lost in the subsequent delayed erythemato-papular response. More rarely the reaction to light is solely that of an urticarial weal and in this instance the term *solar urticaria* is used. The aetiology of this form of chronic urticaria is obscure but the responsible wavelengths tend to fall into certain well-defined parts of the solar spectrum which may, in the future, turn out to have aetiological significance. Repeated irradiation of the skin with appropriate wavelengths of light can result in a suppression of the urticarial response on subsequent exposure to sunlight. This is a similar effect to that obtained in the treatment of polymorphic light eruption. Both these conditions may however respond equally as well, if not better, to pre-seasonal psoralen photochemotherapy (*see* p 363).

Photosensitivity dermatitis

Photosensitivity dermatitis is the commonest presentation of photosensitivity in the male subject (*Plate 24.3*), the skin changes in this photodermatosis being different from those seen in the female with the PLE type of response to light. As the name implies, the morphological changes are those of a dermatitis often in a chronic lichenified form with, however, episodes of activity which may be partly eczematous and partly erythematous. Developing for the first time in adult life, it tends to be confined to the middle and elderly age groups and usually lasts for a number of years. Invariably affecting all exposed skin sites, it has certain distribution features which are of diagnostic help. These are involvement of the rim of the ear, the mastoid area of the neck, and also a straight line at the collar cut-off point; any reaction of the scalp being maximal at sites of constitutional baldness. The skin may also be affected from time to time on covered areas due to penetration of thin fabrics by the responsible wavelengths or as part of the natural history of the dermatitis and the involvement of factors other than photosensitivity. In its most severe form lymphoma-like changes may occur in the skin and the term *actinic reticuloid* is then used for this stage (*Plate 24.4.*).

It is probable that photosensitivity dermatitis is the chronic end stage of a response of the skin to a number of factors acting in association with the abnormal reaction to light. Sometimes a contact irritant or allergic dermatitis is present for months or years before the photosensitivity develops. The association of allergic sensitivity with certain members of the Compositae family of plants and weeds is an important factor and may provide a link between contact dermatitis and photosensitivity. Probably less often the same end point is reached when the dermatitis reaction is due to primary photosensitivity. The responsible wavelengths in most instances involve the short and long wavelength ultraviolet light and sometimes also those of the visible light. The short wavelength ultraviolet light sensitivity can be particularly severe in some subjects. When the action spectrum is broad, i.e. involving ultraviolet and visible wavelengths, and where there may be also exposure to contact allergens, the clinical diagnosis of photosensitivity can be missed by both patient and clinician on account of the affection of the skin being present all the year round and not simply during the sunshine months.

Photocontact dermatitis

Photocontact dermatitis is used to describe the response of the skin to contact with a substance which, following absorption, reacts with wavelengths of ultraviolet or visible light, appropriate to its structure. The subsequent reaction may make use of a phototoxic or photoallergic mechanism (*Figure 24.2*).

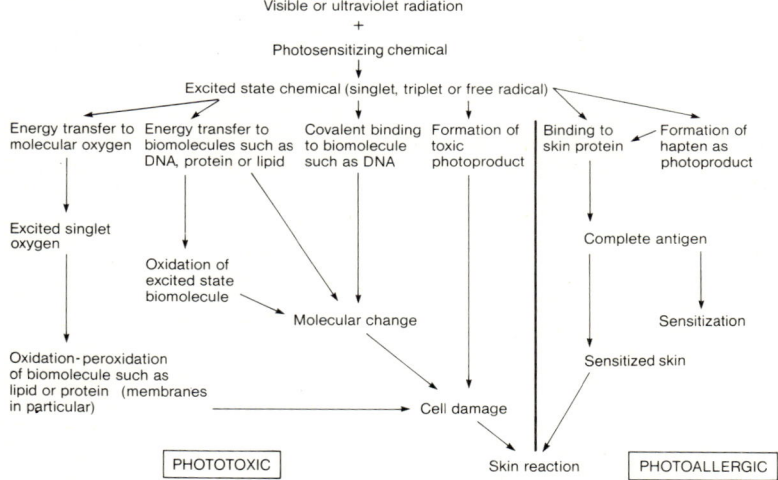

Figure 24.2 *Showing mechanism whereby ultraviolet radiation and chemical agents give rise to phototoxic and photoallergic skin reactions*

The phototoxic response produces changes in the skin which differ from those seen where an immunological mechanism is involved in that there is dusky erythema with or without a variable amount of oedema which may be of only two or three days' duration. The phototoxic response can also be in the form of a more marked erythema and oedema, sometimes with blistering which, as it subsides, leaves the skin dry and flaking and ultimately a variable amount of pigmentation which can persist for some time after the acute episode has passed. A psoralen is a substance which will produce such a phototoxic reaction. The psoralens are a group of substances which play an important role in cutaneous photobiology as illustrated by their use in the photochemotherapy treatment of psoriasis and other dermatoses. They are to be found in certain weeds and plants and as a constituent of perfumes and perfumed cosmetics. The presence of a psoralen (8-methoxypsoralen) in the relatively common weed, the Giant Hogweed, leads to the condition of phytophotodermatitis in those who come in contact with the leaves and stems of the plant and are at the same time exposed to long wavelength ultraviolet light of sunshine. This leads to a phototoxic reaction in the skin which presents in the form of an acute erythema, oedema, vesiculo-bullous lesions, and subsequently pigmentation (*Plate 24.5*). In horticulture the psoralen content of plants such as figs, and fungus infected celery may produce a response in workers similar to that seen in Giant Hogweed dermatitis. The presence of another psoralen, bergapten, (5-methoxypsoralen), in perfumes will produce a similar reaction which is however usually less severe, i.e. erythema followed by pigmentation and sometimes simply pigmentation without the prior development of erythema, a common presentation being that seen in poikiloderma of Civatte (*Plate 24.6*).

The photoallergic response, on the other hand, tends to be essentially a dermatitis reaction which may at some stage have elements of polymorphic erythema and urticaria. Confirmation of these two types of reactions can sometimes be obtained by photopatch testing. In some, the reaction is short-lived, lasting for a few weeks at the most, but in others a chronic dermatitis develops interspersed with episodes of increased activity. This state of 'persistent light reaction' leads to an end stage of a chronic skin response similar to that seen in the photosensitivity dermatitis and actinic reticuloid syndrome.

Certain theories have been proposed to explain the state of persistent light reaction but probably it can arise from more than one sequence of events. The possibilities are that:

(1) A 'photoallergic' reaction to a substance in the skin whereby the protein hapten conjugate formed in the presence of the appropriate wavelengths of light triggers off an immunological response. In some instances a photoproduct may be produced which then acts as a contact allergen leading to a cell mediated allergic response without the necessity for further exposure to light.

(2) Once the photosensitivity reaction has been set in motion the ability to react abnormally to light continues, making use of photobiological mechanisms as yet to be determined.

(3) The chronicity of the dermatitis is in part due to contact allergic sensitivity to certain allergens. Some of these may act both as contact and/or as photocontact allergens or as phototoxic agents.

It is probable therefore that the state of persistent light reaction as demonstrated in photosensitivity dermatitis is due to a range of factors which will vary from subject to subject.

It should also be appreciated that the responsible photoactive substance may reach the skin following ingestion and in this instance any of a number of commonly used drugs can be responsible and especially sulphonamides, sulphonylureas, thiazide diuretics, phenthothiazines (*see Plate 23.5*), tetracyclines, etc. In this instance the response is usually a phototoxic one.

As described in Chapter 23 an abnormal reaction of the skin to a therapeutically administered drug is often in the form of a bilateral symmetrical eruption. The *light-induced drug eruption* differs in that the skin reaction is confined, or is maximal, on the exposed skin. Although immunological mechanisms are sometimes involved, the commonest type of resulting reaction is a phototoxic one. A dusky erythema appears which is burning and irritable leading on to dryness and flaking of the skin and a variable amount of pigmentation which in some instances may be marked and persistent. This pigmentation can develop with minimal and sometimes apparently absent preceding erythema.

In the state of persistent light reaction already referred to the administration of one or other of these drugs may be a relevant factor but in most instances the phototoxic erythema reaction tends to be of relatively short duration providing the responsible drug is withdrawn or the dose reduced along with a reduction in exposure to light.

Bullous lesions appear in a variety of the photodermatoses, e.g. in hepatic porphyria and in hydroa vacciniforme. They are also to be seen in certain drug eruptions which are thought to be light induced. The administration of two such drugs has been associated with a bullous eruption of the exposed skin—nalidixic acid (*see Plate 23.2*) which is used as an antibacterial agent in the treatment of urinary tract infections and the diuretic frusemide. The bullous reaction with the latter is associated with renal failure and high doses of the drug and the relevance of exposure to light has yet to be fully evaluated. Similarly, the photobiological mechanisms involved in the pellagra type of pigmentation of exposed skin developing in some subjects receiving isoniazid remain to be more clearly defined. In the light induced phototoxic drug reaction the action spectrum found on phototesting involves the ultraviolet wavelengths and particularly the long wavelength ultraviolet (UV-A) and this latter involvement can be a useful diagnostic feature.

The porphyrias (*see also Chapter 16*)

In certain abnormalities of porphyrin metabolism excess amounts of porphyrins reach the skin. The structure of these porphyrins (i.e. uroporphyrin, coproporphyrin, protoporphyrin) as distinct from the precursors (delta-amino laevulinic acid and porphobilinogen) is such that they are able to absorb light from the 400 to 600 nm waveband (*Figure 24.1*). The photobiological reaction which results produces certain changes in the skin.

Excess amounts of formed porphyrins are present in the skin in hepatic porphyria, variegate porphyria, congenital porphyria, erythropoietic protoporphyria, and in hereditary coproporphyria, and therefore light induced skin changes will appear in all of these. On the other hand, the structure of the precursors (delta-amino

laevulinic acid and porphobilinogen) is such that they do not absorb
light and this accounts for the absence of photosensitivity in, for
example, acute intermittent porphyria. The symptoms and signs vary
with the type of porphyria. In hepatic porphyria, for example the
exposed skin of the face (including bald scalp) and back of hands,
develop blisters associated with fragility whereby minor trauma
leads to localized loss of surface skin which in time leads to superficial
scarring (*Plate 24.7*). This is associated with varying amounts of
abnormal pigmentation which on the face may be combined with
increased growth of hair. Rarely the degree of skin damage is such
that widespread sclerodermatous changes can develop. Since the
responsible wavelengths are not confined to the sunshine months
the subject is usually unaware of a connection between the skin
condition and exposure to light.

In comparison with hepatic porphyria, where the signs in the skin
are more marked than the symptoms, in erythropoietic protoporphyria the opposite occurs, i.e. the symptoms are more severe than the
signs. This holds true only for temperate climates since the severity
of skin changes in erythropoietic protoporphyria increases with the
amount of light exposure. The presentation of erythropoietic
protoporphyria in Britain is however usually that of a child
complaining bitterly of discomfort of exposed skin, the examination
of which shows only minimal changes. Most sufferers will have
discovered ways of reducing the discomfort and may spontaneously
describe the relief that cold running water brings. At the same time
as the discomfort is felt, the skin may appear to be swollen with
minimal colour change. In time chronic changes develop in the form
of multiple superficial and often thin linear scars of the skin of the
face (*Plate 24.8*) and back or hands, along with a characteristic
thickening with accentuated skin lines over the backs of the
knuckles. However, the condition can be much milder and therefore
go unsuspected into adult life.

Although each case will require the appropriate biochemical and
other tests, the clinical diagnosis can usually be confirmed by the
demonstration of a reaction of the skin on phototesting to the
waveband centred on 400 nm which is the peak of absorption of the
porphyrins.

Treatment of porphyria is directed towards the basic metabolic
abnormality and also to alleviation of the skin photosensitivity. In
hepatic porphyria the treatment of choice lies between repeated
venesection and chloroquine. The latter is safe and effective if given
in small doses of around 77.5 mg twice weekly for a number of months.
Following the demonstration that beta-carotene protects cells in
culture against the damaging combination of haematoporphyrin and
light it has been used with effect in the treatment of erythropoietic
protoporphyria. The use of any appropriate topical photoprotective
agent is referred to on p 362.

The *rare developmental abnormalities* listed in *Table 24.2* all have
a clinical photosensitivity feature which is not always confirmed on
phototesting except in the case of xeroderma pigmentosum. In

Bloom's syndrome in particular, but also in Rothmund–Thomson's syndrome, erythema can occur on skin exposed to sunshine. The subsequent development of pigmentation and telangiectasia (poikiloderma), although often maximal on these exposed skin sites, can appear on covered areas as well (*Plates 24.9* and *24.10*). The study of the clinical photosensitivity in xeroderma pigmentosum has led to a greater understanding of the underlying enzyme defects in this condition and it may be that similar attention to the photosensitivity factor in other examples of this group will also lead to an improved understanding of the basic defect which is affecting the other body systems. In xeroderma pigmentosum the defect in the skin which leads to the development of premature malignancy (basal cell carcinoma, squamous cell carcinoma, malignant melanoma) (*Plate 24.11*), is to be found in the enzyme activity responsible for the control of the ultraviolet induced damage in the cell nucleus. A number of different forms of xeroderma pigmentosum have now been defined with varying degrees of severity of skin damage in association with impairment at different sites of the repair process.

Light can also affect *dermatoses which are not primarily due to photosensitivity*. Some of these involve the skin only, whereas others such as lupus erythematosus have in addition a systemic disease component (*see Table 24.2*). In the group in which the photosensitivity acts essentially as an aggravating factor it tends to be in the form of an ability of the skin to sunburn more easily than normal. As a result of exposure to the sun the resulting sunburn tends to be replaced by the skin changes of the primary dermatoses. Most subjects with psoriasis find that controlled exposure to sunshine improves and even clears the lesions. In photosensitive psoriasis however the lesions are most marked on the face and backs of hands during the sunshine months, a distribution which is unusual in psoriasis.

The form of constitutional eczema in which photosensitivity is occasionally a factor is most often that of the atopic type and is usually seen in the child. Most atopics find their eczema is more severe in the winter, the minority noticing aggravation of exposed skin sites during the summer. During an attack of lichen planus an acute sunburn erythema may be replaced by lesions of the primary eruption. On the other hand, so-called actinic lichen planus (lichen planus tropicus) is morphologically different and confined to the Mediterranean and Middle East countries; the suggested light sensitivity factor as well as the relationship to lichen planus has yet to be adequately evaluated. In Darier's disease and in pemphigus erythematosus the characteristic skin changes can in some instances be produced by exposure of the skin to sunshine or artificial UVR.

Acne aestivalis (Mallorca acne) is included under the photodermatoses although the part played by sunlight in the production of the lesions is uncertain. It affects usually young adult females presenting in the spring and summer as multiple uniform papules, without comedones, on the skin of the face, shoulders, sides of neck, and chest.

Juvenile spring eruption affects mainly young male children during the early spring months and presents as papules and vesicles on the rim of the ears in particular. Climatic factors would appear to be important but whether an abnormal reaction to light is a factor or not is uncertain.

Benign cutaneous lymphocytoma occurring most commonly on the exposed skin of the face can be associated with abnormal photosensitivity. The lesions may be small and numerous as in miliary lymphocytoma or larger and few in number. The photosensitivity may present as one of the photodermatoses such as polymorphic light eruption or solar urticaria. Treatment of the photosensitivity can result in a reduction in the lymphocytomata. Lymphocytic infiltration of the skin described by Jessner and affecting particularly the face, but also sometimes the back, was thought to have a photosensitivity element which has however not been confirmed. The swollen erythematous plaques and annular lesions appear to fluctuate in severity regardless of exposure to light.

In those suffering from pellagra the dermatitis (erythema, hyperpigmentation and desquamation) of the exposed skin sites has been considered to relate to exposure to sunshine. This may be so but attempts to confirm photosensitivity or to explain the photobiological mechanisms involved have been unsuccessful.

In the collagen diseases such as lupus erythematosus and dermatomyositis, photosensitivity is important and particularly so in lupus erythematosus. It may be that the alterations in DNA resulting from absorption of UVR can trigger off the autoimmune process in a predisposed individual. It is necessary therefore for all subjects with systemic lupus erythematosus to minimize exposure of the skin during the sunshine months. It is likely also that the majority of those with cutaneous lupus erythematosus, without any systemic affection, are photosensitive to a variable degree as demonstrated by an ability to produce erythema following exposure to UVR in doses somewhat less than that which will produce the same response in normal individuals.

Investigation

The investigation of a case of light sensitivity will require not only a definition of the responsible wavelengths but also assessment of the general health of the individual to determine whether the light sensitivity is associated with systemic disease or its treatment.

Diagnosis of photosensitivity

It is insufficient to rely on clinical features alone. Certain *phototesting* techniques are required for confirmation of the clinical diagnosis. It would be ideal if the sun's rays were always available and that the solar spectrum remained constant and was not affected, as it is, by climatic and other environmental factors. Since such a solar spectrum is not readily available, phototesting equipment has been developed which provides artificial sources of irradiation which attempt to simulate exposure to daylight. The choice of irradiation equipment will depend on the amount of information required. It is possible to determine whether a subject is sensitive to the shorter wavelength UVR (UV-B, *Figure 24.1*) by using as the irradiation source fluorescent tubes of the 'sunlamp' variety.

Fluorescent tubes providing the longer wavelength UVR (UV-A) are less useful when used to determine UV-A sensitivity on account of the greater amount of energy required to detect UV-A as compared with UV-B sensitivity. The most suitable therefore for simple diagnostic screening procedures is the so-called solar simulator which provides ultraviolet and visible light irradiation from 290 to 850 nm, the ultraviolet mix being similar to that found in sunshine. Using this type of equipment the skin can be exposed to the whole spectrum and photosensitivity confirmed without further definition of the responsible wavelengths. However information can also be obtained as to whether the responsible wavelengths are present in both the UV-B and in the UV-A and visible light by means of a window glass filter inserted between the subject's skin and the source of the irradiation. This filter blocks the UV-B wavelengths below 320 nm. The use of a range of similar cut-off filters will help to define more closely the action spectrum, but this technique has limitations. In using equipment such as this it is necessary to be certain of the purity of the emission so that irradiation with wavelengths in the long wavelength ultraviolet and visible light are free from contamination by the active short wavelength UVR otherwise the results are suspect.

Except when the photosensitivity is of relatively short duration the full action spectrum should be determined. This requires access to an irradiation monochromator which provides a range of selected wavebands throughout the solar spectrum.

The skin patch test is used in the investigation of contact dermatitis to determine whether contact allergic sensitivity of cell mediated type is present. A modification of this test, the '*photopatch test*' is used to determine whether 'photoallergy' or 'phototoxicity' is present. As in the patch test, the suspected substance is applied to the skin by the use of an occlusive patch which is removed after 24 to 48 hours and any skin response recorded. In the photopatch test two such patches are applied, one being used as a closed non-irradiated control and the other irradiated with a minimal response dose, defined for the individual subject, of ultraviolet or visible light. The photopatch test reaction is positive, indicating photoallergy or phototoxicity, if the reaction of the skin differs from that seen at the site of the non-irradiated patch. In a positive phototoxic reaction there is to be seen dusky erythema with or without oedema/blisters and subsequent pigmentation, whereas in the positive photoallergic reaction the morphological changes are usually eczematous (dermatitis).

Treatment

The photosensitive reaction in for example polymophic light eruption and the photosensitivity dermatitis and actinic reticuloid syndrome requires to be suppressed by the application to the skin of steroid-containing preparations, the amounts and strengths of which are reduced in parallel with clinical improvement. The systemic administration of steroid drugs is rarely required and particularly if, while the skin reaction is being suppressed, admittance to hospital is possible, where the subject can be protected by nursing in a special screened bed. Once the skin reaction has subsided, the action spectrum can be defined; this is not usually possible in the presence of a reacting skin. The knowledge of the responsible wavelengths is used to direct attention towards causal factors which may require action separate from the light sensitivity skin response. Once it is known which wavelengths are involved it then also becomes possible to choose the appropriate substance for use as a topical photoprotective agent. Some of these substances are listed in *Table 24.3* along with the wavebands of ultraviolet and/or visible light which they are able to absorb or reflect. Their correct use is important, as well as

Table 24.3 Light screening agents

	UV-B	UV-A	Visible
Para-aminobenzoic acid	+ +	−	−
Para-aminobenzoic acid esters	+ +	−	−
Methoxy cinnamate	+	−	−
Methyl anthranilate	+	+/−	−
Benzophenones	+	+	−
Titanium dioxide	+	+	+

+ + = Very adequate protection
 + = Adequate protection
+/− = Some protection
 − = Inadequate protection

the selection of the one most appropriate for the subject's action spectrum. For example, para-aminobenzoic acid (PABA) has little protective action immediately after application, the protective ability being maximal some two hours later. It is also able to form a depot in the keratin layer of the epidermis and thus to build up its protective ability with repeated application, whereas other agents such as methoxycinnamate have no such build up of protective capacity. Although the vehicle used is often capable of maintaining some protective action after exposure of the skin to water, the majority of preparations available at the present time require reapplication. The exception is a preparation containing octyl dimethyl PABA and an acrylate polymer which provides a protective waterproof film on the skin surface. Similarly the titanium dioxide-containing physical barriers rub off and require to be frequently reapplied. Photosensitivity varies in severity from one person to the next and from one photodermatosis to the next, and a knowledge of the relative protective ability of the various preparations is important. Only those preparations should therefore be prescribed where information as to protective factors for specific wavebands is available. It may sometimes be a disadvantage to 'over protect' a light sensitive subject since the normal protective mechanism of the skin may as a result not develop in those who are only moderately photosensitive, and also the natural 'desensitization' in polymorphic light eruption referred to on p. 353 may be lost.

There is, as yet, little evidence that systemically administered photoprotective agents can play a significant part in the treatment of photosensitivity. The antimalarials such as chloroquine appear to help some patients and in small doses can produce satisfactorily maintained improvement in porphyria cutanea tarda. Beta-carotene appears to ameliorate the cutaneous signs and symptoms of erythropoietic protoporphyria. The effect of its use in the treatment of other photodermatoses is uncertain and awaits controlled studies. The combination of orally administered 8-methoxypsoralen and long wavelength ultraviolet (UV-A) has probably a part to play in the build up of protective melanin pigmentation prior to the sunshine season in the prophylactic treatment of, for example, polymorphic light eruption. It may also have some action on the mechanisms considered to be involved in polymorphic light eruption. Some examples of this latter condition are also helped by a preseasonal radiation course of progressively increasing exposure doses of the relevant ultraviolet wavelengths.

In addition, general guidance should be given as to how exposure to the sun's rays can be minimized; for example particular care to avoid exposure from 10 am to 2 pm. Apparent protection by a beach umbrella or by a brimmed hat is often inadequate because of the UVR from the side in the form of skyshine and reflection from buildings, sand, grass, water and snow. In some of the photodermatoses the response to light is of a delayed type and therefore accumulated small exposures which at the time do not appear to be producing a skin response may do so with unexpected severity during the following days. It is also not always appreciated that for some photosensitive subjects ordinary daylight and sometimes even artificial indoor lighting are important and will cause their skin to react abnormally. It will also be important for contact with defined allergens such as those of the compositae plant family in photosensitivity dermatitis to be avoided or at least minimized.

25 The surgical treatment of skin diseases

Nicholas Breach

The surgical excision of a skin tumour results in the formation of a scar. With benign tumours the resulting scar should be aesthetically superior to the appearance of the lesion itself. The primary objective in the removal of malignant tumours is the eradication of the pathological condition itself; the aesthetics of the repair must of necessity take second place. Knowledge of the anatomy and physiology of the skin contributes to the production of the best possible scar whatever the condition.

The tension lines of the skin have been said to hold the key to the ease and adequacy of surgical repair. The identification of these lines has been attributed to Langer (1861). They are distributed in such a way that a wound made across the lines produces maximum separation of the skin edges; conversely, a wound placed in parallel with Langer's lines will result in minimal deformity and a good aesthetic scar.

Where a scar has to be placed over mobile parts, i.e. joints, some broadening of the scar can be expected as maturation occurs, unless absolute immobilization of the parts is possible and practical while healing takes place. In infancy and early childhood, in specific areas and in certain races, scarring can be excessive and exaggerated, thereby producing either a hypertrophic or keloid scar. The management of these scars is discussed later in the chapter.

The technique of excision and the margin of clearance of skin lesions

An excision of a skin lesion should be done with the knife held at right angles to the skin surface, the depth of excision being dependent upon the extent of penetration of the pathological process. Such an excision technique facilitates accurate coaption of the skin edges in wound closure. In general terms, the extent of the undermining required to achieve easy closure will depend upon the tension at the edges of the wound.

There is a specific margin of clearance for each skin lesion. As far as benign lesions are concerned the excision may literally skirt the

364

tumour margin; the converse is true for malignant tumours. Specific examples will be discussed later in the chapter.

Methods of repairing a skin defect

The best aesthetic result in the repair of a skin defect is achieved when skin adjacent to the defect is used to effect the repair; such skin is the most suitable match for colour and texture.

Skin grafts

Reverdin was the first to record the use of skin grafting to repair skin defects; in those early days he used pinch grafts. The early techniques have been developed so that we can now use both split and full thickness skin grafts. Skin grafts contract: the thinner the graft the greater the contraction, and vice versa, to the extent that full thickness grafts show minimal contraction. Skin grafts themselves cause a contour deformity and their contraction causes tissue deficiency.

Opinions are divided as to whether formal repair should be undertaken immediately following excision of a malignant tumour. Some workers advocate repair by means of a split skin graft so that any subsequent recurrence can be readily observed. Those in favour of primary reconstruction hold that if a tumour is adequately excised and the excision monitored by frozen section, recurrence is unlikely to occur. Most patients will prefer primary reconstruction, thus avoiding a tissue defect which may require a prosthesis to afford adequate cosmetic camouflage.

Flap repair

When a skin flap is principally supplied by one artery from the base of the flap it is known as an 'arterialized flap' or 'axial flap'. When there is no main arterial supply the flap is said to be 'random' or 'cutaneous'. A random flap must comply with certain fundamental principles: that is, the width to length ratio must be more than 1:1.5. This overriding principle can be ignored when an arterial flap is considered.

Simple advancement technique

Most small skin lesions can conveniently be excised by removing an ellipse of skin. Closure of the wound edges can usually be achieved by simple advancement; this generally requires adequate undermining of the edges. The extent of the 'dog ear' formation at either end of the wound depends upon the length to breadth ratio and on skin elasticity. If the breadth of the ellipse is comparatively greater than the length, the 'dog ears' will be more marked. These defects can be lessened by the removal of some of the subcutaneous fat surrounding the point of the ellipse.

As with all skin closures, primary healing can only be achieved by ensuring minimal tension at the wound edges. *Figure 25.1* illustrates the principle of advancement of the skin edges to achieve wound closure.

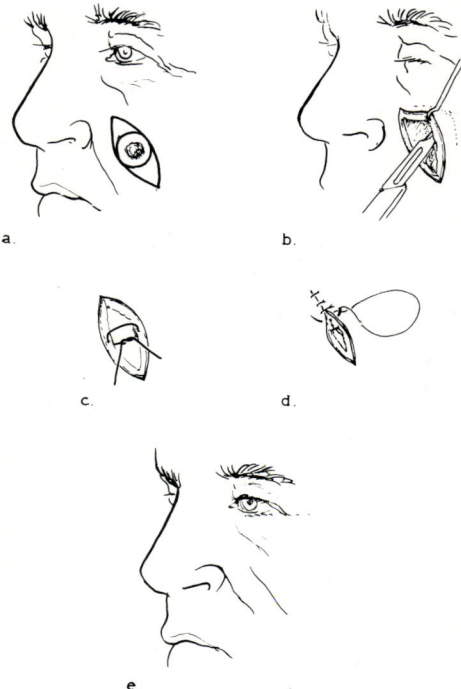

Figure 25.1   *Closure of an elliptical wound by the principle of advancement of the wound edges*

Transposition flaps

When the size of the lesion is such that an elliptical excision would result in an unacceptably long scar or the tissues would not permit closure by simple advancement, an alternative method of repair must be used. The transposition of skin immediately adjacent to the defect may prove an effective method of closure. *Figure 25.2* shows the principles of design and execution of such a technique. Transposition flaps can be moved through an arc of 180 degrees; naturally the greater the arc through which they are moved, the greater will be the resulting 'dog ear', and the more marked the deformity the more likely a secondary correction will be necessary. The transposition of tissue will introduce adjacent skin into the defect; care should be

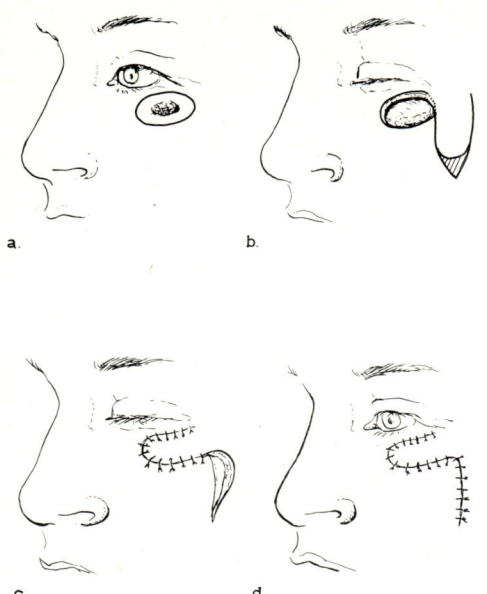

Figure 25.2 *Repair with a transposition flap and primary closure of the secondary defect*

taken not to bring hair-bearing skin into a previously non-hairy area. Various alternative techniques of tissue transposition have been developed in an effort to facilitate repair. Limberg and Dufourmentel have demonstrated the use of angular flaps; bilobed flaps achieve a spread of the tissue gain, and Barron's subcutaneous island pedicle flap also has a place in the repair of tissue defects.

When a small transposition flap is used the secondary defect can usually be closed primarily; when this cannot be done the secondary defect must be repaired by a skin graft.

Rotation flap principle

In certain situations, particularly on the face, the rotation-advancement principle of tissue transfer must be applied to achieve the most satisfactory cosmetic result. The diagrams in *Figure 25.3* show how, by excising a cone shaped piece of skin which equals one-eighth of the area of the rotation flap, primary closure of the defect can be achieved. If, however, extra advancement of the flap is necessary, excision of a Burow's triangle (*see Figure 25.4*) will give that added gain to the flap.

Distant flaps

Where the size of local skin flaps is not adequate or is unsuitable for primary repair, distant skin must be introduced. These distant flaps

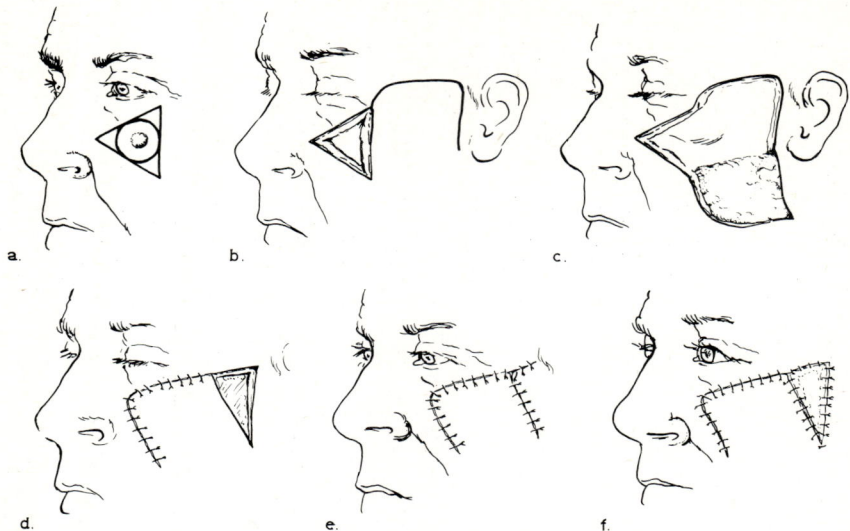

Figure 25.3 *Repair with a transposition flap with skin grafting of the secondary defect*

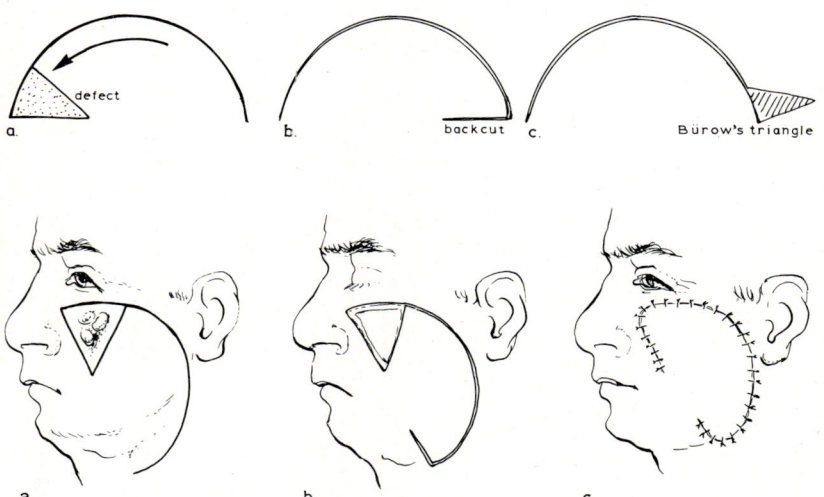

Figure 25.4 *The principle of rotation—advancement to close a skin defect*

are based on similar principles to local flaps. The secondary defect may be closed primarily; if this is impossible, skin grafts must be employed. Repair of defects in the head and neck can be achieved by the following flaps, each one having specific indications: deltopectoral (Bakamjian), epulet (Mutter), acromio-thoracic and the recently developed compound myocutaneous flaps; the sterno-mastoid, pectoralis major and trapezius. In these situations a paddle of overlying skin is carried up on the muscle transfer.

Even more distant flaps may occasionally be required: either the abdominal 'jump' flap or abdominal tubed pedicle. These latter two alternatives are time consuming for the patient, the surgeon and hospital accommodation; consequently they have in the main been superseded by the recent advances.

The transfer of a free composite graft of significant size has only become possible with the use of the operating microscope for the anastomosis of the recipient and donor blood vessels. Neural anastomosis has permitted the re-establishment of sensation; thus totally functional grafts can be transferred. The free transfer of myocutaneous flaps allows for the movement of tissue bulk where bulk is required.

The technique of wound closure and suture materials

The ideal position for the opposed wound edges is slight eversion; no pockets should be present beneath the epithelial surface and there should be only minimal tension at the interface of the wound.

By positioning the skin sutures as shown in *Figure 25.5*, eversion of the skin edges can be achieved. Absorbable dermal sutures maintain the apposition of the wound edges; their presence allows for the early removal of the skin sutures. The presence of subcutaneous sutures and pressure over the wound in the immediate post-operative phase eliminates pocketing and any subsequent haematoma formation.

Skin sutures should be removed as soon as possible, to prevent the formation of 'stitch marks'; the wound can be reinforced by the application of 'steristrips'. The early removal of skin stitches applies particularly to the head and neck. On the trunk and limbs, where healing is not so rapid, skin sutures need to be left *in situ* for longer.

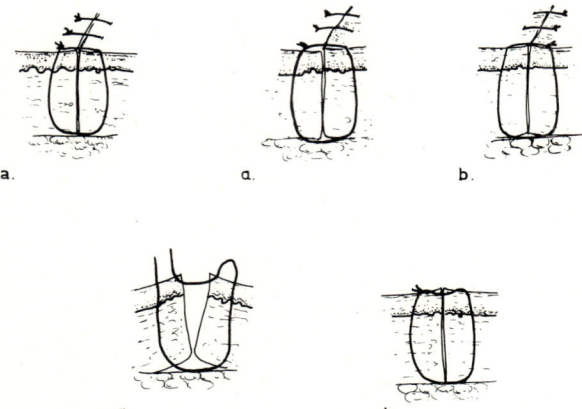

Figure 25.5 *Techniques of skin closure to create the correct apposition of the skin edges*

In such situations it is important to use suture material that is non-irritant, i.e. that causes minimal tissue reaction. Prolene and nylon are satisfactory in this respect. If tension sutures are to be left in place for 12 to 14 days, stitch marks will occur whatever the material used; in such cases a subcuticular suture should be used, for which nylon or prolene are suitable; these sutures may be left *in situ* for several weeks.

Some of the man-made absorbable sutures can cause a hypertrophic-like scar when used in the subcuticular layer. The type of suture used in wound closure is mainly a matter of personal choice; each material has advantages and disadvantages.

Benign tumours

Margin of clearance

The pathological nature of these lesions necessitates an adequate margin of clearance. In cases where recent growth has occurred, the margin must be sufficient to remove the whole lesion. The length of a skin ellipse for excision required to allow easy closure is of necessity greater than the length of the lesion itself. When the size of a lesion is such that a routine elliptical excision would create an unacceptably long scar, an alternative method of repair must be found to achieve an aesthetically acceptable result.

Serial excision

The length of the resulting scar following excision of a lesion can be restricted by using a staged excision technique. This technique is known as serial excision. The first excision is within the length of the lesion; subsequent excisions require removal of the scar and part or the whole of the remaining lesion. Any number of excisions can be undertaken to achieve the final result. This technique is most suitable for benign melanomas, hairy naevi and the occasional angioma. It must be decided whether a better aesthetic result will be achieved by serial excision or by primary excision and grafting. The ultimate result of serial excision will depend upon the degree to which the scar broadens with normal maturation.

Lesions of infancy and childhood

Some skin lesions involute and others resolve. A 'wait and see' policy may be advantageous when dealing with infants and young children, when the main problem is reassurance of the parents during the years of involution. Capillary-cavernous (strawberry) naevi characteristically involute completely during the first few years of life. This delay has the added advantage of leaving the decision to operate to the young adult at a time when he or she is able to understand the problems associated with surgical excision. Capillary haemangiomata (naevus flammeus, port-wine stain) never undergo involution and may subsequently require cosmetic camouflage.

Malignant tumours

Basal cell carcinoma

The margin of clearance of this locally malignant skin tumour should be in accordance with its morphology. By gentle movement of the surrounding skin it can be seen that a cystic type tumour is more localized than the infiltrating lesion; consequently the margin of clearance of the cystic type may be more limited than is required for an infiltrating lesion.

Most basal cell carcinomas can be excised under local anaesthesia, thus causing minimal upset in a relatively aged group of patients. Closure of the wound can be achieved by any of the techniques described above. Surgery is indicated where radiotherapy is specifically contraindicated, e.g. for tumours of the eyelids, nose and ears, where cartilage underlies or is adjacent to the tumour; cartilage is particularly prone to damage following irradiation.

All excision specimens must be examined for the adequacy of tumour clearance; frozen section monitoring for some tumours is the ideal. When a histological report indicates that the tumour has been inadequately excised, it must be decided whether a more radical excision is advisable. Between 5 and 15 per cent of such cases show tumour recurrence, and often in cases where further excision is undertaken, no tumour is identified histologically.

The recurrence rate for primary excision of basal cell carcinomata is ± 3.6 per cent; when radiotherapy is used the recurrence rate is 12–17 per cent. Surgery must be undertaken when recurrence follows radiotherapy; often the whole of the irradiated skin must be excised. The surgeon must decide whether the defect following excision should be repaired by means of a split skin graft or flap cover. The skin graft repair enables early detection of possible recurrences, but where the margin of clearance is adequate, a flap can produce a more cosmetically acceptable result.

Squamous cell carcinoma

The pathological nature of the squamous cell carcinoma demands a wider margin of clearance than for a basal cell carcinoma: 1.0–1.5 cm of skin must be taken from the clinical edge of the tumour. These figures apply equally to the depth of excision. The surgical defect can likewise be repaired with a skin graft or a skin flap, depending upon the site and size of the tumour, and the same general principles apply.

Squamous cell carcinomata metastasize initially to the regional lymph nodes, and these must be examined at each consultation. Secondary deposits from squamous cell carcinomata are not generally sensitive to irradiation; consequently resection of the regional nodes is advisable. Where *en bloc* resection is possible, this is the ideal method. Regular post-operative examination of these patients is necessary for some four to five years after the primary excision.

Malignant melanoma

The margin of clearance for a lentigo maligna (Hutchinson's freckle) is usually dependent upon the site of occurrence. The majority of these lesions are found on the cheeks and temples, where it is not possible to adopt the 5–10 cm margin recommended for the superficial spreading and nodular melanomata. There has been some debate as to whether the deep fascia underlying the skin should be excised; experience has shown that there is no difference in the prognosis when the fascia is left *in situ*.

The size of the defect following excision of a malignant melanoma is such that repair must be effected with a split skin graft; only rarely can primary closure of the wound be achieved. Many feel that closure of the wound does not permit easy examination of the area for recurrence.

Where facilities allow for histological confirmation of malignant melanoma by frozen section, an excisional biopsy can be undertaken without risk of tumour dissemination.

In recent years some authorities have related the overall prognosis in malignant melanoma to the histological staging and tumour thickness. Some doubt has been cast on the accepted criteria for margin of clearance of the primary excision and there appears to be little difference in the prognosis when there is wide excision of tumours less than 0.75 mm thick.

There is no conclusive evidence that routine regional lymph node dissection increases the overall survival in Stage I tumours as compared with an elective node dissection when involved nodes can be palpated.

Only 10 per cent of the metastatic melanotic lesions can be successfully treated with radiotherapy; nor have endolymphatic isotopes proved beneficial in nodal disease. An occasional cure has been claimed with immunotherapy, e.g. BCG.

Chemotherapy has been widely advocated for Stage III disease (i.e. distant metastases); the agent most intensively studied is dimethyl-triazenoimidazole carboxamide (DTIC). This agent has produced tumour regression of 50 per cent in 22 per cent of cases, the duration of the remission being about 16–20 weeeks.

Nodal metastases require elective excision. Many believe that such procedures reduce the bulk of the tumour. Radical lymph node dissection, particularly in the inguinal region, can cause lymphoedema. Isolated limb perfusion with DTIC can control cutaneous disease effectively.

Cryotherapy has been used to treat malignant melanomata; good early results have been reported but long-term results have yet to be assessed.

Other malignant tumours

Tumours of connective tissue usually require removal of the skin overlying the tumour; their removal must of necessity be radical.

There is considerable variation in the mode of repair of the primary defect following the removal of malignant tumours. In certain situations split skin grafts cannot be used because the vascularity of the bed is insufficient to maintain the viability of the graft. Exposed cortical bone, exposed cartilage and tendons denuded of the paratenon, and open joint cavities, all require a skin flap to ensure healing. Care must also be taken when bone has been subjected to irradiation as the vascularity of the overlying periosteum may be inadequate to maintain a skin graft.

Injuries and scars

The scar resulting from an injury is dependent upon the direction of the discontinuity of the skin, the site of the injury and the care taken to repair the defect. The principles of wound repair are identical to those of wound closure after surgical excision.

There will often be a deficiency of tissue following traumatic injuries; under the conditions of wound closure it may appear that there is no loss or that the loss is minimal, and a well performed operation will mask the resulting deformity.

The primary repair of an injury will result in a scar or scars in the direction predetermined by the injury. Scars which are aesthetically displeasing can be revised; the line and direction of the scar may require to be changed to comply with Langer's lines. This can often be done by employing a 'Z' plasty (*see Figure 25.6*); such a technique will mask much of the scar.

Depressed scars can be adjusted into alignment; incongruity is also amenable to correction. Scars do result, whatever technique is used; they must be so positioned as to create the best cosmetic result.

Hypertrophic and keloid scars

Depending on the anatomical site and genetic background, initial normal healing may result in either a hypertrophic or keloid scar formation. Infants and young children frequently form hypertrophic scars as part of the normal healing process; in its most severe form this may follow a burn injury in a child. Central scars of the chest in

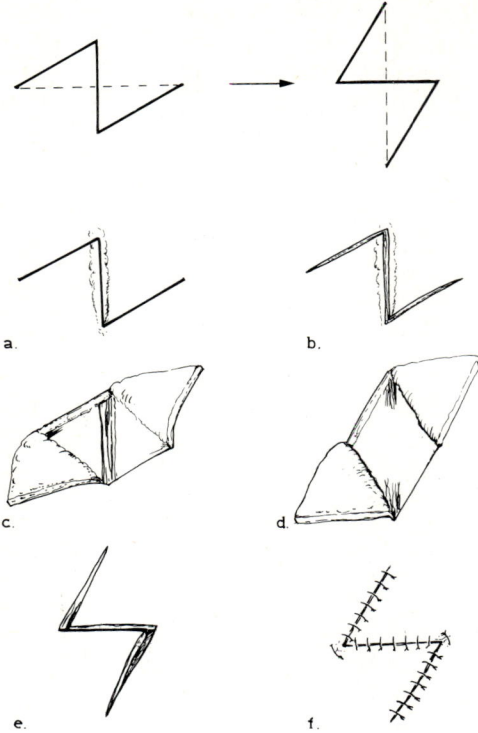

Figure 25.6 *The principle of 'Z' plasty to realign an unsatisfactory scar*

Caucasians frequently result in keloid scars, and in the Negroid races many scars become keloid.

It has recently been demonstrated that continuous pressure inhibits the formation of hypertrophic scars in the post-burn situation. In such cases made-to-measure pressure garments are worn continuously for three to six months. The pressure seems to hasten the normal resolution of hypertrophic scars. Equally success-ful results have been achieved with the use of a 'Zimmer' splint applied to the ear lobe following removal of the post-piercing keloid.

Intralesional injections of triamcinolone often produce some softening of keloid scars. These injections must be given into the scars and not subcutaneously, and they should be repeated three or four times at four-weekly intervals. When placed subcutaneously they cause atrophy of the fat, which can produce scar depression. Radiotherapy may have a limited place in the treatment of the occasional lesion or where a post-operative keloid is considered inevitable. Alternatively, excision of the keloid within the scar may be undertaken, leaving a small rim of the keloid at the periphery of the excision. The defect is then covered with a thin split skin graft. Care must be taken at the skin donor site; with the contracture of the graft an acceptable cosmetic result is achieved. Pre- or post-operative irradiation can be used. Sutures should not be placed outside the original scar, as keloids may arise at the suture sites.

Sebaceous cysts

Primary excision of these cysts is the generally accepted method of treatment; excision of an ellipse of skin overlying the cyst may be necessary with the larger cysts. Excision is relatively straightforward when the cyst has not previously been infected. Following excision, care must be taken to obliterate the resulting cavity, as the formation of a haematoma will complicate healing.

Hyperhidrosis

Excessive axillary sweating requires surgical correction when medical methods of treatment have proved unsatisfactory. The surgical approach requires removal of the axillary eccrine glands. Removal of these glands may be achieved by excision of the hair-bearing skin of the axilla and either primary closure of the wound or re-arrangement of the skin flaps as a 'Z' plasty. As an alternative, the eccrine glands can be dissected from the deep surface of the dermis.

Hidradenitis

This distressing condition of recurring abscesses and persistent sinuses in the axilla, groin and perineum can only be treated effectively by radical excision of the involved skin. The major problem in these cases is to achieve primary healing of the resulting defect. The defect is repaired by the application of a split skin graft.

Acne vulgaris

The 'pock' marks resulting from acne vulgaris present a difficult problem. The major deep scars are best treated by excision and primary closure of the wound. A radical dermabrasion can be achieved by using a high-speed rotating abrasive, which removes the epidermal layer. This compares with a superficial burn. Healing occurs by proliferation of the epithelial cells of the epithelial remnants. Such treatment only achieves a reduction in the contour deformity, improving the overall appearance of the skin in reflected light.

Tattoos

Professional and amateur tattoos present a problem when removal is requested. When the pigments are deposited in the deeper layers of the dermis, only full thickness excision of the pigmented skin will result in the complete removal of the tattoo. Small tattoos can be excised and the wound edges closed primarily; larger tattoos require excision and skin grafting.

Requests for the removal of tattoos may be for cosmetic, social or economic reasons. Patients must be warned of the inevitable scars resulting from the excision of the tattoo.

Age changes of the facial skin

With increasing age there is loss of the elasticity of the skin. Some people find increasing facial lines and laxity of the skin unacceptable and request cosmetic procedures to halt these signs of advancing years.

It must be realized that although much of the laxity of the skin can be removed, crease lines cannot be eliminated. A face lift operation can produce a satisfactory tightening up of the skin of the cheeks and below the jaw-line. The incision is carried from the temporal region in the immediate pre-auricular skin to the lobe of the ear, then on the posterior skin of the ear to the mastoid process and into the hairline. The improvement achieved by a face lift is of the order of five to ten years; the procedure can be repeated if demanded by further skin laxity.

Laxity in the skin of the upper and lower eyelids is treated in a different manner. The upper eyelid can be reduced by excising an ellipse of skin. The lower eyelid, however, requires very accurate assessment of the amount of skin that can be removed without producing distortion of the eyelid. This skin is removed from the eyelid immediately below the eyelashes.

Some of the deformity in 'baggy' eyelids is due to the abnormal protrusion of the intraorbital fat causing herniation of the orbital septum. Judicial excision of some of the intraorbital fat can produce a pleasing contour.

26 Radiotherapy in skin cancer

George Deutsch

Radiotherapy or surgery can cure more than 95 per cent of basal cell and squamous cell carcinoma of the skin. The skill with which either modality is applied is generally more important than the choice of method. Radiotherapists, dermatologists and plastic surgeons working in joint consultation clinics provide the best forum for the optimal treatment of skin cancer. Such factors as the patient's age, fitness for surgery, ease of repairing a surgical defect, the site and size of the tumour and the possible complications can then be considered jointly and a decision taken as to the best form of treatment.

The modern treatment of skin cancer by radiotherapy requires a wide range of equipment, skills and specialized training.

General considerations

Successful radiotherapy of skin cancer is dependent upon a modality of radiation which will, as nearly as possible, provide a homogeneous distribution of radiation throughout the depth of a tumour with an adequate margin of apparently normal skin. The dose must be sufficient to destroy the tumour without preventing the repair of normal tissue and re-epithelialization; it should not cause excessive absorption in underlying bone and cartilage, with consequent necrosis. Where appropriate, vital structures such as the lens must be shielded with lead.

Choice of radiation modality

For the majority of cases superficial x-ray therapy with well filtered beams of 50–150 kV is appropriate, the choice of energy depending on the thickness of the tumour. The risk of necrosis in underlying cartilage and bone can be reduced by the use of higher quality radiation from caesium or cobalt teletherapy units, electron therapy or radium moulds.

The rapid fall off of dose at depth available with radium moulds and electron beam therapy can be useful in minimizing radiation of underlying normal tissues. Electron therapy is therefore particularly useful for treating extensive tumours of the scalp where the underlying brain would otherwise be at risk, and for very large areas of the skin in mycosis fungoides.

Choice of radiation dosage

There is a narrow therapeutic ratio between the dose required to cure a tumour and the dose that so damages normal tissues that repair cannot occur and necrosis results. Several factors can alter this ratio. In general the larger the tumour, the larger the dose required for its cure. As a consequence tumours in excess of 6 cm diameter are very difficult to cure by radiation without causing necrosis, which is particularly likely to result if a large tumour has in itself caused major tissue destruction. Surgery may then be preferable, or it can be used to repair the defect after high dose radiotherapy has removed the tumour.

Spreading, or fractionating, the course of radiotherapy over several days or weeks allows partial repair of the normal tissues between doses or fractions, thus widening the therapeutic ratio. The larger the area irradiated the more prolonged and fractionated the course of radiation should be to ensure final skin healing.

Small lesions up to 1 cm in diameter can often be treated safely by a single dose, though fractionation over several days may give a better cosmetic result by reducing late radiation damage and preventing a sharply defined margin to the irradiated skin. Single treatments are however particularly useful in the elderly.

Complications of radiotherapy

Early and late or delayed skin changes are seen after radiotherapy. The normal early reaction is of erythema followed by dry or moist desquamation with epilation. Healing, often with crusting, then occurs, the time taken depending on the area of skin irradiated and the degree of normal tissue damage caused by the tumour. Whenever possible the irradiated skin should be left exposed to the air and ointments and dressings avoided. If the area needs to be protected by a dressing, a thick bland ointment should be used to prevent the dressing adhering to the irradiated skin. Topical antibiotics are seldom required; steroids should be avoided.

Early necrosis is exceptional but may occur when large tumours, particularly with involved cartilage, are irradiated as a calculated risk in patients who are unfit for or refuse surgery.

Delayed skin changes may develop gradually over months and years, including varying degrees of atrophy and telangiectasia.

Late radiation necrosis can be precipitated many years after therapy by trauma or thermal damage. These lesions often heal, albeit slowly perhaps helped by application of steroid ointments, but failing this plastic surgery may be necessary.

The effects of radiation on the eyelids are described later.

The choice of therapy with regard to tumour type

Basal cell carcinoma

Basal cell carcinomas should not be regarded as a uniform disease as the various morphological types have a characteristic biological behaviour which affects the choice of therapy.

The ulcerating basal cell carcinoma, or rodent ulcer, remains superficial initially, but as it enlarges unsuspected infiltration in depth may occur. Failure to appreciate this accounts for many radiotherapeutic as well as surgical failures in the region of the eye and ala nasi.

The cystic basal cell carcinoma usually remains superficial and well demarcated, so that radiation of only a small margin in depth and of normal skin is required. This lesion is often mistakenly considered to be radioresistant; this impression may be due to the relative bulk of the lesion and the slow regression, which can take several months after completion of radiotherapy. Cure can be expedited by reducing the bulk of the lesion with diathermy prior to irradiating the base.

Morphoeic or cicatricial basal cell carcinomas usually remain superficial; however failure to appreciate the extent to which this variety infiltrates surrounding apparently normal skin accounts for many recurrences following treatment by radiotherapy or surgery. The extent of this infiltration can often be gauged by stretching the skin and viewing with an oblique light. The lesions may have extensive areas of central scarring resembling healing, and in these cases better cosmetic results may be obtained with plastic surgery.

Multiple superficial basal cell tumours are relatively non-invasive and, although they can be treated by superficial x-ray therapy, other methods such as 5-fluorouracil ointment or cryotherapy may sometimes be effective.

Intraepidermal carcinoma

Patches of intraepidermal carcinoma or Bowen's disease are managed in an identical fashion to superficial basal cell carcinoma. This also applies to erythroplasia of Queyrat of the glans penis. Paget's disease of the nipple is an intraepidermal carcinoma but it is always associated with an underlying breast carcinoma and must be treated as such.

Squamous cell carcinoma

Squamous cell carcinoma of the skin is usually of well differentiated type. The ears, dorsa of the hands and the mucosa of the lower lip are the common sites. No difference in radiation dosage or technique from that used for basal cell carcinoma is required, although account must be taken of the infiltrating nature of the tumour by the use of wide margins. The site of the tumour may influence the use of radiotherapy, as discussed later. In general, metastases to the regional lymph nodes are best managed by surgery.

Keratoacanthomas

These lesions are radiosensitive. If they are to be treated, however, they must be irradiated as though they were squamous cell carcinomas. Only a full excision can provide material for a reliable pathology report, and radiotherapy is therefore not the treatment of choice. They respond well to curettage under local anaesthesia.

Cutaneous lymphomas

These lesions are extremely radiosensitive and easily eradicated by low doses of x-ray therapy.

Mycosis fungoides

This disease is radiosensitive and localized tumours can be effectively treated by low doses of x-ray therapy of appropriate energy. Recently excellent results have been obtained in early disease by total body skin irradiation by low energy electron beams.

Malignant melanoma

These tumours are generally radioresistant but useful palliation of inoperable disease can sometimes be obtained. There is some evidence that the use of very large fractions of radiation may increase the radiosensitivity of the tumours.

Kaposi's sarcoma

These tumours are radiosensitive and can usually be controlled although rarely cured by radiation. Mutilating surgery should be avoided; it is rarely curative due to the presence of systemic metastases.

Adnexal tumours

Adenocarcinomas arising from sweat and sebaceous glands are regarded as radioresistant and are the province of the surgeon.

The choice of therapy with regard to tumour site

Flat areas of the face and scalp

The majority of basal cell carcinomas arise on the essentially flat areas of the forehead, temples, cheeks, scalp and upper lip. In these sites radiotherapy and surgery produce identical cure rates and therefore other factors can determine the choice of therapy.

In elderly patients with small lesions a single dose of superficial x-rays gives an acceptable cosmetic result with minimal disturbance to the patient.

With larger lesions fractionated superficial x-ray therapy produces cosmetic results at least equal to and in many cases better than surgery, particularly where a graft or flap would be required for repair.

In young patients, where the cosmetic result is important, radiotherapy should be avoided because of uncertainty regarding the development of late skin changes. In patients with florid facies the pale scar of radiotherapy may result in a poor cosmetic appearance.

Lower eyelid

Radiotherapy and surgery probably produce identical results. Each can cause epiphora due to obliteration or removal of the lacrimal punctum. Ectropion produced by a cicatricial tumour may be increased by the scarring of radiotherapy and therefore expert surgery is preferable. Extensive neoplasms invading the orbital cavity may be better treated by surgery if it proves impossible to protect the eye with lead without shielding the tumour itself.

Upper eyelid

Radiotherapy to the upper eyelid frequently results in keratinization of the tarsal conjunctiva with subsequent corneal damage. Although this can be avoided by the permanent use of contact lens, surgery is generally regarded as the treatment of choice.

Inner canthus area

Accurate superficial x-ray therapy can be difficult due to the curvature of the underlying bone; although radiotherapy is frequently used, local recurrence is common and surgery may be preferable in younger patients.

Nose

Lesions on the flat sides of the nose are easily treated by superficial radiotherapy. The risk of cartilage necrosis has probably been exaggerated in the past. This risk increases if the tumour has invaded the cartilage but even then necrosis is by no means inevitable. Radiotherapy is frequently used if expert surgical reconstruction of the nasal cartilage is not available or feasible. Infiltrating tumours at the junction of the ala nasi and cheek have a tendency to invade deeply and this should be taken into account in planning radiotherapy or surgery. It is technically difficult but not impossible to irradiate lesions extending down both sides of the bridge of the nose, and surgery may be preferable.

Ears

Surgery is generally regarded as the treatment of choice. However, the risk of cartilage necrosis has been exaggerated and it is only likely to occur if the cartilage has been exposed or invaded by tumour. Radiotherapy provides an acceptable alternative for superficial lesions particularly in the elderly and if mutilating surgery would be required.

Lower lip

There is little to choose between the results of radiotherapy and surgery for squamous cell carcinomas of the lower lip. Radiotherapy can produce cosmetic results at least equal to those of surgery even for moderately destructive lesions. However, radiotherapy does produce a painful mucosal reaction which with large lesions can take several weeks to heal. Very bulky destructive lesions and lymph node metastases are best treated by surgery, though cytotoxic therapy may have a part to play in the future.

Trunk and limbs

Lesions here are preferably treated by surgery, particularly as there is generally plenty of available skin for primary closure. Radiotherapy reactions on the trunk and limbs tend to be slow to heal and the resulting atrophic scar is easily damaged by trauma from clothing. However in sites where grafts are frequently lost, such as the midline of the back, radiotherapy may be preferred.

Hands

Although radiotherapy can produce excellent results, surgery is preferable in the active patient as the atrophic skin resulting from radiotherapy is easily damaged by minor trauma. It is considered inadvisable to irradiate the digits.

27 Therapeutic guide and formulary

Patrick Hall-Smith

In dermatology no less than in other branches of medicine the advent of antibiotics and steroids brought about a revolution in the methods and scope of treatment. Clinical experience and correct diagnosis are essential, however, if the best use is to be made of the 'wonder drugs'.

In the preceding chapters specific treatment is recommended for particular diseases. The following is intended as a general guide to the treatment of conditions which most frequently present to the general practitioner and hospital doctor.

Anhidrotics

Anhidrotics are used to diminish sweating in patients with hyperhidrosis. Axillary, palmar and plantar hyperhidrosis, if severe, are embarrassing to the patient and can be disabling. Axillary hyperhidrosis can be controlled by 20% aluminium chloride hexahydrate (Anhydrol Forte) in industrial methylated spirit (IMS) or ethanol. This preparation is best made up by the hospital pharmacist. The patient is instructed to dry under both arms and, with a small paint brush, apply the solution to both axillae; next morning the axillae are washed. This process is repeated each night until sweating ceases during the day. The paint is then applied twice weekly and, if progress is maintained, once weekly. Any irritation is controlled by hydrocortisone cream 1%. The preparation can also be used on the palms and soles, though with less success. Plantar hyperhidrosis also responds to daily painting with 20% formalin, protecting the interdigital skin with vaseline, or 10% glutaraldehyde applications and aluminium hexahydrate.

Direct current iontophoresis using a solution of glycopyrronium bromide once every four to six weeks works well in those experienced in this technique. Severe axillary hyperhidrosis may demand the Shelley–Hurley operation, which entails removing an ellipse of the skin from both axillae, including the underlying sweat glands.

Antipruritics

All agents which act by evaporation, such as wet dressings and shake lotions, have an antipruritic effect; in addition active medicaments

384

with a specific antipruritic effect may be added to shake lotions and creams. Lotions should be avoided in the treatment of acute non-weeping dermatoses when drying and protective action is required. Oozing is a contraindication to the use of shake lotions because caking may occur, leading to retention of debris and bacterial infection. Liniments are lotions containing oil and are therefore less drying. Phenol 0.2 to 2.5%, menthol 0.2 to 1% or camphor 0.2 to 5% may be incorporated. A useful oily calamine lotion is as follows:

Emulsifying wax	7 g
Anhydrous wool fat	5 g
Arachis oil	50 g
Calamine	10 g
Water	to 200 ml

Such applications usually relieve itching but sometimes stronger antipruritics such as crotamiton (Eurax) cream or lotion are used. Crotamiton should not be applied to eczematous or broken skin and a watch should be kept for sensitivity developing. Hydrocortisone preparations are effective in breaking the itch-scratch-itch cycle; the fluorinated steroids are even more effective but are not without risk.

When pruritus is based on skin dryness a water-in-oil type lubricating cream should be used, e.g. Oily cream BP, which leaves an oily residue; a 10% urea cream (Aquadrate or Calmurid) and Boots E.45 cream are also effective emollients. Emulsifying ointment BP can be used as a soap substitute, moisturizer and diluent. Aqueous cream BP, an oil-in-water vanishing cream, is cooling and cosmetically acceptable.

Antihistamines and trimeprazine (Vallergan) are frequently given by mouth as a supplement to local therapy for pruritic dermatoses. Antihistamine and local anaesthetic creams should be avoided on the skin because of the risk of topical sensitization.

Antibacterial agents

Oxytetracycline (Terramycin) and chlortetracycline (Aureomycin) are broad-spectrum antibiotics with a low sensitizing capacity. However, it is common to meet with organisms which are tetracycline resistant, and especially so in hospitals. Neomycin, and in particular Cicatrin ointment (neomycin–bacitracin) is valuable in impetigo, where it will not be used for more than a week; this lessens the risk of sensitization developing.

Gentamicin (Genticin or Cidomycin) is effective against Gram-positive and Gram-negative organisms. This antibiotic is used systemically and resistance develops rapidly, so it should only be used in a selective fashion.

Penicillin, chloramphenicol and streptomycin possess a high sensitizing risk and should be avoided.

Antiseptic agents have an advantage over antibiotics because they do not produce organism resistance, nor do they sensitize.

Crystal violet paint 0.5% aqueous solution is a drying paint useful in leg ulcers. It is effective against Gram-positive bacteria and yeasts.

Eusol (chlorinated lime and boric acid solution BPC) and eusol, liquid paraffin, of each equal parts, are a useful and time honoured application for infected leg ulcers. Steroxin (chlorquinaldol 3% ointment), Vioform (clioquinol 3%) and Betadine ointment (povidone–iodine) possess Gram-positive and antibacterial and antifungal properties; the latter may stain.

Cleansing agents

Cetrimide solution is useful for removing adherent crusts and can be used as a shampoo (Cetavlon PC). Betadine skin cleanser (povidone–iodine 4% solution) and Phiso-Med (hexachlorophane 3%) are useful skin cleansers in superficial staphylococcal infections and acne.

Baths

The fear held by many skin patients that water will worsen their condition must be dispelled. Dry and inflamed skin is helped by bath oils such as Oilatum emollient or emulsifying ointment BP. A sachet of Aveeno colloidal or oilated protein fraction of oat is also comforting. Pyococcal infections are helped by potassium permanganate solution NF or Ster-Zac bath concentrate. Tar baths (coal tar solution BP or Polytar emollient) are used in psoriasis.

Covering agents

Several proprietary cosmetic agents are available to blend with various skin shades. Covermark, Keromask or Ardena covering cream are effective.

Depigmenting agents

Most preparations contain hydroquinone 2–5%. The Sheffield formulation is effective:

Hydroxyquinone	5%
Hydrocortisone BP	1%
Retinoic acid	0.1%
Butylated hydroxytoluene	0.5%
Polyethylene glycol	47%
Methylated spirit 74 op	to 100%

Hyperpigmenting agents

Methoxypsoralen 0.15% in spirit may be applied to the skin followed by short exposure to ultraviolet light. An alternative regime is tabs. methoxypsoralen tablets 10–20 mg daily by mouth two hours before exposure to long-wave ultraviolet light.

Fungicides

The relatively new imidazole preparations, clotrimazole 1% cream (Canesten) and miconazole 2% cream (Daktarin, Dermonistat) and econozole nitrate 1% (Ecostatin) are effective and seldom irritate; they are effective against Candida as well as dermatophytes.

Pigmentum magenta (Castellani's paint) used full strength or in a quarter to a half strength dilution, the diluent being acetone 4%, IMS 8%, water to 100%, has the disadvantage of staining the skin and underwear. It is however effective in intertriginous areas and, like the imidazole preparations, has a wide spectrum of activity.

Benzoic acid ointment compound (Whitfield's ointment) has its limitations and can irritate the skin. It works well in tinea versicolor, as does selenium shampoo (Selsun, Lenium) smeared over the trunk at night and washed off in the bath in the morning on three successive occasions.

Nystatin and amphotericin have limited value against Candida and are useless against other fungal infections.

Griseofulvin is the only effective treatment for scalp ringworm and for dermatophyte nail infections. It is the treatment of choice for widespread tinea corporis, cruris and manuum, and in animal ringworm. It has no value in Candida or versicolor infections or in interdigital tinea pedis. The dose is 500 mg (one tablet) daily for four weeks for an adult. In fingernail infections griseofulvin must be continued for six to nine months. The drug is disappointing in toe nail infections.

Antiparasitics and repellents

Benzyl benzoate applications BP and crotamiton cream (Eurax) are highly effective in scabies. Sulphur ointment, though effective, is no longer used because it is messy and may cause dermatitis.

Gamma benzene hexachloride 1% (Lorexane cream, Quellada lotion) is now often preferred in scabies, especially in children, as it is non-stinging.

Benzyl benzoate emulsion 25% and gamma benzene hexachloride must be applied to the whole body surface, except the head and neck, on two successive days, followed by a bath. All members of the household should be treated at the same time.

Pediculosis capitis and pubis is best treated with malathion lotion 0.5% (Prioderm, Derbac). It is rubbed into the hair and left to dry naturally; after 12 hours shampoo, preferably using malathion 1% cream shampoo, and comb out with a fine nit comb.

Carbaryl lotion 0.5% (Carylderm) is equally effective and can be used in resistant cases.

Protective agents

Silicone preparations such as dimethicone cream help to protect the skin from maceration by urine and faeces. Siopel and Vasogen are effective proprietary preparations.

Aluminium compound paste BPC (Baltimore paste) which contains aluminium powder 20% and zinc oxide and liquid paraffin of each 40%, is effective around colostomies, as is the proprietary Ostomy Plus.

For protection against short-wave ultraviolet light mexenone cream 4% (Uvistat) and padimate 2.5% in alcoholic solution (Spectraban) are helpful. Sometimes a combination of both these light protectives, the Spectraban being applied first, proves more effective than either alone or either used singly.

Dundee cream:

titanium dioxide	20%
zinc oxide	6%
kaolin	2%
brown and oblique red ferric oxide	1%
mexenone cream	4% to 100%

is more effective than mexenone cream alone.

Scalp preparations

Suitable applications for the hairy scalp are lotions and emulsifying agents, preferably of the oil in water type. For psoriasis and seborrhoea capitis coal tar and salicylic ointment BPC, or salicylic acid and sulphur cream BPC are useful, though not always cosmetically acceptable, especially in women. The following formulation for compound coconut ointment is often used in scalp psoriasis:

coal tar solution	12%
precipitated sulphur	4%
salicylic acid	2%
lavender oil	2%
coconut oil	60%
emulsifying wax	13%
yellow soft paraffin	7%

as is dithranol 0.4%, liquid paraffin 74.6%, emulsifying wax 25%. The ears should be protected with vaseline. Women patients may only consent to using these greasy preparations when it is feasible for them to shampoo their hair the following morning. Betnovate scalp lotion, Locoid scalp lotion and Synalar Gel are aesthetically more acceptable. If used intermittently and not extravagantly, the dangers of rebound are lessened. For shampooing the hair, Polytar liquid, Ceanel, Cetavlon PC or Lenium and Selsun have stood the test of time.

Wart removers, keratolytics and caustics

There is no single effective application in the treatment of viral warts. Salicylic acid 16.7%, lactic acid 16.7% in collodion (Salactol) or glutaraldehyde 10% solution (Glutarol) are popular proprietary applications. Salicylic acid 10% in spirit, podophyllin 10% in spirit can be used, as can 0.7% cantharadin in acetone and collodion flex in equal parts. This last is a powerful vesicant and should not be given to the patient. Formalin 5% foot soaks for 15 minutes each night, protecting the surrounding skin with vaseline, has been used for plantar warts since the Second World War.

Plane warts on the face are a problem. Salicylic acid 3% in ung. aquosum or calamine lotion may be used; they have a placebo effect if nothing else. The very careful application of the cautery point or liquid nitrogen can be effective in expert hands. Liquid nitrogen, when available, is favoured by most dermatologists for warts of hands and feet, though it is by no means 100 per cent effective.

Acuminate, perianal, penile and vulval warts are treated by applying 20% podophyllin in spirit or liquid paraffin to the lesions. The surrounding skin may be protected with zinc oxide paste. After four hours the area is washed, and the application may be repeated after 48 to 72 hours, depending on the reaction sustained. Cryotherapy may be given a trial for perianal warts; some cases require removal under local or general anaesthetic.

Recalcitrant warts in adults are most effectively dealt with by curettage under local anaesthetic.

Topical corticosteroid preparations

In order to use topical steroids effectively and safely it is important to know something about their pharmacological action.

Unfortunately, with the advent of more potent, inflammatory agents has come a realization that the more effective the steroid, the more undesirable, usually, are the side effects.

Locally applied steroids have both vasoconstrictive and anti-inflammatory actions, and the more powerful fluorinated steroids have an additional antiproliferative action which renders them liable to cause epidermal thinning and dermal atrophy.

Another problem is percutaneous absorption which may result in depression of the hypothalamic pituitary adrenal axis, and, again this problem of adrenal suppression arises mainly with the fluorinated steroids which are more rapidly absorbed into the circulation.

From the practical standpoint, therefore, the practitioner should have in mind the major groups of steroids classified according to potency. It is convenient to assemble them into four groups listed in terms of decreasing potency (*see Table 27.1*). Groups I and II are the potent synthetic fluorinated derivatives. It is obviously impossible to include all the steroids, so only the better known ones are included.

With certain preparations greasy bases appear to enhance the activity and when applied under occlusion the steroid is 'promoted' to the group above.

Table 27.1   Topical steroids

	Pack size
Group I—very potent	
Dermovate = clobetasol propionate 0.05%	25 g
Halciderm = halcinonide 0.1%	30 g
Nerisone Forte = difluocortolone valerate 0.3%	15 g
Propaderm Forte = beclomethasone dipropionate 0.5%	5 g
Synalar Forte = fluocinolone acetonide 0.2%	5 g
Group II—potent	
Betnovate = betamethasone valerate 0.1%	15 g
Metosyn = fluocinonide 0.05%	25 g
Nerisone = difluocortolone valerate 0.1%	30 g
Propaderm = beclomethasone dipropionate 0.025%	15 g
Synalar = fluocinolone acetonide 0.025%	15 g
Topilar = fluclorolone acetonide 0.025%	30 g
Group III—moderately potent	
Adcortyl = triamcinolone acetonide 0.1%	15 g
Eumovate = clobetasone butyrate 0.05%	25 g
Haelan = flurandrenolone 0.0125%	60 g
Locoid = hydrocortisone 17-butyrate 0.1%	30 g
Ultradil = fluocortolone pivalate 0.1% / hexanoate 0.1%	50 g
Group IV—weak	
Alphaderm = hydrocortisone 1% / urea 10%	30 g
Dioderm = hydrocortisone 0.1%	30 g
Efcortelan = hydrocortisone 1%	15 g

There are certain principles or guidelines for the use of topical steroids.

Know your steroids and how to use them safely. Always be on the look-out for the first sign of side effects, such as local atrophy or systemic changes.

Fluorinated steroids are contraindicated in many dermatoses and on certain sites. These include: rosacea, perioral dermatitis, acne vulgaris; skin ulcers, mucous membranes, flexures and eyelids; viral infections—herpes simplex, zoster, varicella, vaccinia, warts, molluscum contagiosum; fungal infections—candidiasis, dermatophytosis;

bacterial infections—boils, impetigo, erysipelas, secondarily infected eczema; scabies and other ectoparasitoses.

Group I fluorinated steroids are best avoided in infancy and early childhood.

So long as the diagnosis is certain and topical steroids are indicated, use the most effective steroid for a short, sharp burst of three to five days and then wean on to a weaker steroid. Palliative treatment before a confirmed diagnosis has been made may be a disaster course involving spread of the original disorder, masking of the diagnosis, topical addiction and systemic absorption.

Give the patient or parent precise instructions.

If favourable control does not occur promptly, then the steroid should be discontinued.

In the event of a rebound following cessation of therapy, reconsider the diagnosis.

Learn to move up and down the table of steroids and so side-step the side effects.

Avoid giving repeat prescriptions without closely re-examining the patient. In any event, limit the amount given to an adult to 50 g a week of a Group I or II steroid.

Always keep a record of which steroids have been applied, how much and for how long, and supply these details in any letter of referral for a second opinion.

Refer to hospital if you think the patient may have adrenal suppression.

Remember infants and children are particularly liable to show side effects.

Topical antibiotic preparations

Penicillin must never be used as a topical application on the skin; it has a strong sensitizing potential. The broad spectrum antibiotic compounds, with the exception of chloramphenicol, are relatively safe and are speedily effective in pyococcal infections. Neomycin and framycetin are effective also but are potential sensitizers. Sodium fusidate ointment (Fucidin) and gentamicin sulphate (Genticin and Cidomycin) are useful in tetracycline-resistant cases; the latter antibiotic is effective also against Gram-negative infections—e.g. infected leg ulcers—though again a watch should be kept for allergic reactions. Clindamycin lotion is effective in acne—i.e. clindamycin 600 mg, isopropyl alcohol 70% 48 ml, water 6 ml, propylene glycol 6 ml. In recurrent aphthous ulceration of the mouth a mouthwash of tetracycline 250 mg in 5 ml of water four times daily is useful.

Systemic therapy
Antibiotics

Tetracyclines (chlortetracycline, oxytetracycline and tetracycline) are widely used in the treatment of acne vulgaris in a dosage of 250–500 mg daily. At least two months continuous therapy is required to effect improvement; recalcitrant cases may require up to 1000 mg daily for as much as a month. Alternatively erythromycin sometimes works well when tetracycline fails. Cotrimoxazole (Septrin) twice daily may be used in those intolerant of tetracycline and erythromycin. Clindamycin is effective, but there are dangers of mucomembranous colitis, though this side effect is uncommon in young people.

Photosensitivity reactions are particularly liable to occur with demeclocycline (Ledermycin, Deteclo). The use of tetracyclines in pregnancy is contraindicated because of deposition in fetal teeth.

Tetracyclines are indicated in superficial staphylococcal infections when the organism is sensitive to this drug, though the incidence of tetracycline resistant staphylococci is increasing rapidly. In these resistant cases erythromycin or cephalexin (Ceporex) can be used when indicated by antibiotic sensitivity tests.

Penicillinase resistant penicillins, when indicated, are preferable for most mixed streptococcal-staphylococcal infections. Flucloxacillin (Floxapen) should be given six-hourly for seven to ten days. This form of therapy is indicated in impetigo in children because of the dangers of glomerulonephritis and toxic epidermal necrolysis. In erysipelas and cellulitis penicillin G is the drug of choice: 1 million units of penicillin G three times daily for one to two days, followed by benzathine penicillin V 250 mg six-hourly, continued for two weeks. Penicillin is also indicated in erysipeloid, anthrax and fusispirochaetal diseases. Erythromycin or cephalexin (Ceporex) can be used in patients allergic to penicillin.

In summary, systemic antibiotics should be used in the following circumstances:

(1) When lymphangitis, lymphadenopathy or fever are present.
(2) When the infective process is spreading or unduly destructive.
(3) When infections appear with systemic steroid therapy.
(4) When pus is present in the skin lesions.
(5) When the immune mechanism is depressed by immunosuppressive therapy or systemic disease is present, e.g. diabetes, leukaemia, etc.
(6) As a preventive measure in certain denuded dermatoses, e.g. pemphigus.

Initial treatment of a severe infection must be prompt even when culture and sensitivity tests have not yet been performed.

Corticosteroids

Prednisolone is the drug of choice. A single daily morning dose is preferred, though alternate day dosage has few side effects and long-term cases should follow an alternate day schedule.

For acute severe dermatoses of expected short duration:

5 mg tablets: 4 daily for seven days,
    3 daily for seven days,
    2 daily for seven days.

To wean long-term cases:

After courses lasting a year or more spontaneous revival of adrenal cortical activity will usually occur within 48 hours, but in rare cases it may fail completely. During the weaning period corticotrophin will assist the revival, but its value is short-lived and it will not effect subsequent maintenance. The pituitary adrenal axis continues to be subdued for up to five months after weaning though its activity is usually adequate for ordinary maintenance purposes.

When corticosteroids are to be discontinued, either because the underlying disease is quiescent or because of steroid complications, a repository ACTH preparation should be given by intramuscular injection once a day in a dose of 60 units for at least a week. Alternatively Synacthen depot can be given in a dose of 1 mg daily. It is advisable to continue with the ACTH injections in these patients until there is unequivocal evidence from estimations of steroids in plasma or urine that a satisfactory adrenal response has been obtained.

When initiating corticosteroid therapy for severe dermatoses, e.g. pemphigus vulgaris or pemphigoid, a high dosage of prednisolone may be necessary, e.g. 180 mg (36 tablets) daily for some weeks until blistering is controlled; the dosage should then be reduced rapidly at first and later more slowly until a maintenance dose is reached.

Some ACTH intraveous drip 40 units daily for three days produces dramatic results when prednisolone is relatively ineffective. The dose of ACTH can then be gradually reduced.

When steroids are reduced to maintenance level azathioprine in a dose of 2.5 mg/kg body weight may allow gradual complete withdrawal of prednisolone.

In some cases morning injections of tetracosactrin depot (Synacthen or Cortrosyn) 1 mg daily for three days, then on alternate days for one week, is useful to cover withdrawal.

With higher dosage if the total duration exceeds three weeks a stress dose of steroid must be given (e.g. pre-operatively) for up to one year. The serum cortisol level may be normal yet unable to rise to stress. Physiological doses up to 10–15 mg daily are unlikely to cause pituitary adrenal suppression.

Immunosuppressive agents

The most widely used immunosuppressive agents in dermatological conditions are folic acid antagonists (e.g. methotrexate) and purine analogues (e.g. azathioprine). Methotrexate is used in widespread and intractable psoriasis when other therapy has failed. A satisfactory dosage schedule is ten 2.5 mg tablets (25 mg) taken in a single dose at weekly intervals; alternatively 25 mg im can be administered as a weekly injection. Many side effects have been reported with methotrexate, including mouth ulcers, gastrointestinal haemorrhage, leucopenia, low platelet count and liver cirrhosis. A weekly blood count and a six-monthly liver biopsy are essential when using this drug. Methotrexate has been used in pemphigus but azathioprine (*see above*) is preferred. Azathioprine has also been used in psoriasis employing similar precautions as with methotrexate.

Procarbazine (Natulan) in a dose of 50 mg thrice daily is being used in mycosis fungoides. A dose of even 50 mg daily may be sufficient to cause regression of tumours, lymphadenopathy and enlargement of the liver and spleen. Procarbazine is an MAO inhibitor and caution is needed with foods and local anaesthetics.

Index

Figures in italics refer to pages on which illustrations or tables appear.